So you want to be a brain surgeon?
The medical careers guide

Third edition

Career development titles from Oxford

More books to help guide your career are available from Oxford, including:

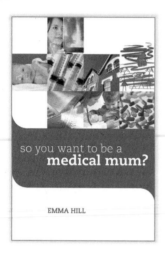

so you want to be a
medical mum?

The first and only guide for mothers and mums-to-be aimed directly at doctors, providing 'one-stop' practical advice on issues such as coping with your job whilst pregnant, managing your finances, and your legal rights.

248 pp | February 2008 | Paperback

So you want to be a brain surgeon?

The medical careers guide

Third edition

Edited by

Simon Eccles
Stephan Sanders

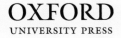

OXFORD
UNIVERSITY PRESS

OXFORD
UNIVERSITY PRESS

Great Clarendon Street, Oxford OX2 6DP

Oxford University Press is a department of the University of Oxford.
It furthers the University's objective of excellence in research, scholarship,
and education by publishing worldwide in

Oxford New York

Auckland Cape Town Dar es Salaam Hong Kong Karachi
Kuala Lumpur Madrid Melbourne Mexico City Nairobi
New Delhi Shanghai Taipei Toronto

With offices in

Argentina Austria Brazil Chile Czech Republic France Greece
Guatemala Hungary Italy Japan Poland Portugal Singapore
South Korea Switzerland Thailand Turkey Ukraine Vietnam

Oxford is a registered trade mark of Oxford University Press
in the UK and in certain other countries

Published in the United States
by Oxford University Press Inc., New York

British Library Cataloguing in Publication Data
Data available

Library of Congress Cataloging-in-Publication-Data
Data available

ISBN 978–0–19–923196–6

10 9 8 7 6 5 4 3 2 1

Typeset in ITC Charter
by Cepha Imaging Private Ltd., Bangalore, India
Printed in Great Britain
on acid-free paper by
Ashford Colour Press Ltd., Gosport, Hampshire

Dedication

to Ramanie (SE)

to Imogen, my wonderful wife (SS)

Foreword

Choosing your specialty is always going to be a hard decision for any doctor. The ability to make this key choice is made far easier by having a really good understanding of what each possibility may mean. This excellent book brings together experts from every field to provide very clear accounts of why they chose their particular specialty. The contributors have provided frank accounts of what their job entails and what an average day is really like.

As a practising surgeon whose career now takes me all over the NHS, I have had the privilege of seeing the amazing breadth of choices that a career in medicine offers doctors. There are few other professions which offer this choice and it can be hard to truly appreciate it even with the broader based foundation training schemes. This book offers insights into the full range of career options both mainstream and alternative. The editors have succeeded in including many smaller specialties to give a feel for emerging new careers as they evolve from their larger parent specialties.

This third edition includes timely and helpful advice on how an individual can make their CV or application forms stand out from their peers and how to ensure they always present the best of themselves. I have enjoyed reading the book, and have no doubt it will prove invaluable in helping medical students and young doctors to find a career path which suits them.

Professor The Lord Darzi of Denham KBE
Hon FREng, FMedSci

Preface

This third edition of *So You Want To Be A Brain Surgeon*? has been a long time in gestation and we offer our apologies to those who've written asking us to get on with it! Our problem, shared with all doctors, has been the constantly moving goalposts of UK postgraduate medical training. Whilst the final details of training in the post-Tooke report era are still not clear (see p77), the essential ideas and key structures are now apparent allowing us to write this guide. Some details and names may change but the shape and key points along the route are fixed and therefore the necessary decisions for doctors in training should remain constant for the next few years.

The biggest change from the last edition has been the change in editors. Stephan Sanders has joined having helped write the best-selling *Oxford Handbook of the Foundation Programme*. He has brought his boundless enthusiasm and energy to the challenge of coordinating over 100 contributors without whom the book would not be possible. Chris Ward has 'retired' to Oxford and we wish him and Wendy every happiness in their retirement.

There have been many other changes since the second edition: we have given the chapters a consistent format and arranged them alphabetically to make it easier to find the information you want (and hopefully to encourage serendipitous discoveries of unexpected alternatives); the guidance on the career pathways through Specialty Training have been rewritten and now sit together; finally we have bolstered the initial chapters offering advice on choosing, and getting, the career you want.

Feedback from readers has helped shape this book since the first edition over ten years ago. Please do keep sending in comments and suggestions, we remain grateful for all contributions.

Simon Eccles
Stephan Sanders
2008

Acknowledgements

This book would never have been possible without the help of many kind people and organizations who gave their time and energy for our benefit. In particular:

All the authors of the individual chapters who have produced such lovely vignettes that we both wondered if we'd chosen the right specialties.

Dr Chris Ward for the original idea, the first two editions and his ongoing interest and support.

Catherine Barnes from OUP for her continued support and dedication to this book.

Sara Chare from OUP for her help in getting this project started.

Kate Wanwimolruk from OUP for her excellent work as production editor.

Dr Mary Docherty for her input into the prison medicine chapter.

Professor Elizabeth Paice for helping us find the authors for the initial chapters on the organization of medical careers under MMC.

Dr Andrew Long for his three excellent chapters on the organization of medical careers which gave an extremely useful insight into a complicated subject.

Claire Chapman, the General Medical Council (GMC) and Healthcare Knowledge Ltd (creators of http://www.SpecialistInfo.com) for providing us with data about the number of doctors in each specialty.

The Medical Women's Federation.

Merlin (Medical Emergency Relief International).

Voluntary Services Overseas (VSO).

Finally, anyone who helped us find an author for a chapter of this book.

Three people deserve special mention since their input has been absolutely vital:

Anna Winstanley our loyal and dedicated assistant commissioning editor from OUP who tirelessly sought out chapter authors and answered our endless queries.

Dr Imogen Hart for her grammatical excellence and wise comments on the entire manuscript, along with maintaining the sanity of one of the authors.

Captain Piers Page for proof-reading the entire manuscript.

Contents

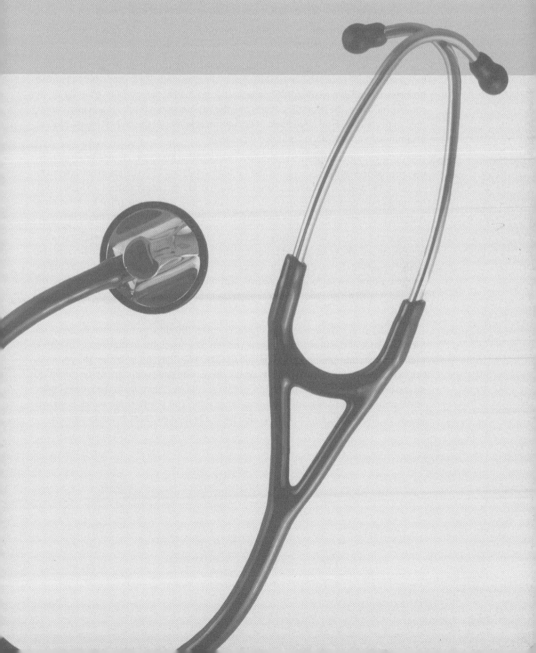

Introduction

Using this book

Welcome to the third edition of *So you want to be a brain surgeon*? This book is split into five sections, each covering a different aspect of medical careers:

Part 1 Career routes. These chapters describe the basic progression from a medical student to a fully qualified consultant or GP under the new Modernising Medical Careers (MMC) system. They are split into two subsections:

> **The 'usual' route** describes the career route that the vast majority of doctors take including an overview of the MMC careers system and membership exams

> **Alternative routes** describes the other career options such as academia, working overseas or jobs outside the NHS

Part 2 Specialty overviews. A group of chapters describing the career progression in the major specialties under the new MMC system. For example, if a doctor wanted to train in obstetrics and gynaecology, this page would show them the specialist training application procedure, the necessary exams and the subspecialties available as a final career (e.g. maternal and fetal medicine). Every option available at the end of the foundation programme under MMC is discussed separately.

Part 3 How to get a job. Along with changes to career paths, MMC has changed the application procedures and working practices for junior doctors. This section gives a detailed description of the application procedure for foundation programmes and specialist training and tips on how to do well. It also describes how competitive each training route is, provides interview tips and explains how to take a break from medicine.

Part 4 The organization of medical careers. This section summarises the major changes that have occurred under MMC and following the Tooke Report, along with outlining the likely changes in the near future. It also describes the new institutions governing junior doctor training (useful for interview preparation) and systems for changing career and concludes with a discussion of discrimination in medicine, particularly with regard to women.

Part 5 Career chapters. These two-page chapters cover 100 different medical careers and form the bulk of the book. Each one is written by a specialist in that career to give a unique insight into what their life and job are like. The first page describes the patients, the work and the job in that specialty whilst the second page summarises the specialty, giving an example of 'a day in the life' of that specialist, the route to the career under MMC and scales to compare the job to other jobs. The key to these scales is shown opposite. The chapters are arranged alphabetically to make them easier to look up.

Key to the summaries

myth	The popular myths about each job ...
reality	... and the reality
personality	Personality traits found in each specialty; these are not absolutes, just a guide
best aspects	Why being a doctor in this specialty is better than sliced bread
worst aspects	The bits of the job that can make a doctor's blood boil
route	The route through the new MMC system to get to the specialty, and the necessary membership exams
numbers	The number of trained doctors in the UK and the percentage of these posts filled by women where known
locations	Whether the job is based in the community, all hospitals, larger hospitals, teaching hospitals or specialist centres

uncompetitive	Ranked according to MMC competition ratios; graded 1 to 5	**competitive**
life	Graded according to the overall impact of the job on life outside medicine; 1 to 5	**work**
boredom	Graded according to the risk of boredom or burnout; a score of three is a good balance with a risk of boredom at 1 and of burnout at 5	**burnout**
quiet on-call	Graded according to the 'severity' of on calls including number of calls and need to come into hospital; from 1 to 5	**busy on-call**
low salary	Most doctors earn a similar amount (p 71); this scale shows potential earnings on a scale of 1 to 5. It is important to realize that the majority will not get this and those who do will need to work very hard	**high salary**

Medical careers terminology

The medical hierarchy

Consultant The boss in each specialty (p 13)

General practitioner (GP) Equivalent of a consultant, but in primary care (p 12)

Associate specialist Consultant experience without the accountability (p 14)

ST3–8 A doctor in specialist training beyond basic training (p 8)

Staff Grade ST3–8 experience but not in specialist training (p 14)

ST1–3 A doctor in a specialist training programme (p 8)

CT1–3 A doctor on a core-training programme (p 8)

Fixed-Term Specialty Training Appointment (FTSTA) Equivalent to ST1–3, but not in specialist training (p 14)

F2 Foundation training year 2 (p 6)

F1 Foundation training year 1 (p 6)

Old names

Specialist registrar (SpR) Equivalent to ST3/4 and above

Senior house officer (SHO) Equivalent to F2, ST1–3 and CT1-3

Pre-registration house officer (PRHO) Equivalent to F1

Other terms

Academic clinical fellowship (ACF) Academic equivalent of ST1–3 (p 16)

Certificate of Completion of Training (CCT) Awarded at the end of specialist training to allow the doctor to work as a consultant (p 13)

Core-training Basic specialist training in an uncoupled specialty (p 8)

Flexible training Foundation or specialist training in a part-time job (p 72)

Foundation programme The two years of training after medical school (p 6)

General Practice Certificate of Completion of Training (GPCCT) Awarded at the end of GP vocational training to allow the doctor to work as a GP (p 12)

Modernising Medical Careers (MMC) Series of changes aimed at reforming junior doctor training (p 76)

Non-consultant career grade (NCCG) A doctor who is not on the career path to becoming a consultant; the old name for staff and associate specialist grade (p 14)

Postgraduate Medical Education and Training Board (PMETB) Regulatory body responsible for junior doctors' training (p 81)

Run-through Training that starts at ST1 and continues through to CCT (p 8)

Specialty training Training that leads to a CCT/GPCCT award and being a consultant or GP (p 8)

Staff and specialist associate grade (SASG) An experienced doctor in either a staff grade or associate specialist post; the term also covers other non-training posts at a similar level (p 14)

Tooke Report Independent inquiry into MMC by Professor Sir John Tooke, commissioned by the Secretary of State for Health (p 77)

Uncoupled Training with a break and reapplication between basic core-training and specialist training (p 8)

GP vocational training scheme (GPVTS) GP training equivalent to specialty training (p 32)

Contributors

Working abroad
Ms Jo Waterfield
Head of International Development
British Medical Association
BMA House
Tavistock Square
London WC1H 9JP

Flexible training
Dr Anne Hastie
Director of Postgraduate General Practice
Education
London Deanery
Stewart House
32 Russell Square
London WC1B 5DN

Switching specialist training pathways
Overseeing education
Alternative routes (Articles 14 and 11)
Dr Andrew Long
Associate Dean
London Deanery
Stewart House
32 Russell Square
London WC1B 5DN

Women in medicine
Mrs Scarlett McNally
Consultant Orthopaedic Surgeon
Medical Women's Federation
Tavistock House North
Tavistock Square
London WC1H 9HX

Academic GP
Prof Mike Pringle
Head of School of Community Health Sciences
Floor 13, Tower Building
University of Nottingham
Nottingham NG7 2RD

Academic medicine
Prof Iain Carpenter
Professor of Human Ageing
Centre for Health Services Studies
George Allen Wing
University of Kent
Canterbury
Kent CT2 7NF

Acupuncture
Dr Penny Brougham
Specialist in Complementary Medicine
141 Mulgrave Road
Sutton
Surrey SM2 6JX

Acute medicine
Dr Veronica White
Consultant Acute and Respiratory Physician
Barts and the London NHS Trust
Whitechapel
London E1 1BB

Anaesthesia
Dr Justin Richards
Consultant Anaesthetist
Nottingham City
Hospital Huchnall Road
Nottingham
NG5 1PB

Army medicine
Capt Piers Page
Clinical Research Fellow
Department of Academic Emergency
Medicine
James Cook University Hospital
Middlesbrough TS4 3BW

Audiovestibular medicine
Dr Tony Sirimanna
Consultant Audiological Physician
Great Ormond Street Hospital for Children
London WC1N 3JH

Dr Katherine Harrop-Griffiths
Consultant Audio-Vestibular
Physician
Royal National Throat Nose and Ear Hospital
Grays Inn Road
London WC1X 8EE

Breast and oncoplastic surgery
Mr Douglas Macmillan
Consultant Surgeon
Nottingham Breast Institute
City Hospital Campus
Hucknall Road
Nottingham NG5 1PB

Cardiology
Dr Mark Dayer
Consultant Cardiologist
Musgrove Park Hospital
Taunton
Somerset TA1 5DA

Cardiothoracic surgery
Mr Jon Anderson
Consultant Cardiothoracic Surgeon
Hammersmith Hospital
Du Cane Road
London W12 0HS

Chemical pathology
Dr Adrian Park
Consultant Chemical Pathologist
West Suffolk Hospital
Hardwick Lane
Bury St Edmunds
Suffolk IP33 2QZ

Civil Service medicine
Dr Erika Denton
Consultant Radiologist and National Clinical
Lead for Diagnostic Imaging
Radiology Department
East Block level 2
Norfolk and Norwich University Hospital
NHS Trust
Colney Lane
Norwich NR4 7UY

Clinical genetics
Dr Helen Firth
Consultant Clinical Geneticist
Addenbrookes Hospital
Cambridge CB2 2QQ

Clinical oncology
Dr Martin Scott-Brown
Specialist Registrar in Clinical Oncology
Oxford Radcliffe Trust
Churchill Hospital
Headington
Oxford OX3 7LJ

Clinical pharmacology
Dr Jeff Aronson
Reader in Clinical Pharmacology
Department of Primary Health Care
Rosemary Rue Building, Old Road Campus
Headington
Oxford OX3 7LF

Community paediatrics
Dr David Lewis
Consultant in Community Paediatrics
Worcestershire Primary Care Trust
Wyre Forest Locality
Kidderminster Health Centre
Kidderminster
Worcs DY10 1PG

Dermatology
Dr David de Berker
Consultant Dermatologist
Bristol Royal Infirmary
Bristol BS1 3NU

Ear, nose and throat (otolaryngology)
Mr Grant Bates
Consultant ENT Surgeon
Radcliffe Infirmary
Woodstock Road
Oxford OX2 6HE

Mr James Ramsden
Specialist Registrar in ENT
Radcliffe Infirmary
Woodstock Road
Oxford OX2 6HE

Elderly medicine
Dr Jeremy Snape
Consultant Geriatrician
Kings Mill Hospital
Mansfield Road
Sutton in Ashfield
Notts NG17 4JL

Emergency medicine
Dr Jonathan Wyatt
Consultant in Accident and Emergency
Medicine
Royal Cornwall Hospital
Treslinke
Truro TR1 3LJ

Endocrinology and diabetes
Dr John Anderson
Consultant Endocrinologist
Homerton Hospital
Homerton Row
London E9 6SR

Expedition medicine
Dr Jon Dallimore
Medical Director, Wilderness Medical
Training
The Coach House
Thorny Bank
Garth Row
Kendal
Cumbria LA8 9AW

Forensic medical examiner
Dr Meng Aw-Yong
Principal Forensic Medical Examiner
Metropolitan Police
New Scotland Yard
Broadway
London SW1H 0BG

Forensic pathology
Prof Christopher Milroy
Chief Forensic Pathologist of the Forensic
Science Service
University of Sheffield
Home Office Pathology
The Medico Legal Centre
Watery Street
Sheffield S3 7ES

Forensic psychiatry
Dr Darryl Gregory
Consultant Forensic Psychiatrist
The John Howard Centre
Centre for Forensic Mental Health
12 Kenworthy Road
Homerton
London E9 5TD

Gastroenterology
Dr Mark Anderson
Consultant Gastroenterologist
City Hospital, SWBH NHS Trust
Dudley Road
Birmingham B18 7QH

Dr Brian Cooper
Consultant Gastroenterologist
City Hospital, SWBH NHS Trust
Dudley Road
Birmingham B18 7QH

General practice
Dr Hilary Audsley
General Practitioner
The Fort House Surgery
32 Hersham Road
Walton On Thames
Surrey KT12 1UX

General surgery (colorectal surgery)
Mr Ian Scott
Consultant Colorectal Surgeon
Ipswich Hospital NHS Trust
Heath Road
Ipswich
Suffolk IP4 5PD

Genitourinary medicine (GUM)
Dr Mary Poulton
Consultant HIV/GUM
King's College Hospital
Denmark Hill
London SE5 9RS

GP in a rural setting
Dr Jon Macleod
General Practitioner
Tigh-na-Hearradh
Lochmaddy
Islew od North Uist
Western Isles PA82 5AE

GP with a special interest
Dr Pauline Brimblecombe
General Practitioner
Newnham Walk Surgery
Wordsworth Grove
Cambridge CB3 9HS

Gynaecological oncology
Dr Eugene Kuzmin
Research Fellow in Gynaecological Oncology
Department of Oncology and Molecular
Therapeutics
Imperial College School of Medicine
Hammersmith Campus
6th floor
Cyclotron Building
Du Cane Rd
London W12 0HS

Gynaecology
Ms Samantha Chinnakotla
Specialist Registrar in Obstetrics and
Gynaecology
Queen's Medical Centre
Nottingham University Hospitals
Derby Road
Nottingham NG7 2UH

Haematology
Dr John Hanley
Consultant Haematologist
Royal Victoria Infirmary
Queen Victoria Road
Newcastle upon Tyne NE1 4LP

Hand surgery
Mr David Warwick
Consultant Hand Surgeon
Southampton University Hospitals
Southampton SO16 6UY

Histopathology
Dr Lisa Browning
Clinical Lecturer and Honorary SpR in
Histopathology
Nuffield Department of Clinical Laboratory
Sciences
John Radcliffe Hospital
Oxford OX3 9DU

Homeopathic medicine
Dr Bob Leckridge
Specialist in Homeopathic Medicine
Glasgow Homeopathic Hospital
Glasgow G12 OYN

Immunology
Dr Matthew Helbert
Consultant Immunologist
Immunology
Manchester Royal Infirmary
Oxford Road
Manchester M13 9WL

Infectious diseases and tropical medicine
Dr Robert Davidson
Consultant in Infectious Diseases
Lister Unit, Northwick Park Hospital
Harrow HA1 3UJ

Intensive care
Dr Mike Celinski
Consultant in Intensive Care
Southampton General Hospital
Tremona Road
Southampton SO16 6YD

Journalism and medical writing
Dr David Delvin
Director of the Medical Information
Service
Brighton BN2 7GP

Locuming
Dr Heiko Kindler
Specialist Registrar in Cardiology
MRC Clinical Sciences Centre
Hammersmith Hospital
London W12 0NN

Maternal and fetal medicine
Prof Mark Kilby
Birmingham Women's Hospital
Metchley Park Rd
Edgbaston
Birmingham B15 2TG

Maxillofacial surgery
Mr Graham I Smith
Consultant Maxillofacial Surgeon
St George's Hospital
Blackshaw Road
Tooting
London SW17 0QT

Medical defence organizations
Dr Angelique Mastihi
Medicolegal advisor
Medical Protection Society (MPS)
33 Cavendish Square
London W1G 0PS

Medical education
Dr Adam Feather
Senior Lecturer in Medical Education
Centre for Medical Education
Queen Mary College
University of London
London E1 4NS

Medical entrepreneur

Dr Mike Stein
Medical Director, Map of Medicine
First Floor, Clerkenwell House
67 Clerkenwell Road
London EC1R 5BL

Medical ethics

Dr Daniel Sokol
Lecturer in Medical Ethics
Centre for Medical and Healthcare
Education
4th Floor, Hunter Wing
St George's
University of London
London SW17 0RE

Medical law

Dr Michael Fertleman
Consultant in Geriatrics and Barrister
St Mary's Hospital
London W2 1NY

Medical management consulting

Dr Sally Getgood
Getgood Solutions
5 Ainsworth Place
Cambridge
CBI 2PG

Medical manager

Dr Ian Scott
Consultant Surgeon and former Medical
Director
Ipswich Hospital NHS Trust
Heath Road
Ipswich
Suffolk IP4 5PD

Medical microbiology

Dr Anne Marie Karcher
Consultant Microbiologist
Western Infirmary
Department of Microbiology
Glasgow G11 6NT

Medical oncology

Dr Pauline Leonard
Consultant Medical Oncologist
Southend University Hospital
Prittlewell Chase
Westcliff-on-Sea
Essex SS0 0RY

Medical politics

Dr James Johnson
Past Chairman of Council
BMA House
Tavistock Square
London WC1H 9JP

Merlin

Dr Alex Bolo
Merlin Placement in Liberia
Merlin
12th Floor, 207 Old Street
London EC1V 9NR

Metabolic medicine

Dr Rob Cramb
Consultant Chemical Pathologist
University Hospital Birmingham NHS
Foundation Trust
Queen Elizabeth Hospital
Edgbaston
Birmingham B15 2TH

Neonatology

Dr Shu-Ling Chuang
Consultant Neonatologist
Chelsea and Westminster Hospital
369 Fulham Road
London SW10 9NH

Neurology

Prof Phil Smith
Consultant Neurologist
University Hospital of Wales
Cardiff and Vale NHS Trust
Cardiff CF14 4XW

Dr Rhys Thomas
Specialist Registrar in Neurology
University Hospital of Wales
Cardiff and Vale NHS Trust
Cardiff CF14 4XW

Neurosurgery

Mr Peter Richards
Consultant Paediatric Neurosurgeon
Radcliffe Infirmary
Woodstock Road
Oxford OX2 6HE

Nuclear medicine

Dr John Buscombe
Consultant in Nuclear Medicine
Royal Free Hospital
Pond Street
London NW3 2QG

Obstetrics

Mr Guy Thorpe-Beeston
Consultant in Obstetrics and Gynaecology
Chelsea and Westminster Hospital
369 Fulham Road
London SW10 9NH

Occupational medicine

Dr Paul Grime
Consultant in Occupational Medicine
Royal Free Hospital
Pond Street
Hampstead
London NW3 2QG

Ophthalmology

Mr Nicholas Evans
Consultant Ophthalmologist
Royal Eye Infirmary
Aspley Road
Plymouth PL4 6PL

Orthopaedic surgery

Mr Andrew Carr
Consultant Orthopaedic Surgeon
Nuffield Orthopaedic Centre
Windmill Road
Oxford OX3 7LD

Overseas aid

Dr Mark Wilson
Specialist Registrar in Neurosurgery and
Pre-Hospital Care
Royal London Hospital
Whitechapel
London E1 1BB

Paediatric surgery

Dr Mervyn Griffiths
Consultant Paediatric and Neonatal
Surgeon
Southampton General Hospital
Tremona Road
Southampton
SO16 6YD

Paediatrics

Dr Louise Wells
Consultant Paediatrician
Queen's Medical Centre
Nottingham University Hospitals
Derby Road
Nottingham NG7 2UH

Pain management

Dr Peter Evans
Consultant in Pain Medicine
Charing Cross Hospital
Fulham Palace Road
London W6 8RF

Palliative medicine

Dr Andrew Hoy
Medical Director
Princess Alice Hospice
West End Lane
Esher KT10 8NA

Pharmaceutical physician

Dr Hugh Boardman
Pharmaceutical Physician
Boardman Clarke
Medical Services Consultancy
6 Stanton Road
London SW20 8RL

Plastic and reconstructive surgery

Mr Per Hall
Consultant Plastic Surgeon
Addenbrooke's Hospital
Hills Road
Cambridge CB2 2QQ

Pre-hospital medicine

Dr David Hillebrandt
General Practitioner
Derriton House
Derriton
Holsworthy
Devon EX22 6JX

Prison medicine

Dr Brian Docherty
Medical Director Durham Cluster of
Prisons
HMP Durham
Old Elvet
Durham DH1 3HU

Psychiatry: child and adolescent
Dr Tim Hughes
Consultant Child Psychiatrist
CAMHS
Heart of Hounslow Health Centre
92 Bath Road
Hounslow
Middlesex TW3 3EL

Psychiatry: general adult
Dr Peter Trigwell
Consultant in Liaison Psychiatry
Leeds General Infirmary
Great George Street
Leeds LS1 3EX

Psychiatry: old age
Dr John Holmes
Senior Lecturer in Liaison Psychiatry
of Old Age
University of Leeds
Institute of Health Sciences
101 Clarendon Road
Leeds LS2 9LJ

Psychiatry of learning disability
Dr Tim Andrews
Consultant in Learning Disability Psychiatry
Ridgeway Partnership NHS Trust
Slade House
Horspath Driftway
Headington
Oxford OX3 7JH

Psychotherapy
Dr John Hook
Consultant Psychiatrist in Psychotherapy
Specialist Psychological Therapies Service
Farnham Road Hospital
SABP NHS Foundation Trust
Guildford GU2 7LX

Public health
Dr Jackie Spiby
Head of School Public Health
London KSS Deaneries
Stewart House
32 Russell Square
London WC1B 5SN

Radiology: diagnostic
Prof Philip Robinson
Consultant Radiologist
Department of Clinical Radiology
St James's Hospital
Leeds LS9 7TF

Radiology: interventional
Prof Anthony Watkinson
Professor of Interventional Radiology
The Peninsula Medical School
The Royal Devon and Exeter Hospital
Exeter
Devon EX2 5DW

Rehabilitation medicine
Dr Angela Gall
Royal National Orthopaedic Hospital
Spinal Cord Injury Centre
Brockley Hill
Stanmore HA7 4LP

Renal medicine
Dr Vijayan Suresh
Consultant in Renal Medicine
Glaxo Renal Unit
Birmingham Heartlands Hospital
Bordesley Green
Birmingham
West Midlands B9 5SS

Reproductive medicine
Prof Neil McClure
Professor of Obstetrics and Gynaecology
Queen's University Belfast
Institute of Clinical Science
Grosvenor Road
Belfast BT12 6BJ
Northern Ireland

Respiratory medicine
Dr Jonathan Corne
Consultant in Respiratory Medicine
Queen's Medical Centre
Nottingham University Hospitals
Derby Road
Nottingham NG7 2UH

Rheumatology
Dr Marwan Bukhari
Consultant Rheumatologist
University Hospitals of Morecambe Bay
NHS Trust
Royal Lancaster Infirmary
Ashton Road
Lancaster LA1 4RP

Royal Air Force medicine
Wing Commander Rich Withnall
Department of GP Training (RAF)
Building 170
RAF Halton
Aylesbury HP22 5PG

Royal Navy medicine
Surgeon Commander Funmi Daramola
Principal Medical Officer
HMS Illustrious BFPO 305

Sexual and reproductive health
Mr Babatunde Gbolade
Consultant Gynaecologist and Director of
Fertility Control Unit
Leeds Teaching Hospitals NHS Trust
St James' University Hospital
Beckett's Street
West Yorkshire
Leeds LS9 7TF

Dr Lesley Bacon
Consultant in Sexual and Reproductive
Health
Lewisham PCT
Suite 10
Waldron Health Centre
Stanley Street
London SE8 4BG

Ship's doctor
Dr Philip Brooks
Ship's Doctor – Emerald Princess
Carnival UK
Richmond House
Terminus Terrace
Southampton SO14 3PN

Spinal surgery
Mr Paul Thorpe
Spinal Surgery
Musgrove Park Hospital
Taunton TA1 3PX

Sports and exercise medicine
Dr Pippa Bennett
Team Doctor, England Women's Football
Team
Football Association
25 Soho Square
Westminster
London W1D 4FA

Transfusion medicine
Dr Edwin Massey
Consultant Haematologist
NHS Blood and Transplant
Southmead Road
Bristol BS10 5ND

Transplantation surgery
Mr Andy Weale
Specialist Registrar in Vascular and
Transplant Surgery
Southmead Hospital
Westbury-on-Trym
Bristol BS10 5NB

Mr Paul Lear
Consultant Vascular and Transplant
Surgeon
Southmead Hospital
Westbury-on-Trym
Bristol BS10 5NB

Trauma surgery
Mr Thomas Konig
Trauma Fellow
The Royal London Hospital
Whitechapel
London E1 1BB

Urogynaecology
Dr Louise Webster
Specialist Training Registrar in Obstetrics
and Gynaecology
Chelsea and Westminster Hospital
369 Fulham Road
London SW10 9NH

Urology
Mr John Beatty
Specialist Registrar in Urology
Charing Cross Hospital
Fulham Palace Road
London W6 8RP

Vascular surgery
Mr Chris Imray
Consultant General and Vascular Surgeon
Coventry and Warwickshire County
Vascular Unit
University Hospital Coventry and
Warwickshire
Clifford Bridge Road
Coventry CV2 2DX

Virology
Dr Mark Zuckerman
London South Specialist Virology Centre
3rd Floor, Rayne Institute
King's College Hospital NHS Trust
123 Coldharbour Lane
London SE5 9NU

Voluntary Service Overseas (VSO)
Dr Catherine Atkins
VSO Placement in Namibia
Voluntary Services Overseas
317 Putney Bridge Road
London SW15 2PN

Career routes

The 'usual' route

Alternative routes

Career routes

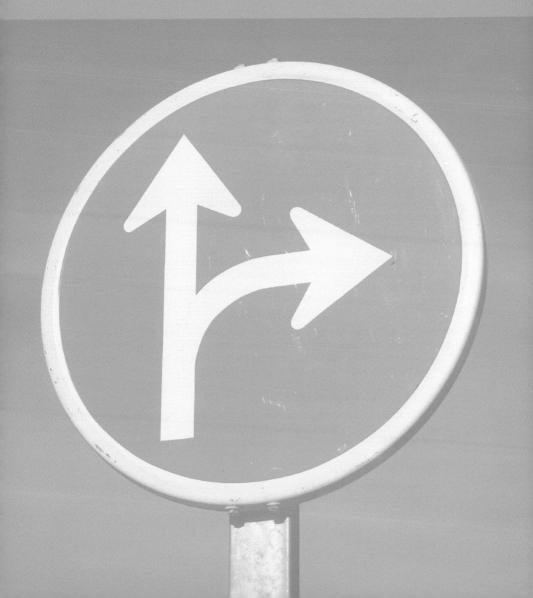

Career overview

The vast majority of medical careers follow a similar basic pattern, shown in the figure on the opposite page. This chapter describes the main stages of a medical career in greater detail, followed by the main alternatives to the standard medical career, such as academia. The next chapter (specialty overviews, p 26) describes how to pursue a career path in a specific specialty (e.g. paediatrics).

Medical school

To work as a doctor it is essential to have a medical degree. Applications to medical school are made online through the Universities and Colleges Admissions Service (UCAS, http://www.ucas.ac.uk). There are two main types of medical school:

Undergraduate schools These account for the majority of medical schools; the courses take five to six years, depending on the school and whether there is an intercalated year leading to an extra degree (e.g. BSc). Graduate students, i.e. those who have already completed a university degree, can also apply to these schools.

Graduate schools These are purely for graduate students. The courses are four to five years long and competition for places at these schools is more intense.

Foundation programme (p 6)

At the end of medical school the graduate registers with the General Medical Council (GMC) and becomes a junior doctor. Training continues in salaried jobs within the NHS starting with the two-year foundation programme. All UK medical graduates are guaranteed a foundation job, however they are allocated competitively so that the 'best' doctors get their first choice of location and placements, whilst those with lower-scoring applications might only be offered jobs in regions of the UK they did not choose (see p 55 for more details on this allocation process).

Early specialty training (p 8)

In the second year of the foundation programme doctors must apply for a particular specialty (e.g. general practice, surgery, obstetrics and gynaecology). Application is competitive and this time there is no guarantee of getting a job.

Membership exams (p 10)

These are essential to progress in almost all medical careers. They are difficult to pass and one of the main limiting factors in doctors' careers. There is now considerable time pressure to complete these exams and failure to do so may result in the loss of a job and career path.

Further specialty training (p 8)

Depending on the specialty these jobs may be guaranteed or may require another competitive application. At this stage many doctors have to choose a particular specialty or subspecialty. These posts are still new under Modernising Medical Careers (MMC) so there are likely to be changes, probably including the total length of training.

General practitioner (p 12)

This is a final career equivalent to consultant, but based in the community rather than in hospital. General practitioners are responsible for their patients' health, acting as their advocate in their interaction with other services. GP partners also run their GP practices as small businesses.

Consultant (p 13)

This is the final career stage of all hospital-based, and some community-based, specialties. The role carries responsibility for the patients, the team members and the department itself.

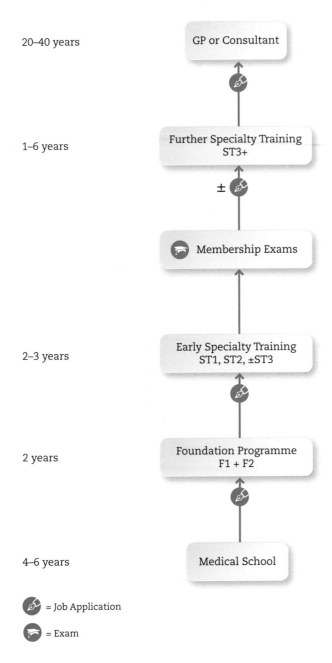

20–40 years — GP or Consultant

1–6 years — Further Specialty Training ST3+

± Membership Exams

2–3 years — Early Specialty Training ST1, ST2, ±ST3

2 years — Foundation Programme F1 + F2

4–6 years — Medical School

= Job Application

= Exam

Foundation programme

After completing medical school, junior doctors start the foundation programme (FP). This typically lasts two years and has replaced the pre-registration house officer year (PRHO) and the first year as a senior house officer (SHO).

F1 year This is a 12-month internship that must include 3 months of medicine and 3 months of surgery. Most jobs feature three placements of four months: medicine, surgery and a specialty, so an example F1 year could include four-month placements in cardiology, vascular surgery and paediatrics. The order of the placements varies.

F2 year These jobs can be in almost any specialty: 80% of FP jobs will include a four-month placement in general practice, usually in the F2 year. Most F2 jobs feature three placements of four months, e.g. anaesthetics, general practice and histopathology.

Applying for foundation programmes

Foundation programme applications take place in the autumn of the final year of medical school through a nationwide online applications service: http://www.foundationprogramme. nhs.uk. The application form features several different components. Many of these are self-explanatory: name, age, education, qualifications, references, etc., however, there are two difficult sections:

Questions There are about seven questions requiring short written answers of 150–250 words; they carry the majority of marks on the application form.

Preferences The applicant needs to rank the 26 foundation schools in order of preference. It is not possible to choose specific hospitals or placements at this stage—these will be allocated by the specific foundation school, often using a similar ranking system.

Techniques to help complete this form and to get a high score are discussed on p 62.

Does the specific foundation programme matter for a career?

The main objective of the FP is to ensure that all doctors reach a basic level of competency in being a doctor. All doctors who complete the foundation programme are eligible to apply for any specialty training post (except oral and maxillofacial surgery, which requires a dentistry degree). It is not the end of the world, or end of a career plan, if a particular specialty is not included as a placement. However, medicine is competitive and having spent four months in a specialty is usually an advantage at job interviews.

Provisional GMC registration

Once a medical student successfully completes medical school they should obtain provisional registration with the General Medical Council (GMC) to allow them to practice as a doctor. During the last two years of medical school a GMC representative will visit the medical school on a specific date to confirm each student's identity. A GMC reference number and PIN are then posted to the student while a password is sent by email; this allows access to the MyGMC website (via the home page of http://www.gmc-uk.org).

During the last three months of medical school the university will inform the GMC which students will graduate. Students must visit MyGMC to complete an online application form and a declaration of fitness to practice form (questions about convictions, health and disciplinary action; this can be seen on the GMC website under the section on 'Applying to join the register'). They also need to pay a £135 fee. If successful, the student should receive an email and a certificate in the post and be able to see their provisional status when they check their name on the register. Failure to register will prevent the medical student from beginning work as a junior doctor.

Assessments, reviews, and forms

Junior doctors face many obstacles between medical school and their final careers, but fortunately foundation programme assessments pose few problems. While they might be a hassle to complete, very few people fail to pass them and achieve competency. There are four formal types of assessment:

1) **Direct observation of procedural skills (DOPS)** A senior doctor observes the FP doctor performing a procedure (e.g. taking blood): at least six should be completed each year.

2) **Mini-clinical evaluation exercise (Mini-CEX)** A senior doctor observes the FP doctor clerking a patient: at least six should be completed each year.

3) **Case-based discussion (CbD)** Presenting a patient to a senior doctor and discussing the clerking, investigations and management: at least six should be completed each year.

4) **Multisource feedback (MSF)** 10–12 health professionals (consultants, F2s, nurses, occupational therapists [OTs], etc.) complete a form about the FP doctor's performance: at least one should be completed each year.

Alongside these assessments there should be regular meetings with an educational supervisor, ideally once every two months, but at the very least these must take place at the start and end of each placement. All these reviews and assessments involve completing specific forms found in the Foundation Learning Portfolio that are available online: http://www.foundationprogramme.nhs.uk.

There are three forms that are absolutely vital to 'passing' the foundation programme:

1) **End of placement final review form** Signed by the educational supervisor at the end of each four-/six-month placement to prove the FP doctor has completed the placement.

2) **5.1 Attainment of F1 competency form** Completed by the educational supervisor at the end of the F1 year (after reviewing the end of placement final review forms and the forms for the assessments described above). The original should be sent to the local Deanery, often with a certificate of experience from the GMC website. The Deanery will then submit these to the GMC. It is essential to keep a copy of this form in the portfolio.

3) **5.2 Foundation achievement of competency document (FACD)** Completed by the educational supervisor at the end of the F2 year upon reviewing the entire portfolio. Again the original should be sent to the local deanery whilst a copy must go into the portfolio. It is this form that shows that the FP doctor has passed the foundation programme.

Taster weeks

These are week-long 'tasters' during the F2 year spent in a specialty of the FP doctor's choice. Their purpose is to give the doctor a feel for specialties that they are considering for their final career, especially if their foundation programme has not included a placement in this specialty. These weeks should be taken as study leave, though some trusts insist (inappropriately) that annual leave is used instead. FP doctors can be imaginative in choosing tasters; so long as their educational supervisor and another senior doctor agree, they can do taster weeks in any specialty in the Trust.

Full GMC registration

At the end of the F1 year, doctors who have successfully completed all the F1 competencies can apply for full registration with the GMC. This is done by signing into MyGMC and completing another on-line application form and declaration of fitness to practice form along with paying a fee of £390. Alongside the application it is necessary to print and complete a Certificate of Experience from the GMC website. This should be posted to the deanery of the university of graduation (often with the Attainment of F1 competency form, above, and a stamped addressed envelope) where it will be signed and sent to the GMC. Failure to obtain full registration will prevent the F1 doctor from starting their first F2 placement.

Specialty training

After completing the foundation programme, the next stage of training is specialty training. As its name suggests, this is the when a junior doctor chooses a particular specialty and is trained to act independently at consultant level. The training takes between three and eight years depending on specialty. The career path through specialty training differs between specialties, however there are three broad types of training:

1) GP vocational training This is the most common career path and about 50% of doctors will opt for this route. Training is relatively straightforward, consisting of a single application during F2, followed by two years of training in hospitals (ST1 and ST2) and one year of training in a GP practice (ST3/GP registrar). Successful completion of the ST3 year and nMRCGP exam (p 10) leads to the award of General Practitioner Certificate of Completion of Training (GPCCT) entitling the doctor to apply for salaried or partner GP posts (p 12).

2) Specialty training This is also called **'Run-through training'**. After a successful application during the F2 year the doctor is guaranteed a training post in the same deanery until they have finished training, so long as they pass the necessary exams and assessments. While they may still need to apply for certain posts within specialty training (e.g. subspecialties), whatever the outcome they will have a job that leads to a Certificate of Completion of Training (CCT) award allowing them to apply for consultant jobs.

3) Core-training These career paths are also called **'Uncoupled'** because there is a lack of continuity between early training and later training. The doctor applies for initial training during F2 just in the same way as for the other types of training and this lasts for two to three years (CT1, CT2, ± CT3) depending on the specialty. At the end of core-training they apply for a specialty training post in a particular specialty. This application is competitive and a job is not guaranteed; however, those who are successful will then be guaranteed a job in the same deanery until the completion of training (and a CCT award) so long as they pass the necessary exams and assessments.

Do these different routes matter?

For those who have their hearts set on a particular specialty there is usually only one route to reach it. If several specialties are of interest then it is worth considering the advantages and disadvantages of the different types of specialty training when making a career decision:

- *General practice*
  - **Good points** Short training; clear training route; good job security.
  - **Bad points** Final career decision immediately after the foundation programme.

- *Run-through training (specialty training)*
  - **Good points** Good job security; stay in a single region of the UK for at least four years; training is usually slightly shorter than the uncoupled route.
  - **Bad points** Subspecialty options and routes can be unclear; difficult to change location; final career decision immediately after the foundation programme.

- *Uncoupled training (core-training)*
  - **Good points** More choice over exact specialty; longer time to decide before choosing a final career; opportunity to change location midway through training.
  - **Bad points** Less job security; few options for those who fail to get a specialty post; may be forced to change deanery between core-training and specialty training; training is usually longer.

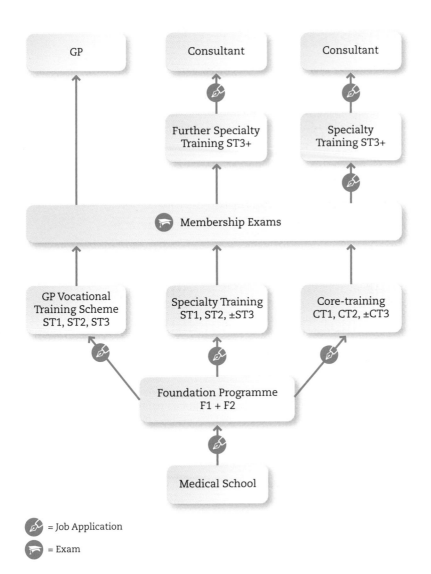

= Job Application

= Exam

Run-through (specialty training)		Uncoupled (core-training)	
Neurosurgery	p 50	Academia	p 16
Obstetrics and gynaecology	p 36	Anaesthetics	p 30
Ophthalmology	p 50	Medicine	p 34
Oral and maxillofacial surgery	p 50	Other surgical specialties	p 48
Paediatrics	p 38	Psychiatry	p 42
Pathology	p 40		
Public health	p 44		
Radiology	p 46		

Membership exams

Passing the dreaded membership exams is an essential step to becoming a consultant or GP. Most doctors find these exams are the hardest that they ever take in their lives. There are a number of factors that make them unpleasant:
- There are several exams (often three) for each membership
- Low pass rates, often 35–40% per exam; most candidates fail at least one
- Expensive
- Months of intense revision alongside a full-time job

On the good side the exams have become more relevant to the job than previously and there is no doubt they improve a doctor's knowledge base and clinical skills.

Many colleges are also adding an exit exam at the end of specialist training to prove the trainee has reached the expected level of ability. This is likely to become more common.

Exams available

Membership exams are available from the following Royal Colleges, Colleges and Faculties ('M' stands for 'Member', 'F' for 'Fellow' and 'n' for 'new'):
- Anaesthetics (FRCA)
- Emergency medicine (MCEM)
- General practitioners (nMRCGP)
- Obstetrics and gynaecology (MRCOG)
- Occupational medicine (MFOM)
- Ophthalmology (MRCOphth)
- Paediatrics and child health (MRCPCH)
- Pathologists (FRCPath)
- Physicians (MRCP)
- Psychiatry (MRCPsych)
- Public health (MFPH)
- Radiology (FRCR)
- Surgeons (MRCS)

Exam formats

Every membership exam has its own unique structure: some involve dissertations, laboratory skills, videoed consultations or vivas. However, the majority of exams are in two formats:
- Written exams These are usually multiple choice (MCQ), extended matching (EMQ) or best-of-five (BOF) questions on the science behind the specialty or clinical cases within the specialty. They are often time-pressured and the questions may be ambiguous (like patients).
- Clinical exams These involve multiple stations with real patients, actors or videos to test the candidate's history taking, communication and examination skills. Each station will test a specific skill, for example cardiovascular examination, and most are time-pressured. Passing the exam is about looking like a doctor and demonstrating core abilities—candidates need excellent clinical skills along with confidence.

Costs

The exact costs vary between specialty and type of exam. The following gives an idea of the costs per exam; bear in mind there are often three exams, not counting the common retakes:
- Exam £170–£1260 with clinical exams costing the most. There is debate as to whether these are tax deductible; they are essential to career progression.
- Courses £250–£1200 depending on duration and type. Trainees are entitled to study leave and funding for these, though actually getting these benefits can be very difficult.
- Travel costs up to £1000 for a course and exam if these are not commutable. This can be claimed from study leave funds.
- Websites and books £150 though this is very variable.

When to take exams

This varies between specialties—some can be taken straight after medical school, others require more experience (see Career overviews, p 28–50, for more details). Membership exams are essential to apply to, or progress through, specialty training and failure to pass at the right stage might necessitate switching to an FTSTA (p 14) or Staff and Associate Specialist Grade (SASG) post, see p 14.

Important points for planning exams

1) Do not 'try out' a membership exam without really revising; this often starts a pattern of repeated failure. Make each exam a top priority and aim to pass each one first time.

2) Avoid taking exams alongside other big events (e.g. weddings, buying a house).

3) Take exams at the earliest opportunity, having attained sufficient clinical experience to pass.

Revision

The exams are hard and will stretch even the best candidates. As an absolute minimum they require 2 months of intense revision (at least 20 hours a week). Many people need more than this (e.g. 3–4 months per exam). Doctors often take annual leave for revision before critical exams. Written exams require web- or book-based question banks with feedback, alongside reading around each subject. Clinical exams necessitate patient examination and presenting findings to colleagues/seniors, though a reasonable degree of reading is also required.

Exam resources

There is a competitive market for revision books, courses and websites so it is worth shopping around and asking colleagues for recommendations (they may even have books or revision notes to pass on). Courses are expensive, but might allow study leave; they also give a good idea of what might come up. Two websites have question banks for multiple membership exams: http://www.onexamination.com and http://www.pastestonline.co.uk.

Failing exams

Doctors generally lack experience at failing exams, however membership exams are difficult and failing is common. Failing does not make someone a bad doctor or not clever enough, it simply means that their social life and bank balance are in for more damage.

Once the initial shock of failing has passed it is important to try to be objective about the reasons for failure. Common problems include:

- Poor exam technique The questions are ambiguous and may sometimes seem impossible to answer. Remember that an exam board has passed this question so there must be a logical reason to select one answer over another. It is not about knowing the answer, but picking the correct response. Rule out wrong answers and try to think from the writer's perspective.
- Wrong revision Try to focus revision towards the exam. While it is important to have a good background knowledge of the specialty, this knowledge can continue to develop throughout the career. Focus on the subjects that come up regularly.
- Insufficient revision Retaining a social life suggests the need to hit the books harder!
- Bad luck Keep trying: eventually most people get through.

Look at any feedback from the exam board, talk to colleagues who have taken the exams and discuss methods of revision. Consider using revision websites or enrolling on courses.

Recurrent failure

If you really cannot pass an exam, for example after three attempts, then it is important to take a step back and think about your career. Are you doing a specialty that you enjoy and are good at? Do you need a break? Without membership, hospital-based careers are limited to staff grade posts (p 14); in a good department this can still be a good career.

General practitioner

This page describes the process of becoming a fully registered general practitioner (GP) after training. For details of the GP career pathway see p 32. For a description of the job and lifestyle of a general practitioner see the following pages:
* General practitioner (p 144)
* GP in a rural practice (p 150)
* GP with a special interest (GPwSI) (p 152)
* Academic GP (p 92)
* Prison medicine (p 236)
* Pre-hospital medicine (p 234)

Certificates and registration

General Practitioner Certificate of Completion of Training (GPCCT) At the end of the GP registrar year those who have completed the entire nMRCGP examination should be eligible for the GPCCT award issued by the Postgraduate Medical Education and Training Board (PMETB). To receive this certificate the trainee must complete two steps:

1) Register online with the Royal College of General Practitioners (RCGP) at the start of the GP Vocation Training Scheme (GPVTS, p 8); this will allow the trainee to complete the ePortfolio and provide the College with proof that the trainee has completed the training posts.

2) In the final six months of training the Royal College will inform PMETB Certification Unit which trainees are nearing completion of training. PMETB will send the trainees a GPCCT application form which they must complete, along with a photograph, full CV and a cheque for £750.

Certificate confirming Eligibility for General Practitioner Registration (CEGPR) It is possible to register as a general practitioner in the UK even for those who have not completed a UK GPVTS scheme. The applicant has to demonstrate equivalent training and experience to PMETB under Article 11; see p 82 for more detail on this process.

Inclusion on the GP register Following the award of a GPCCT or CEGPR certificate, a doctor's name should be automatically added to the GP register managed by the GMC. It is essential that a doctor's name is on this list before they practice as an independent GP; there are contact details and an application form on the GMC website (http://www.gmc-uk.org) for those whose name is not present on this list despite having received one of these certificates. There is no further charge for being added to this register.

GP jobs

GP jobs are advertised in a variety of locations including *BMJ Careers* (p 55). There are three main types of GP job:

1) **Partnership** These are GPs who 'own' their surgery, along with the other partners, and have a contract with the Primary Care Trust (PCT) to provide services to their patients. They are responsible for the management of the surgery and their salary is partly determined by how well the surgery functions; it usually ranges between £80000 and £120000.

2) **Salaried GP** These GPs are employed directly by the PCT; their salary is mostly determined by their number of years of GP experience and ranges from £50000 to £100000. Their salary is not affected by the income of the surgery that they work in and they have no official management role in the surgery.

3) **Locum GP** Employed to cover specific sessions or a period of absence by a permanent member of staff. Pay rates vary between jobs.

Consultant

This page describes the process of becoming a fully registered consultant. For the consultant career pathway see p 9. For the pathway for a particular specialty see pp 26.

Certificates and registration

Certificate of Completion of Training (CCT) At the end of specialist training, doctors who have completed all the necessary assessments and exams should be eligible for the CCT award issued by the Postgraduate Medical Education and Training Board (PMETB). The application to PMETB is made via the trainee's College (e.g. Royal College of Physicians), usually in the last six months before completion of training. The trainee needs to provide the following:
- Annual Review of Competency Progression Form G from the postgraduate deanery, issued following a final review of training and the portfolio.
- College notification form (available from the College)
- PMETB CCT application form (sent to the applicant by PMETB)
- Passport photograph
- Full CV
- Cheque for £750

Certificate confirming Eligibility for Specialist Registration (CESR) This is an alternative route for doctors to join the specialist register without completing PMETB-approved specialty training posts (e.g. associate specialists and those who have trained overseas). The applicant has to demonstrate equivalent training and experience to PMETB under Article 14; see p 82.

Inclusion on the Specialist Register Following CCT or CESR, doctors' names are added to the GMC specialist register automatically without further costs. Only those on this register can practice as a consultant specialist; there are contact details and a form on the GMC website (http://www.gmc-uk.org) for those awarded a certificate but whose name is not the register.

Consultant jobs

There are two ways to obtain a consultant post: by responding to an advert in *BMJ Careers* (p 55) or by being told when the advert for 'your' post will be placed in the *BMJ Careers*. This latter route is not the old-boy network: it is the result of careful preparation by the trainee allowing them to write the ideal CV for that job and perform at their best at interview.

Trainees are eligible to apply to consultant posts for six months prior to their CCT date, by which time the trainee should know their intended field ± subspecialty. By talking to as many consultants/clinical directors as possible, trainees should know where upcoming posts will be and the competitiveness. It is important to visit these departments and meet the senior consultants. If a post may be available soon, but not immediately, it is possible to locum as a consultant (p 174). If no post is likely in the foreseeable future the trainee needs to rethink their particular field or subspecialty interest.

Application is competitive, often involving interviews and presentations; posts are given to those who are 'best' on the day. It is important to find out who will be on the interview panel (often: lay chair, hospital chief executive or a representative, medical director/representative, College representative, consultant from the department, ± several others) and what will be expected. The question in the panel's mind is: 'Do we wish to work with this person for the next 30 years?'

It is common to negotiate the terms and conditions of service (including starting salary) after accepting the post. Do not sign any contract until completely happy. Ask the BMA and colleagues for advice. Some hospitals, sadly, try to start consultants on disadvantageous terms.

Staff and associate specialist grade (SASG)

Alternative names non-consultant career grade (NCCG), staff grade, clinical fellow, Trust doctor, Trust fellow, non-training grade, clinical assistant, hospital practitioner

Not every doctor wants to become a GP or consultant; a proportion will stay in hospital-based medicine in service positions. These doctors perform similar clinical activities to other senior doctors, but do not have management accountability and are not on a training path towards becoming a consultant. For some people SASG posts offer the ideal career structure with all the excitement of clinical medicine but less of the administration or responsibility of a consultant position. The hope of MMC is that these jobs will be seen as an attractive career option for many doctors.

Doctors can move from SASG posts to consultant posts by joining the specialist register. To do this they must prove they have the experience and competencies of doctors who have been through specialist training and be granted the certificate of eligibility for specialist training by PMETB under Article 14 (see p 82 for more details). In practice this is a difficult and slow route with no guarantee of success.

Good points Chance to be established in a department and hospital instead of moving every six months; no time pressure to take exams or assessments; can still gain excellent experience; can undertake full range of clinical activities; markedly reduced administrative functions

One of the main questions that junior doctors ask about MMC changes is 'What happens if I don't get a specialty training post?' The answer may include these non-training jobs. This is also the case if doctors in specialty training cannot pass membership exams or assessments within the required timeframes. Even if these jobs seem attractive as a career it is worth considering trying to complete a specialist training job and achieve the Certificate of Completion of Training (CCT) then apply for these jobs afterwards.

Bad points Hard to transfer to a Specialty Training/Consultant job; worse access to training opportunities; perceived as lower status; less pay (p 71); less independence; less control over working conditions; potentially less job security

Training

Foundation Foundation posts are guaranteed for all graduates from a UK medical school. There are 5% more foundation posts than UK medical school graduates; these extra posts are for doctors who need to retake the F1 year or, more commonly, for overseas medical graduates.

FTSTA applications same format as the equivalent specialty training application, p 26

Fixed-Term Specialty Training Appointment (FTSTA) Year-long jobs equivalent to early specialist training; they allow doctors to gain competencies and improve their CV to allow them to apply for specialist training the next year. It is important to note that entry to specialist training is more competitive at higher levels, e.g. ST2 is more competitive than ST1. These posts are only found in Run-through specialties (p 8); there is no equivalent for core-training.

Staff and Associate Specialist Grade The exact job varies between specialties, hospitals and departments. There are few fixed standards so the exact role is open to negotiation. There is considerable pressure to ensure formal access to training within this grade.

Exams

Unlike every other hospital-based medical specialty, membership exams are not always required. There is still benefit in taking membership exams or diplomas to allow subspecialty interests or to help demonstrate competencies for Article 14 (p 82) to transfer to consultant jobs.

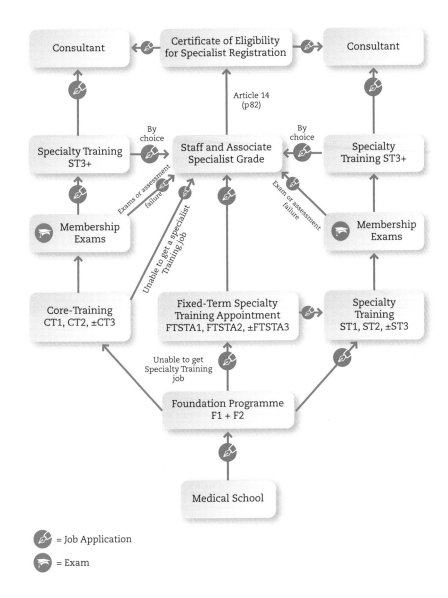

Consultant ←✐ Certificate of Eligibility for Specialist Registration ✐→ Consultant

Article 14 (p82)

Specialty Training ST3+ ✐ By choice → Staff and Associate Specialist Grade ← By choice ✐ Specialty Training ST3+

Exams or assessment failure

Unable to get a specialist Training job

Exam or assessment failure

Membership Exams

Membership Exams

Core-Training CT1, CT2, ±CT3

Fixed-Term Specialty Training Appointment FTSTA1, FTSTA2, ±FTSTA3 ✐→ Specialty Training ST1, ST2, ±ST3

Unable to get Specialty Training job

Foundation Programme F1 + F2

Medical School

✐ = Job Application

📖 = Exam

For further information:

Non-Consultant Career Grade Doctors Committee: http://www.rcplondon.ac.uk/college/committee/nccg
BMA: http://www.bma.org.uk, search for 'SAS'

Academic career

Academics are found in every specialty from general practice (p 32) to medicine (p 34); they are the doctors who push the boundaries of medical practice by pioneering new treatments, investigations and practices. One of the major developments from Modernising Medical Careers (MMC) was to formalize the academic career structure. In the past there was no clear academic route and junior doctors had to seek out research opportunities alongside full-time clinical training, then take career breaks to undertake the research.

The career route described is not the only way into academia, it is simply the most direct route. Any doctor who has sufficient research qualifications and clinical experience will be able to get an academic job. It is also possible to transfer between the clinical and academic routes.

Academic jobs tend to be highly competitive and require proof of academic excellence (e.g. distinction in medical degree, publications, first class intercalated BSc).

Training

Foundation There are special Academic Foundation Programmes (AFPs) available; the F1 year is no different from other FP jobs while the F2 year has two four-month specialty placements and a four-month academic placement that will involve doing research (e.g. in a laboratory). The research will often be based on one of the other specialty placements in the F2 year (e.g. renal medicine followed by renal research).

ST applications These are sent to the specific deanery, but all deaneries use a standard application form based on a standard CV created by the National Co-ordinating Centre for Research Capacity Development (NCCRCD). See contact details opposite.

Specialty training After the FP all trainees can apply for academic clinical fellowships (ACFs) in a specific specialty (e.g. haematology). These are equivalent to early specialty training or core-training but 25% of the trainee's time is devoted to academic activities (e.g. research, PhD/MD project design, funding applications). They last 2–3 years.

Training fellowship During the academic clinical fellowship the trainee should have designed a PhD/MD research project and applied to funding bodies. The training fellowship is when the PhD/MD is undertaken; a small amount of time will be spent in clinical practice to maintain skills. Fellowships usually last three years.

Clinical lectureship After completing a PhD/MD the trainee continues clinical training (equivalent to the later stages of specialty training) alongside further postdoctoral research; their time should be split 50:50 between clinical and research activities. In some specialties there may need to be a period of full-time clinical work to allow specialty training to be completed. These posts last up to four years and at the end of the post the trainee should have completed their entire specialty training programme and be ready for a consultant or senior lecturer position.

Exams and funding

The concept of the academic career path is that the trainee completes all the requirements of specialty training alongside research; this includes membership exams in the chosen specialty. The timing of these will be determined by the particular exams (see Specialty overviews p 26).

Academics also have to apply for funding to support their research. In practical terms they must find a funding source to support their training fellowship and their clinical lectureship. One advantage of the new career path is that there should be mentors and supervisors to help trainees through this process.

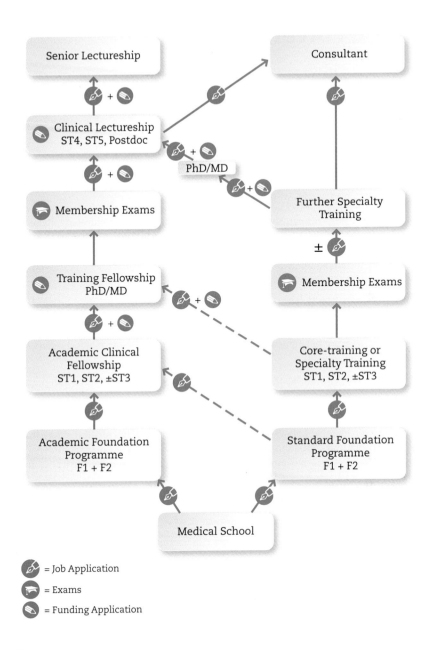

Senior Lectureship

Consultant

Clinical Lectureship
ST4, ST5, Postdoc

PhD/MD

Membership Exams

Further Specialty
Training

Training Fellowship
PhD/MD

±

Membership Exams

Academic Clinical
Fellowship
ST1, ST2, ±ST3

Core-training or
Specialty Training
ST1, ST2, ±ST3

Academic Foundation
Programme
F1 + F2

Standard Foundation
Programme
F1 + F2

Medical School

= Job Application

= Exams

= Funding Application

For further information:

National Co-ordinating Centre for Research Capacity Development (NCCRCD), Leeds
Innovation Centre, 103 Clarendon Road, Leeds, LS2 9DF
Tel: 0113 346 6260   Fax: 0113 346 3272   Web: http://www.nccrcd.nhs.uk

Armed Forces career

Doctors in the Armed Forces are trained as officers alongside their medical training. Like their civilian counterparts, the majority of military doctors train as GPs; this role can be very diverse since the doctor will follow their patients to wherever they are stationed, including warzones. There are three services within the armed forces and training follows a similar pattern in each:

- Army (p 102)
- Royal Air Force (p 264)
- Royal Navy (p 266)

Training

Medical student Students can apply for medical cadetships whilst at university; these will pay a salary for the last three years of medical school (about £14000 to £17000 per year) and payment of university tuition fees (effectively a further £3000 per year). In return the doctor must work for the armed forces for at least five years after the end of the F2 year. While the money is attractive the commitment is binding and expensive to buy out of.

Foundation Medical cadets can apply for a military FP. These follow the same format as the normal foundation programme (p 6) except they are based in one of five Military of Defence hospital units (MDHU) at Derriford, Frimley Park, Northallerton, Peterborough and Portsmouth. These are not compulsory and there are currently more medical cadets than military foundation jobs.

> **ST applications** These are made to the West Midlands Deanery which works with the Defence Postgraduate Medical Deanery (DPMD)

Specialty training After the end of the F2 year military training begins with medical officer training (about 6 months) followed by 12 months as a general duties medical officer (a role similar to a GP registrar). After this trainees must choose a specialty; the options are restricted to those required by the armed forces (e.g. it is not possible to train in paediatrics). Military specialist training jobs are set aside for military doctors so despite applying through MMC they are only in competition with other military doctors, not civilian doctors. If they leave the armed forces during specialty training they will lose their training number so hospital doctors will often need to sign up for a further two to four years of service to complete training.

Specialists After completing training, doctors can continue to work in the armed forces; there are two main options:

1) As a GP usually working as the registered medical officer of a regiment and following that regiment on all its activities including training and deployment.

2) As a consultant working in a Ministry of Defence hospital unit.

Doctors can also join the armed forces as a specialist (i.e. having completed training independently); it is necessary to sign up for at least three years.

Exams

It is essential to pass the membership exams for the given specialty. There is no difference in the specific exams between the armed forces and other medical careers. See p 10 for more details or look at the overview for a specific specialty (p 26).

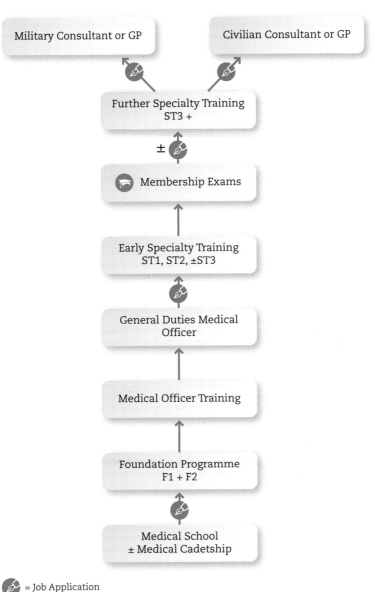

Military Consultant or GP

Civilian Consultant or GP

Further Specialty Training
ST3 +

± Membership Exams

Early Specialty Training
ST1, ST2, ±ST3

General Duties Medical
Officer

Medical Officer Training

Foundation Programme
F1 + F2

Medical School
± Medical Cadetship

 = Job Application

= Exam

ℹ️ *For further information:*

Defence Postgraduate Medical Deanery, ICT Centre, Birmingham Research Park, Vincent Drive, Edgbaston, Birmingham, B15 2SQ
Tel: 0121 415 8158   Fax: 0121 415 8161
Hospital-based specialties: Squadron Leader Jon Gregory
Tel: 0121 415 8165   Email: jonagreg@dsca.mod.uk
General practice vocational training: Major Debbie Butterworth
Tel: 0121 415 8158   Email: debrbutt@dsca.mod.uk

'Off the beaten path' career

While a medical degree allows graduates to work as doctors in hospitals or in general practice, it does not limit them to these jobs. There are many jobs where medical training can provide a unique insight that is highly valued. There are also jobs that require the skills of doctors in different situations (e.g. expedition doctors). It is difficult to describe a career path for these jobs since they are diverse and uncommon, however these two pages attempt to give suggestions. The jobs are described in more detail on the following pages, it is not an exhaustive list:

• Acupuncture	p 96	• Journalism	p 172	• Medical management	p 192
• Civil Service	p 114	• Law	p 188	• Medical politics	p 198
• Entrepreneur	p 184	• Medical consultant	p 190	• Pre-hospital medicine	p 234
• Expedition doctor	p 134	• Medical defence organizations	p 180	• Pharmaceutical medicine	p 230
• Forensic medical examiner	p 136	• Medical education	p 182	• Prison medicine	p 236
• Homeopathy	p 164	• Medical ethics	p 186	• Ship's doctor	p 270

There are three important points of guidance when considering these types of jobs:

1) Very few doctors manage to make a full-time career out of these jobs; it is much more common to undertake one of them alongside a 'standard' medical career.

2) Generally the more advanced a doctor is in their medical training, the more capable they are at one of these jobs. Completing the foundation programme is basically essential, membership exams are a huge benefit and completing specialist training is advantageous.

3) Training for these jobs needs to occur alongside clinical training; often it will be a personal interest that develops with courses, qualifications and experience.

Training

Foundation While medical school gives the title of doctor it is the foundation programme that makes graduates think and act like one. The specific placements are unlikely to have a great bearing on a career, but consider what may be useful (e.g. general practice, emergency medicine).

Specialty training The choice of training programme will depend on personal interests; think about what skills will be useful for a future career, but make sure it is a specialty worth working in for itself rather than just for a future goal.

Experience Many of the jobs above will require the trainee to develop skills and experience outside of their normal medical careers (e.g. writing skills, politics, problem-solving skills, ethical analysis). These skills are usually cultivated alongside medical training outside working hours; it is often necessary to have developed such skills highly before someone will pay for them.

Courses There are many courses which may help training towards one of these careers. It may be possible to secure study leave and funding for some of these.

Exams and qualifications

Completion of membership exams is an important marker of ability and experience within a specialty. People are much more likely to take a medical opinion seriously if it is backed by membership-level experience and qualifications. The process of passing the exams also forces the doctor to learn the key knowledge (and lots of less key knowledge) for their specialty. Alongside taking membership exams it is important to consider what qualifications will help in a future career; these can often be taken as part-time courses:

• **Degrees** e.g. law, management, education
• **Diplomas** e.g. mountain medicine, tropical medicine and hygiene, acupuncture, homeopathy, remote medicine, forensic.

Unlike other career paths these two paths need to be undertaken together

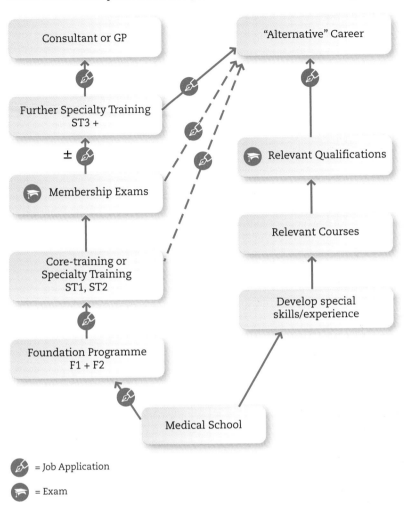

Consultant or GP		"Alternative" Career

Further Specialty Training ST3 +

Membership Exams

Relevant Qualifications

Relevant Courses

Core-training or Specialty Training ST1, ST2

Develop special skills/experience

Foundation Programme F1 + F2

Medical School

= Job Application

= Exam

ℹ️ For further information:

See individual career chapters p 90.

Overseas career

Medicine offers fantastic opportunities to travel round the world. There are three broad categories of overseas career that doctors might undertake:

1) Voluntary/aid work In countries with less developed medical services or recent disasters a doctor can have a huge impact on people's lives and health. Alongside making a difference there is the chance to live and work within a different culture; it can be a life-changing experience. Three examples of this type of work are included in this book:
* Merlin, an emergency relief organization (p 200)
* Overseas aid an overview of working for aid organizations (p 220)
* Voluntary Services Overseas (VSO) (p 290)

2) Training/practicing in a foreign country A UK medical degree is accepted as proof of medical training in most countries, though the doctor may need to prove they can speak the local language and pass the equivalent of medical school finals (e.g. USA and Canada). Every country has a different training path and describing each of these is beyond the scope of this book. It is especially common to undertake a period of training (e.g. one year, though it will probably not count towards UK training times) in Australia or New Zealand since there is no need to take further exams.

3) Travelling as an expert Specialists may be invited to share their expertise in foreign countries at conferences or specific hospitals and universities. This is more common amongst academics.

Training

Foundation It is essential to complete the foundation programme to work as a doctor in a foreign country; it also enables the trainee to re-enter the UK training system in the future. Try to include placements that cover broad areas, for example general practice, emergency medicine, paediatrics, obstetrics and gynaecology, acute medicine.

Specialty training Many doctors take a break between the foundation programme and specialty training to work in Australia or New Zealand. The training usually does not count towards UK training (unless pre-approved by PMETB), however the experience will be useful and may help to secure a job. Voluntary and aid organizations prefer doctors with general experience and at least three years' experience after medical school.

Long-term It is possible to devote an entire career to overseas aid (p 220); while the initial jobs are often voluntary or offer a minimal stipend, with increasing experience it is possible to earn a salary whilst doing this sort of work. Examples include the World Health Organisation (WHO), United Nations (UN) or organizations such as Merlin or Médecins Sans Frontières.

Exams and qualifications

It is well worth completing membership exams prior to undertaking voluntary or aid work overseas. They will help to develop the experience and knowledge necessary to deal with difficult situations and also make it much easier to obtain a job upon return. It is also worth considering other qualifications which may help. The most common of these is the diploma in tropical medicine and hygiene; this is a full-time three-month course in London or Liverpool that costs just over £4000.

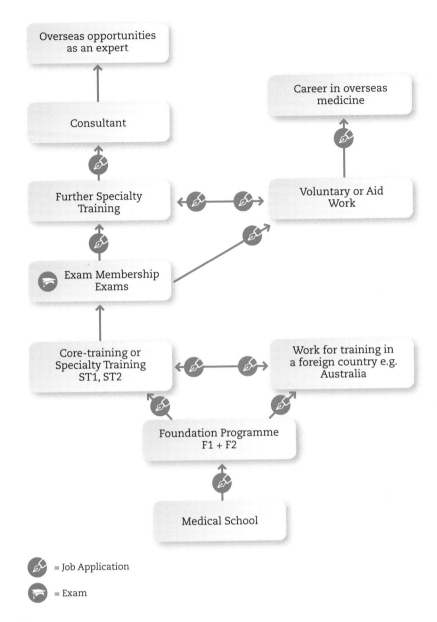

Overseas opportunities as an expert

Consultant

Career in overseas medicine

Further Specialty Training ← → Voluntary or Aid Work

Exam Membership Exams

Core-training or Specialty Training ST1, ST2 ← → Work for training in a foreign country e.g. Australia

Foundation Programme F1 + F2

Medical School

= Job Application

= Exam

ℹ️ For further information:

Voluntary Services Overseas (VSO), 317 Putney Bridge Road, London, SW15 2PN
Tel: 020 8780 7200   Web: http://www.vso.org.uk
Merlin, 12th Floor, 207 Old Street, London, EC1V 9NR
Tel: 020 7014 1600   Fax: 020 7014 1641   Web: http://www.merlin.org.uk
Australia Department of Health and Ageing for information about working in Australia
Web: http://www.doctorconnect.gov.au
New Zealand Government website on moving to New Zealand
Web: http://www.newzealandnow.info

Leaving clinical medicine

Medicine is not a life sentence. For doctors who do not enjoy a medical career, or simply feel that they've had enough, there are many options available. While a medical degree is a vocational qualification it also counts as a normal degree and it is highly regarded as such.

Before you leave consider the following:

* Is the problem clinical medicine or just the current job/hospital/city/country?
* Would changing to a different specialty help? Look at all the options in this book.
* Would a break be sufficient? Look at the chapter on time out, p 68.
* Is there a chance of wanting to return to clinical medicine? Don't burn bridges.
* What are the financial implications of taking a break from a medical career?
* Signing on with a locum agency provides a great source of fast cash, but takes 2–3 months.
* Are any qualifications or courses required before starting a different career?
* Will a different career lead to greater happiness?

When considering a change of career try to establish what aspects of a job matter and how the new career matches these. Consider taking a part-time/low-banded clinical job or some locum shifts to cover life expenses whilst planning a career change. Talk to people doing the job about the good and bad aspects and ensure that the new career is better than a medical career. Think about:

* Income
* Location (e.g. small towns vs major cities)
* Competition and qualifications
* Lifestyle and free time
* Flexibility
* Travel opportunities/requirements
* Career progression
* Opportunity for part-time work
* Benefits (e.g. cars, pensions)

Careers related to medicine

There are many non-clinical jobs where medical experience will be a huge asset, or even an essential requirement, to fulfil the role. The jobs are likely to be advertised outside of *BMJ Careers* and it is essential to find out where the adverts will be. This book presents some of the more common options, however the list is not exhaustive:

* Civil Service p 114
* Entrepreneur p 184
* Journalism p 172
* Law p 188
* Medical consultancy p 190
* Medical education p 182
* Medical ethics p 186
* Medical management p 192
* Medical politics p 198
* Research p 94
* Pharmaceutical medicine p 230

Careers unrelated to medicine

Alongside diagnostic skills and the ability to cannulate whilst half asleep, medicine teaches many transferable skills. It is important to highlight these in a CV whilst removing all medical jargon. Key skills include: time management, prioritization, communication (both written and oral), presentations, management, team work, decision-making, coping with stress and teaching.

Try to make contacts with people in the new career to help guide the changeover and suggest ways to find employment. Few organizations function like the NHS so be careful not to assume things will be done in the same way.

Specialty overviews

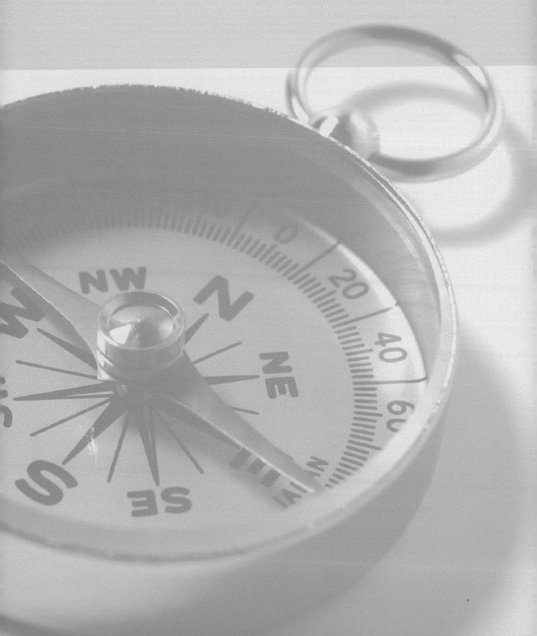

Part 2

Specialty overviews

Acute care common stem (ACCS)

This is the training route for three specialties:

1) Acute medicine (p 98) Doctors who oversee the critical 24–72 hours at the start of a patient's medical admission. They generally work on medical admission units (MAU) and manage patients referred from the emergency department (ED) or by GPs.

2) Anaesthetics (p 100) Doctors who provide general or regional anaesthetic for patients undergoing surgery. This is not the only training route for anaesthetics; it is possible to apply directly to an anaesthetics programme (p 30).

3) Emergency medicine (p 130) Doctors who work in the emergency department (ED); formerly called accident and emergency (A+E). They manage patients who require immediate treatment and self-referring patients.

ACCS is also a starting point for a career in intensive care (see p 170).

Training

Foundation There is a strong emphasis on acute care in the foundation programme so most jobs will include at least one of the above specialties; also consider tasters in the F2 year.

ACCS CT applications These are made directly to the deanery of choice.

Specialty training These specialties all start with a period of core-training followed by competitive entry to specialty training after two to three years. Despite having a common stem, each specialty has different core-training, making it difficult to change between them:

- Acute medicine Two years of core-training (CT1, CT2) followed by competitive entry to acute medicine ST3. The core-training is equivalent to core medical training (p 34) so also allows application to any medical specialty at ST3.
- Anaesthetics Three years of core-training (CT1, CT2 and a further CT2 in anaesthetics) followed by competitive entry to anaesthetics ST3.
- Emergency medicine Three years of core-training (CT1, CT2, CT3) followed by competitive entry to emergency medicine ST4.

Subspecialties The training path for intensive care has not been formalized at the time of writing, but it is likely to be an option during specialist training in anaesthetics, acute medicine and some general medical specialties, for example respiratory medicine.

Exams

- Acute medicine MRCP part 1 required for ST3 application, see p 34
- Anaesthetics Primary FRCA required for ST3 application, see p 30
- Emergency medicine Completion of the Membership of the College of Emergency Medicine (MCEM) exam is required for application to ST4. There are three parts which must be passed within four years from the first attempt of part A:
  - Part A Basic science MCQs, usually taken in CT1 or CT2
  - Part B Data interpretation written paper usually taken in CT2 or CT3
  - Part C 18 station OSCE usually taken in CT2 or CT3

Fellowship (FCEM) is a separate exam required by the end of specialist training to obtain a CCT; trainees can attempt this exam from the end of ST5

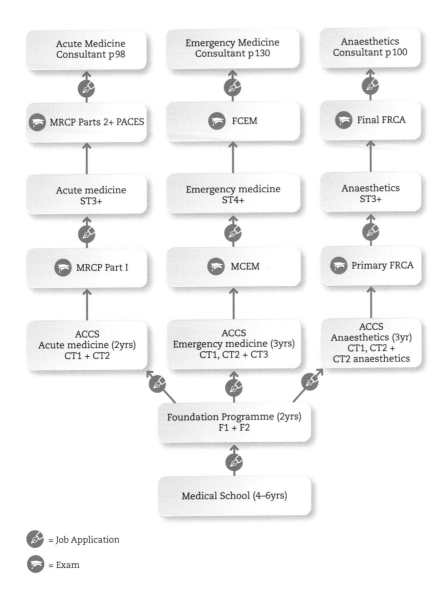

Acute Medicine
Consultant p 98

Emergency Medicine
Consultant p 130

Anaesthetics
Consultant p 100

MRCP Parts 2+ PACES

FCEM

Final FRCA

Acute medicine
ST3+

Emergency medicine
ST4+

Anaesthetics
ST3+

MRCP Part I

MCEM

Primary FRCA

ACCS
Acute medicine (2yrs)
CT1 + CT2

ACCS
Emergency medicine (3yrs)
CT1, CT2 + CT3

ACCS
Anaesthetics (3yr)
CT1, CT2 +
CT2 anaesthetics

Foundation Programme (2yrs)
F1 + F2

Medical School (4–6yrs)

= Job Application

= Exam

ⓘ For further information:

College of Emergency Medicine, Churchill House, 35 Red Lion Square, London, WC1R 4SG
Tel: 020 7404 1999   Fax: 020 7067 1267   Web: http://www.emergencymed.org.uk
Society for Acute Medicine (UK), Royal Infirmary of Edinburgh, 51 Little Frances Crescent,
Edinburgh, EH16 4SA
Web: http://www.acutemedicine.org.uk

Anaesthetics

Anaesthetics is the largest single specialty in hospital-based medicine. The training route leads to three main roles:

1) Anaesthetics (p 100) The majority of anaesthetics trainees will work with surgeons and occasionally medics to provide adequate pain relief, sedation or anaesthesia for procedures and operations. They may also be involved in intensive care, pain clinics, post-operative pain relief and as a key member of the crash team.

2) Intensive care (p 170) Some anaesthetists will specialize in intensive care with only occasional anaesthetic lists. ACCS anaesthesia provides the most direct route, but it is also possible to reach this career via medical training (e.g. acute medicine or respiratory medicine).

3) Pain medicine (p 226) These are anaesthetists who specialize in chronic pain relief; it is a clinic-based specialty, though they may be involved in ward-based pain teams.

Training

Foundation Four-month placements in anaesthetics or intensive care are available. Placements in acute medicine, general medicine and surgery will also be of benefit. Those who do not have anaesthetics or intensive care placements should consider an F2 taster attachment.

Anaesthetics CT/ST applications These are made directly to the deanery.

Core-training Anaesthetics can be reached by two routes:
- Anaesthetics core-training (CT1 and CT2), which takes two years
- Acute care common stem in anaesthetics core-training (CT1, CT2 and CT2 in pure anaesthetics), which takes three years with two years of acute care training followed by a further year that is the same as the second year of anaesthetics core-training.

Choosing between anaesthetics and ACCS anaesthetics

For those who are sure that they want a career in anaesthetics it is possible to avoid an extra year of training by applying to anaesthetics directly. There are three main reasons to consider the longer ACCS route instead:

1) The extra experience makes training and getting jobs in intensive care easier

2) The benefit of extra experience prior to the responsibility of being an anaesthetist

3) ACCS would allow the trainee to change to a medical specialty after CT2 if anaesthetics was not the right career choice; note that MRCP part 1 is required for ST3 medical specialties.

Specialist training After completing one of the above core-training programmes and the primary FRCA exam (below), trainees can apply for anaesthetics ST3. If successful they begin a five-year training programme that leads to a CCT in anaesthesia.

Subspecialists Some anaesthetists subspecialize during specialist training based on training opportunities (e.g. paediatrics, neurosurgery). It is also possible to specialize in pain medicine and intensive care; at present these careers are also reached via specialist training in anaesthetics.

Exams

The Fellowship of the Royal College of Anaesthetists (FRCA) exam is required for an anaesthetic career:
- **Primary** MCQ; those that pass attend an objective structured clinical examination (OSCE) and viva exam one month later. Passing all these components is required to apply for anaesthetics ST3.
- **Final** Short answer questions and MCQ; those that pass attend a viva two months later. Passing all these components is required to progress to ST5.

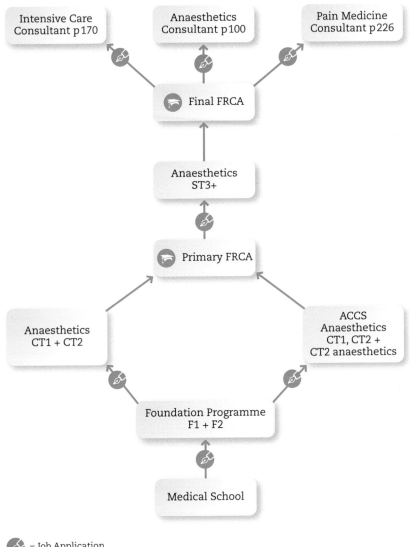

Intensive Care
Consultant p170

Anaesthetics
Consultant p100

Pain Medicine
Consultant p226

Final FRCA

Anaesthetics
ST3+

Primary FRCA

Anaesthetics
CT1 + CT2

ACCS
Anaesthetics
CT1, CT2 +
CT2 anaesthetics

Foundation Programme
F1 + F2

Medical School

= Job Application

= Exam

ⓘ For further information:

Royal College of Anaesthetists, Churchill House, 35 Red Lion Square, London, WC1R 4SG
Tel: 020 7092 1500 Fax: 020 7092 1730 Web: http://www.rcoa.ac.uk

General practice

About 50% of doctors will choose a career in general practice (p 144), making it the largest specialty within medicine. The job is diverse and there are opportunities to develop specific roles:

- **GP with special interests** (GPwSI, p 152) This is when a GP has developed particular skills in a specialty, for example paediatrics, cardiology. It provides the chance to run dedicated specialty clinics in a similar manner to hospital consultants.
- **Minor operations and procedures** Many GP surgeries have a small theatre run by GPs for operations or procedures that can be performed under local anaesthetic.
- **Academia** (p 92) Like all specialties there is an opportunity to work in an academic setting to advance the methods and practice of medicine.

Training

Foundation 80% of FPs should include a four-month placement in general practice which provides an excellent opportunity to experience the GP career. Those keen on being a GP should consider using their F2 tasters to experience GP practices in different settings (e.g. inner city vs rural) or GPs with special interests.

> **GPVTS applications** There are three stages:
>
> 1) Nationwide online application
>
> 2) MCQ exam covering clinical knowledge and situational judgements (a GP aptitude test)
>
> 3) Assessment centre (if shortlisted from the first two assessments); includes a simulated patient consultation, a group discussion exercise and a written test of prioritizing tasks and ability to reflect on decisions.

Specialty training GPs need to complete the GP vocational training scheme (GPVTS). This lasts three years: the first two are spent in hospital-based specialties (e.g. paediatrics, obstetrics and gynaecology, psychiatry) and the last is spent as a GP registrar working in general practice under supervision.

Switching tracks Doctors can apply to GPVTS from other specialty training posts; some ST experience may be credited by GPVTS allowing them to apply for ST2 or ST3, though this may be more competitive. It remains easier to switch from hospital specialties to GP than vice versa.

Subspecialists GPwSI schemes are for fully trained GPs and entail further training by working with a hospital consultant to develop skills to meet specific competencies. The availability of this training is determined by local need, as decided by the PCT.

Exams

GP trainees must pass the new Membership of the Royal College of General Practioners exam (nMRCGP). The pass rate for the nMRCGP exams is higher than for many other membership exams, however this may change. It has three components:

- **Workplace-based assessment** (WPBA) This is basically the outcome of educational supervisor reviews and the trainee's portfolio assessments over the entire three years of GPVTS. The information and assessments required for the portfolio are similar to those in the FP portfolio.
- **Applied knowledge test** (AKT) An MCQ exam taken in the GP registrar year.
- **Clinical skills assessment** (CSA) A twelve-station objective structured clinical examination (OSCE) taken in the GP registrar year.

Diplomas Alongside the membership exam many GPs take diplomas during training. While these are not essential they help in the increasingly competitive world of GP job applications. Common examples include the diploma in child health (DCH) and the diploma of the Royal College of Obstetricians and Gynaecologists (DRCOG). The exams are similar in format to membership exams (e.g. MCQs and OSCEs) with GP specific content and a higher pass rate.

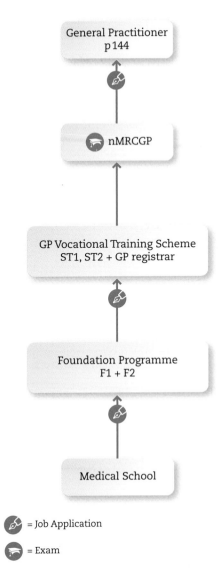

General Practitioner
p144

nMRCGP

GP Vocational Training Scheme
ST1, ST2 + GP registrar

Foundation Programme
F1 + F2

Medical School

= Job Application

= Exam

ℹ️ For further information:

Royal College of General Practitioners, 14 Princes Gate, Hyde Park, London, SW7 1PU
Tel: 0845 456 4041   Fax: 020 7225 3047   Web: http://www.rcgp.org.uk
For details of GPVTS applications see also: http://www.gprecruitment.org.uk

Internal medicine

Internal medicine, also called 'general medicine' or 'simply medicine', covers a large range of hospital-based jobs and gives the trainee great flexibility in choosing a career. The jobs range from the generalist, who deals with all medical admissions, to the subspecialist who is an expert in their particular field. There is a tendency towards greater subspecialization, though the generalist attitude is still required when on-call or dealing with multiple pathologies.

Most medical jobs are a mixture of ward-based and clinic-based medicine; some doctors also spend time in theatre (e.g. cardiology) or in laboratories (e.g. haematology). For more details on specific medical specialties see the following pages:

Training

Foundation Four months of internal medicine is compulsory during the F1 year. Many placements will include a further four months in a specific medical specialty; placements in emergency medicine and acute medicine will also offer useful experience. If a particular specialty is of interest then request a taster attachment during the F2 year.

Medicine CT and ST applications These are run by local deaneries; usually based on CV and interview.

Core-training Medical specialties are reached via two years of core medical training (CT1 and CT2) during which the MRCP part 1 should be completed (see below). Most core-training programmes involve four placements of six months in different medical specialties. Alternatively core-training in acute care common stem (ACCS) acute medicine entitles the trainee to apply for medical specialty training.

Specialty training Completion of core-training and MRCP part 1 entitles doctors to apply for ST3 in a specific medical specialty (see table above). This training lasts between four and six years, varying between specialties. There may be an option to qualify in general (internal) medicine (G(I)M) alongside the specialty; this usually adds a year to training.

Exams

To progress through medical specialties it is essential to pass the membership of the Royal College of Physicians exam (MRCP). Part 1 can be taken 18 months after completing a medical degree (i.e. midway through F2) and is essential for applying for all medical specialties at ST3 level; a few specialties require the complete MRCP at this stage and this may also be necessary for the more competitive jobs.

* Part 1 A written exam in best-of-five (BoF) format; it tests knowledge of clinical science and common or important diseases. There is a published syllabus.
* Part 2 A written clinical exam in best-of-five (BoF) or extended matching questions (EMQ) format. It tests diagnosis, investigation, management and prognosis of patients.
* PACES A clinical exam with five stations (some with multiple parts) with patients or actors covering clinical examination, history-taking, communication and ethics.

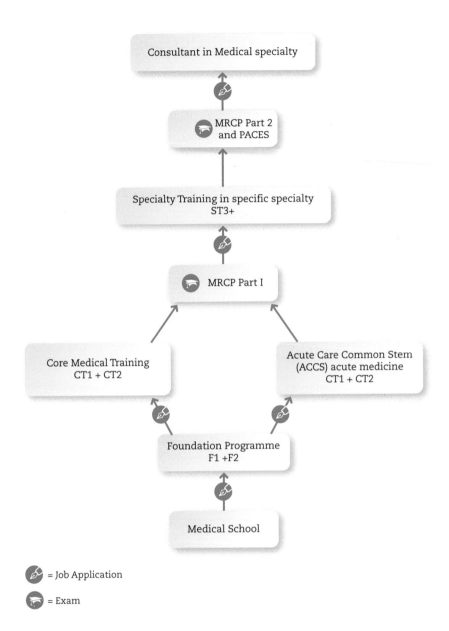

Consultant in Medical specialty

MRCP Part 2 and PACES

Specialty Training in specific specialty ST3+

MRCP Part I

Core Medical Training CT1 + CT2

Acute Care Common Stem (ACCS) acute medicine CT1 + CT2

Foundation Programme F1 +F2

Medical School

= Job Application

= Exam

ⓘ *For further information:*

Royal College of Physicians of London, 11 St Andrews Place, Regent's Park, London, NW1 4LE
Tel: 020 7935 1174   Fax: 020 7487 5218   Web: http://www.rcplondon.ac.uk
For further information about exams: http://www.mrcpuk.org

Obstetrics and gynaecology

Obstetrics and gynaecology training is the starting point for a number of specialties and sub-specialties. Many of them combine surgical techniques with medical care:

- Gynaecology (p 156) General care for disorders of the female reproductive system and the management of uncomplicated pregnancies below 20 weeks gestation.
- Obstetrics (p 212) Management of pregnancy from 20 weeks gestation (earlier if there are complications in current or previous pregnancies), childbirth and post-childbirth care.
- Gynaecology oncology (p 154) A surgical specialty focusing on the management of cancer of the female reproductive tract.
- Maternal and fetal medicine (p 176) Care of complicated pregnancies and diagnosis and treatment of fetal abnormalities.
- Sexual and reproductive health (family planning) (p 268) Providing advice on contraception, management of sexually transmitted diseases and psychosexual health.
- Reproductive medicine (fertility) (p 258) Assisting couples who have difficulty conceiving naturally.
- Urogynaecology (p 282) Managing disorders of the female urinary tract.

Training

Foundation Four-month placements in obstetrics and gynaecology are relatively common. Placements in general surgery and emergency medicine would also be of benefit. Week-long tasters can be requested in all of the above specialties.

Obstetrics and gynaecology ST applications Made using a nationwide online form. The form asks for CV details along with short answer questions about teamwork, communication skills, personality, etc; it is similar to the foundation programme form.

Specialty training After the FP, doctors must apply for a seven-year training programme. This is a run-through training programme (p 8) so after securing this position a training post should be guaranteed until the CCT is attained, as long as the trainee passes the necessary exams and assessments.

Subspecialists Entry to the five subspecialties shown above (e.g. maternal and fetal medicine) requires competitive entry to a three-year training programme after ST5. This training will include a year of research. This route is for full subspecialization; it is possible to develop an interest in these specialties through the conventional training route by completing advanced training skills modules (ATSMs).

Exams

The MRCOG exam is split into three parts. The syllabuses are available on the college website:

1) Part 1 This is a written exam of MCQs that can be taken any time after finishing medical school though it is usually taken after FP/ST experience in obstetrics and gynaecology.

2) Part 2 written This is taken at least five years after finishing medical school (i.e. ST3 and beyond) and at least two years of full-time obstetrics and gynaecology after passing part 1. The paper is made of MCQs, EMQs and short answers.

3) Part 2 oral This must be taken two months after passing Part 2 written. There are ten stations covering communication, diagnosis, management and critical appraisal.

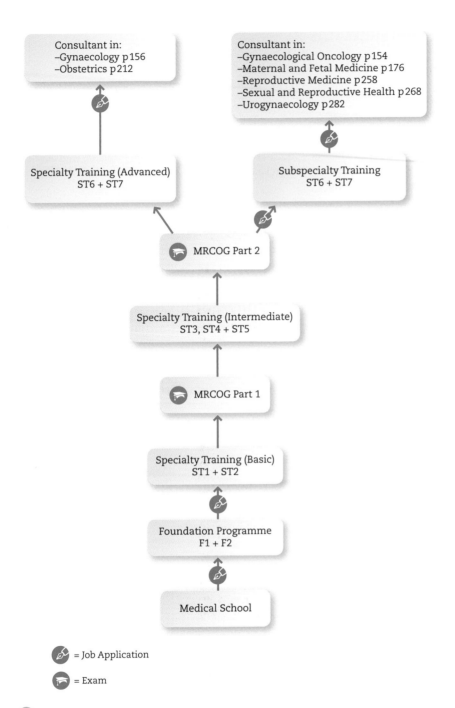

Consultant in:
–Gynaecology p156
–Obstetrics p212

Consultant in:
–Gynaecological Oncology p154
–Maternal and Fetal Medicine p176
–Reproductive Medicine p258
–Sexual and Reproductive Health p268
–Urogynaecology p282

Specialty Training (Advanced)
ST6 + ST7

Subspecialty Training
ST6 + ST7

MRCOG Part 2

Specialty Training (Intermediate)
ST3, ST4 + ST5

MRCOG Part 1

Specialty Training (Basic)
ST1 + ST2

Foundation Programme
F1 + F2

Medical School

= Job Application

= Exam

ⓘ For further information:

Royal College of Obstetricians and Gynaecologists, 27 Sussex Place, Regent's Park, London, NW1 4RG
Tel: 020 7772 6200   Fax: 020 7723 0575   Web: http://www.rcog.org.uk

Paediatrics

Paediatrics is divided into three main specialties:
- General paediatrics (p 224) This accounts for the majority of paediatricians. It is a hospital-based job covering children from birth to the age of 16 years. In district general hospitals the job may also include elements of neonates or community paediatrics.
- Neonatology (p 204) This is the specialty of newborn babies. It is usually based in an intensive care unit looking after premature babies or babies with problems at birth.
- Community paediatrics (p 122) These paediatricians look after children with developmental, social or behavioural problems and those with physical disabilities outside the hospital environment.

Training

Foundation Four-month placements in paediatrics are relatively common and give an excellent insight into the job. While these are not essential, they will make the ST interview and application process much easier. Alternatively, consider week-long tasters in the specialties above.

Paediatric ST applications These are coordinated nationwide by the college. Applicants fill in a CV-based application form and a list of deanery preferences. The preferences list is sent to the college whilst the application form is sent directly to the first two choices of deaneries on the list. Applicants are interviewed at these deaneries using three 10 minute stations: communication skills station, a presentation and a structured interview.

Specialty training Doctors can apply to specialty training in paediatrics at the end of the foundation programme. The initial years are split between general paediatrics and neonatology with some posts offering time in specialty posts (e.g. community paediatrics). This is a run-through training programme (p 8) so once the trainee secures this position a training post should be guaranteed until the CCT is attained, as long as the necessary exams and assessments are passed.

Subspecialists After completing five years of paediatrics specialty training (i.e. at the end of ST5) trainees can apply for competitive specialist positions (e.g. neonatology, endocrine, paediatric emergency medicine) via the national training number (NTN) grid system. This is for those who want to specialize completely (i.e. in a tertiary centre); many paediatricians develop a special interest whilst working as a general paediatrician.

Exams

The MRCPCH exam is split into four parts, though the first two are usually taken together. The first exam can be taken straight after medical school, although most people wait until they have completed at least six months of paediatrics (e.g. ST1).
- Part 1a This is a written exam testing common paediatric clinical and non-clinical knowledge; GP trainees also take this exam towards a diploma in child health (DCH).
- Part 1b This covers more complex clinical and non-clinical paediatric knowledge.
- Part 2 written This is a written clinical exam that tests diagnostic and patient management skills using photos, case histories and data interpretation questions.
- Part 2 clinical There are ten stations with patients or actors and a video station. Highlights include development, communication and history/management.

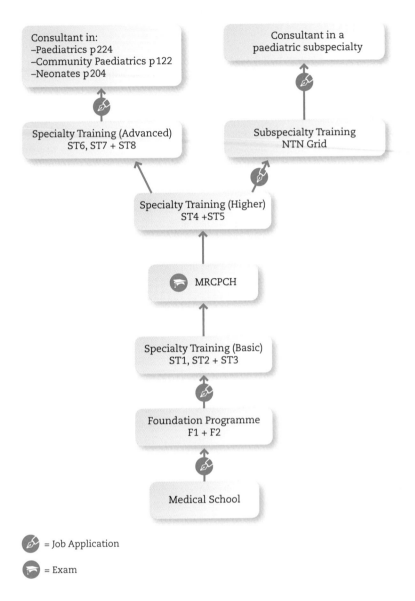

Consultant in:
–Paediatrics p 224
–Community Paediatrics p 122
–Neonates p 204

Consultant in a
paediatric subspecialty

Specialty Training (Advanced)
ST6, ST7 + ST8

Subspecialty Training
NTN Grid

Specialty Training (Higher)
ST4 + ST5

MRCPCH

Specialty Training (Basic)
ST1, ST2 + ST3

Foundation Programme
F1 + F2

Medical School

= Job Application

= Exam

ℹ️ For further information:

Royal College of Paediatrics and Child Health, 50 Hallam Street, London, W1W 6DE
Tel: 020 7307 5600   Fax: 020 7307 5601   Web: http://www.rcpch.ac.uk

Pathology

By 'pathologist' most people understand 'histopathologist', however the term encompasses many specialties. These are mostly laboratory-based, though many involve patient contact. All of the jobs require a very broad and detailed knowledge of medicine. This book focuses on the most common specialties, but there are options to subspecialize, for example in paediatrics or neuropathology:

- **Chemical pathology** (clinical biochemistry) (p 112) Doctors who run the biochemistry laboratory interpret complex biochemical tests and advise on, or manage, patients with metabolic disturbance (e.g. dyslipidaemias, artificial nutrition) on the wards or in clinic.
- **Forensic pathology** (p 138) Subspecialty of histopathology; perform autopsies where a death has legal implications (e.g. murder)
- **Haematology** (p 158) and **Immunology** (p 166) are clinical jobs with strong laboratory components. They are entered via internal medicine see (p 34).
- **Histopathology** (p 162) Diagnose diseases from tissue samples using a range of techniques and microscopes; a few perform autopsies if there are no legal concerns.
- **Medical microbiology** (p 194) Run the microbiology laboratory to identify disease-causing microbes from fluid/tissue samples; provide advice on antimicrobial therapy and ward rounds of unusual cases and high-risk areas, e.g. the intensive therapy unit (ITU).
- **Virology** (p 288) Subspecialty of microbiology focusing on viruses.

Training

Foundation Four-month placements are available in the main pathology specialties, though they are not common. As pathology is diverse any specialty will be of benefit. Those who are interested in pathology should consider a taster week in one of the above specialties.

> **Pathology ST applications** Histopathology applications are made to the London deanery who coordinate the applications for all deaneries. All other pathology applications are made to the deanery of choice.

Specialty training At the end of the foundation programme doctors can apply directly to ST1 posts in chemical pathology, histopathology, medical microbiology and virology. These are all run-through posts (p 8) so that once a job is secured a training post should be guaranteed until CCT is attained, as long as the necessary exams and assessments are passed. Haematology and immunology are uncoupled specialties (p 8) so trainees need to apply to core medical training (p 34), complete two years of training and pass the MRCP Part 1 before reapplying for an ST3 post in haematology or immunology.

Subspecialists It is possible to subspecialize within pathology specialties (e.g. forensic pathology, neuropathology); subspecialty training begins after completing the Part 1 FRCPath exam for the specialty, usually after two or three years.

Exams

There is a unique FRCPath exam for each specialty within pathology. The exams are made up of written papers and laboratory/practical skills relevant to that specialty:

- **Chemical pathology, histopathology, microbiology** Exams are taken early in specialist training, ideally Part 1 during ST2 and Part 2 during ST3.
- **Haematology, immunology** Taken after MRCP and entry at ST3.
- **Forensics, virology** Part 1 is taken as for histopathology and microbiology respectively but Part 2 is unique to the subspecialty.

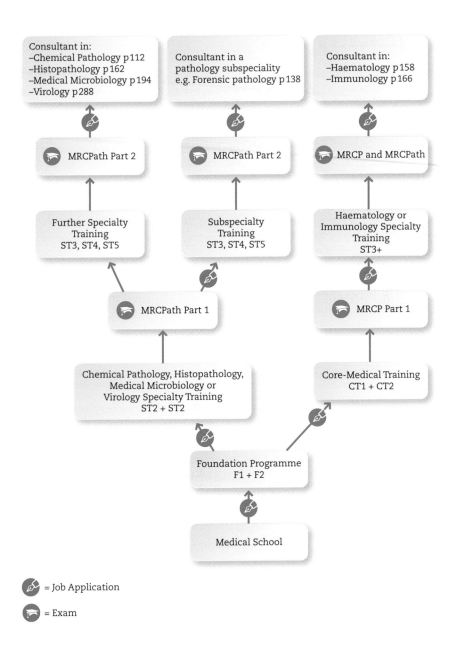

Consultant in:
–Chemical Pathology p 112
–Histopathology p 162
–Medical Microbiology p 194
–Virology p 288

Consultant in a
pathology subspeciality
e.g. Forensic pathology p 138

Consultant in:
–Haematology p 158
–Immunology p 166

MRCPath Part 2

MRCPath Part 2

MRCP and MRCPath

Further Specialty
Training
ST3, ST4, ST5

Subspecialty
Training
ST3, ST4, ST5

Haematology or
Immunology Specialty
Training
ST3+

MRCPath Part 1

MRCP Part 1

Chemical Pathology, Histopathology,
Medical Microbiology or
Virology Specialty Training
ST2 + ST2

Core-Medical Training
CT1 + CT2

Foundation Programme
F1 + F2

Medical School

= Job Application

= Exam

For further information:

Royal College of Pathologists, 2 Carlton House Terrace, London, SW1Y 5AF
Tel: 020 7451 6700   Fax: 020 7451 6701   Web: http://www.rcpath.org

Psychiatry

Psychiatry is a very diverse specialty which includes many different roles:

- General adult psychiatry (p 240) This is the largest group of psychiatrists; they manage psychiatric disease in patients aged 18–65 years in inpatient and outpatient settings.
- Child and adolescent psychiatry (p 238) Psychiatrists who specialize in managing those under 18 years of age. This includes neurodevelopment disorders (e.g. autism) in the younger ages and similar diseases to adult populations in teenagers (e.g. depression, schizophrenia).
- Old age psychiatry (p 242) Psychiatrists who deal with patients aged over 65 years. Psychiatric disease is more common in this age group, especially depression and dementia.
- Psychiatry of learning disability (p 244) Psychiatric illness is common in those with learning disability. These psychiatrists specialize in this very diverse group of patients; the job is largely community-based.
- Forensic psychiatry (p 140) Provide psychiatric care to prison inmates and those in secure hospitals. Acting as an expert witness in court is also common.
- Psychotherapy (p 246) Specialize in the diagnosis and treatment of psychiatric disorders through psychotherapy.

Training

Foundation Many foundation programmes include four months in psychiatry; experience in general practice and emergency medicine will also be of benefit. Alternatively trainees can use F2 tasters to gain experience of psychiatry in any of the roles described above.

Psychiatry ST applications These are run by local deaneries; usually based on CV and interview.

Core-training Psychiatric training begins with a three-year core-training programme (CT1, CT2 and CT3) to give a wide range of experience in the different psychiatric specialties.

Specialty training Trainees who have completed CT3 psychiatry and MRCPsych parts 1 and 2 (see below) can apply for an ST4 post in one of the psychiatric specialties listed above. Those who are successful in attaining one of these posts will train for a further three years until they attain their CCT in that specialty.

Subspecialists Psychiatric specialties are chosen during application to ST4. There is some scope for subspecialization within these specialties; for example, addiction psychiatry (alcohol, substance misuse) and liaison psychiatry (patients in non-psychiatric areas of the hospital, e.g. the emergency department or ward reviews) can be reached via general adult psychiatry.

Exams

It is essential to pass the membership of the Royal College of Psychiatrists exam (MRCPsych) during core and specialty training. The exam has four parts:

- Paper I A written MCQ and EMI paper that covers psychiatric evaluation and diagnosis, psychiatric theory and ethics. It can be taken after the end of CT1.
- Paper II A written MCQ and EMI paper that covers psychiatric treatment, statistics and psychiatric pathology. It is taken after Paper I and must be passed before the end of CT3.
- Paper III A written MCQ and EMI paper that covers psychiatry in each of the psychiatric specialties along with research methods, statistics and critical appraisal. It should be taken during the ST4 year.
- Clinical assessment of skills and competencies (CASC) A twelve-station clinical examination. It is usually taken in the ST5 year.

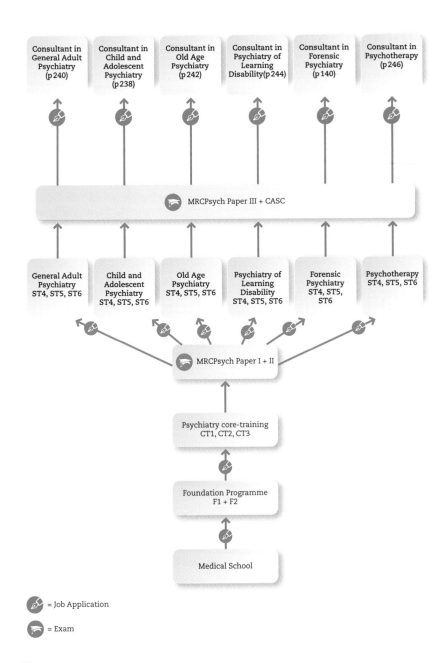

Consultant in General Adult Psychiatry (p 240)

Consultant in Child and Adolescent Psychiatry (p 238)

Consultant in Old Age Psychiatry (p 242)

Consultant in Psychiatry of Learning Disability (p 244)

Consultant in Forensic Psychiatry (p 140)

Consultant in Psychotherapy (p 246)

MRCPsych Paper III + CASC

General Adult Psychiatry ST4, ST5, ST6

Child and Adolescent Psychiatry ST4, ST5, ST6

Old Age Psychiatry ST4, ST5, ST6

Psychiatry of Learning Disability ST4, ST5, ST6

Forensic Psychiatry ST4, ST5, ST6

Psychotherapy ST4, ST5, ST6

MRCPsych Paper I + II

Psychiatry core-training CT1, CT2, CT3

Foundation Programme F1 + F2

Medical School

= Job Application

= Exam

ℹ️ For further information:

Royal College of Psychiatrists, 17 Belgrave Square, London, SW1X 8PG
Tel: 020 7235 2351 Fax: 020 7245 1231 Web: http://www.rcpsych.ac.uk

Public health

In the 2007 applications for ST1 Public health had the most competition per place of all the specialties available (alongside clinical radiology). Public health is also unique because competition is not only presented by other doctors; non-medical graduates with relevant experience can apply to train as a consultant in public health. For more details on the role of a public health doctor see p 248.

Training

Foundation A few foundation programmes will include a four-month placement within public health, however this is uncommon. Those who are considering this specialty should undertake an F2 taster week to make them familiar with the role of a public health doctor and to establish whether it is a suitable career for them.

Public health ST applications There is a national application procedure:

1) Online application

2) Half-day at an assessment centre for numerical critical reasoning and verbal critical reasoning test

3) Half-day at a selection centre for those shortlisted from the assessment centre; includes interviews, a group exercise and giving a presentation.

Specialty training Public health features a five-year training programme starting at ST1. Once a position is secured, a training post should be guaranteed until the CCT is attained, as long as the necessary exams and assessments are passed.

Alternative routes The Faculty of Public Health states that it welcomes applicants with extra clinical experience and postgraduate qualifications. While it would be necessary to start again at ST1, passing other membership exams, e.g. MRCP, would be likely to be a great asset in succeeding against the strong competition.

Exams

To complete the public health training it is necessary to pass the membership of the Faculty of Public Health exams (MFPH). There are two parts:
- **Part A** This is a written exam composed of two papers, each with two parts (IA, IB, IIA and IIB). It is taken over two days and includes questions on statistics, critical paper analysis, economics and management. The exam is usually taken during ST2.
- **Part B** This is an objective structure public health exam (OSPHE) with six stations. It is usually taken during ST3.

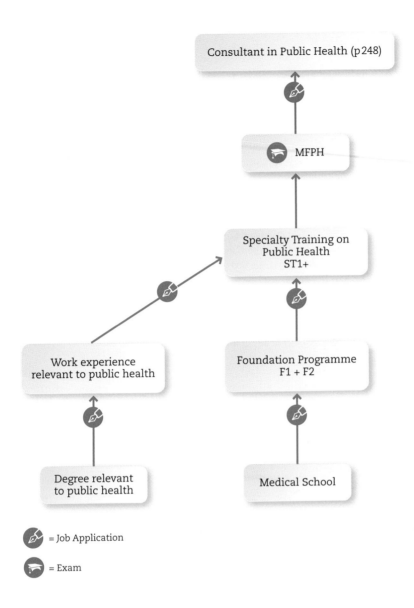

Consultant in Public Health (p248)

MFPH

Specialty Training on Public Health ST1+

Work experience relevant to public health

Foundation Programme F1 + F2

Degree relevant to public health

Medical School

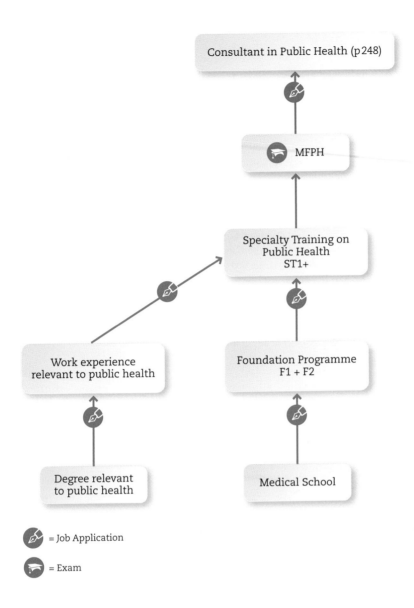 = Job Application

= Exam

ℹ️ For further information:

Faculty of Public Health, 4 St Andrews Place, London, NW1 4LB
Tel: 020 7935 0243   Fax: 020 7224 6973   Web: http://www.fphm.org.uk

Radiology

In the 2007 applications for ST1, radiology had the most competition per place of all the specialties available (alongside public health). There are four specialties related to radiology:

- Diagnostic radiology (p 250) Interpretation of images obtained through a variety of techniques including X-rays, contrast imaging, ultrasound, CT and MRI. For the more complicated imaging techniques the radiologist is actively involved in taking the images; they may also perform procedures under imaging guidance.
- Interventional radiology (p 252) Radiologists who specialize in invasive procedures requiring imaging guidance.
- Clinical oncology (p 118) Doctors who treat cancer using radiotherapy alongside other treatments; medical oncologists (p 196) cannot give radiotherapy. Training is via core medical training (p 8) along with the MRCP exam (p 34) and FRCR exam (below).
- Nuclear medicine (p 210) Doctors who perform investigations involving radioactive tracers (e.g. radio-labelled iodine); there is also a treatment role (e.g. radioactive iodine for hyperthyroid). This specialty is reached via core medical training (p 8).

Training

Foundation Some foundation programmes include a four-month placement in radiology, but this is not essential for a specialist training position. Alternatively, trainees can use F2 tasters to gain experience of radiology in any of the roles described above.

> **Radiology ST applications** These are run by local deaneries; usually based on CV and interview.

Specialty training ST1 posts in radiology can be applied for immediately after the foundation programme. As mentioned above, the competition is intense; applicants will need an above-average CV and to demonstrate an interest in radiology. Once a position has been secured, a training post should be guaranteed until CCT is attained, as long as the necessary exams and assessments are passed. The training lasts five years.

Subspecialists Many radiologists have a special interest (e.g. interventional radiology, neuroimaging) and these can be developed in the last two years of training. This may involve transferring to a specialty centre, which is likely to be competitive.

Exams

During specialty training it is essential to pass the Fellowship of the Royal College of Radiologists exam (FRCR). The exam has three parts:

- First FRCR This is a short written paper in an MCQ format. It largely concentrates on the science behind radiology (i.e. lots of physics) along with how radiology equipment works and UK legislation regarding ionizing radiation. It can be taken any time after starting a radiology specialty training post, but it must be passed by the fourth attempt.
- Final FRCR Part A This can be taken after completing the first FRCR, but is usually taken during the ST3 year. It consists of six written MCQ papers (called modules) on clinical radiology and lasts for two consecutive days.
- Final FRCR Part B This can be taken after passing Part A and completing the ST3 year. It consists of a written reporting session, a rapid spot diagnosis session and two 30-minute oral exams.

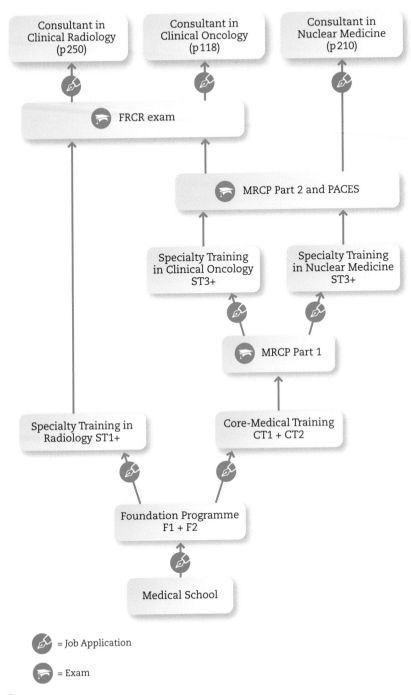

Consultant in Clinical Radiology (p250)

Consultant in Clinical Oncology (p118)

Consultant in Nuclear Medicine (p210)

FRCR exam

MRCP Part 2 and PACES

Specialty Training in Clinical Oncology ST3+

Specialty Training in Nuclear Medicine ST3+

MRCP Part 1

Specialty Training in Radiology ST1+

Core-Medical Training CT1 + CT2

Foundation Programme F1 + F2

Medical School

= Job Application

= Exam

For further information:

Royal College of Radiologists, 38 Portland Place, London, W1B 1JQ
Tel: 020 7636 4432   Fax: 020 7323 3100   Web: http://www.rcr.ac.uk

Surgery

Surgical training is one of the more complex routes in the new system, since it varies dramatically between different surgical specialties. Most careers in surgery are discussed on this page except for maxillofacial surgery, neurosurgery, and ophthalmology, which are discussed on p 50. To add to the confusion the exact route into many surgical careers has yet to be defined beyond starting with general surgery. The situation is developing rapidly so it is important to check with the Royal College to get the latest information before committing to a specific route.

Training

Foundation Four months of general surgery is compulsory during the F1 year and some placements will feature a further four months in a specific surgical specialty; placements in emergency medicine and anaesthetics will also offer useful experience. If a particular surgery specialty is of interest then request a taster attachment during the F2 year.

> **Surgery CT applications** These are run by local deaneries; usually based on CV and interview.

Core-training Most surgical specialties are reached via two years of surgery in general (CT1 and CT2). There are three types of surgical training in the first two years:
- **Generic training** Core-training in a range of surgical specialties without specifying one in particular; useful for those who are unsure which specialty to choose.
- **Specific training** There are core-training programmes specifically for general surgery, otolaryngology (ENT), paediatric surgery, plastic surgery, trauma and orthopaedic surgery and urology. Specific core-training may limit the trainee's ability to change to other surgical specialties. Note that there is no core-training specific to cardiothoracic surgery.
- **Specialty training** For maxillofacial surgery, neurosurgery and ophthalmology, trainees enter specialty training at ST1 instead of core-training (see p 50).

Specialty training Completion of core-training and the MRCS exams (below) entitles trainees to apply for ST3 in a specific surgical specialty (see list above). This training lasts between five and six years, varying between specialties.

Exams

To apply for ST3 in surgical specialties it is essential to pass the membership of the Royal College of Surgeons exam (MRCS). There is considerable time pressure as candidates must pass all sections within 3 years of their first attempt at part A.
- **Part A** Applied basic sciences MCQ and principles of surgery-in-general MCQ.
- **Part B** Six structured interviews; successful candidates will go on to take another exam a month later with four objective structured clinical examination (OSCE) stations and two communication skills stations.

FRCS Surgical specialties have an exit exam taken towards the end of specialty training prior to receiving the certificate of completion of training (CCT) necessary to be a consultant. These exams are specific to the particular surgical specialty and have a relatively high pass rate.

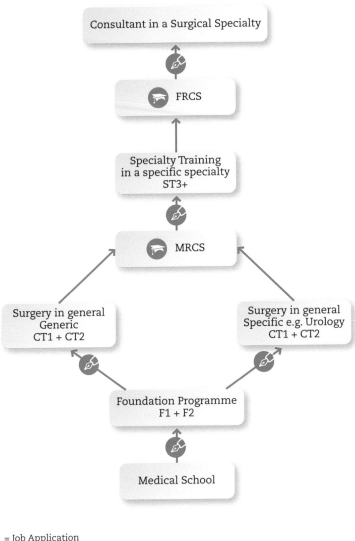

Consultant in a Surgical Specialty

FRCS

Specialty Training
in a specific specialty
ST3+

MRCS

Surgery in general
Generic
CT1 + CT2

Surgery in general
Specific e.g. Urology
CT1 + CT2

Foundation Programme
F1 + F2

Medical School

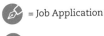 = Job Application

= Exam

For further information:

Royal College of Surgeons of England, 35–43 Lincoln's Inn Fields, London, WC2A 3PE
Tel: 020 7405 3474   Web: http://www.rcseng.ac.uk
Note there are also surgical colleges in Edinburgh, Glasgow and Ireland.

Surgery continued

Oral and maxillofacial surgery

Training

Foundation Maxillofacial surgery placements are very rare within the foundation programme, however all surgical specialties will be useful experience and it is possible to request a taster attachment during the F2 year.

Dental degree This is required alongside a medical degree. Most doctors entering maxillofacial surgery have trained in dentistry before medical school, however it is possible to train in medicine followed by dentistry. Dental school takes four years full-time.

Specialty training Trainees can apply to ST1 Oral and maxillofacial surgery once they have a medical degree and a dental degree and have completed their foundation programme.

Exams

The MRCS exam needs to be completed during specialty training (see p 48 for details) and there is a specific FRCS exit exam in oral and maxillofacial surgery.

Neurosurgery

Training

Foundation Neurosurgery placements are uncommon within the foundation programme; experience in surgical specialties and F2 taster attachments will help job applications.

Specialty training Trainees can apply to ST1 Neurosurgery (core neuroscience training) having completed the foundation programme. Training takes eight years as long as the trainee completes the necessary exams and assessments.

Exams

The MRCS exam needs to be completed during core neuroscience training (see p 48 for details) and there is a specific FRCS exit exam in neurosurgery.

Ophthalmology

Training

Foundation Ophthalmology placements are uncommon within the foundation programme; experience in surgical specialties and F2 taster attachments will strengthen job applications.

Specialty training Trainees can apply to ST1 Ophthalmology after the foundation programme; training then continues for six years, as long as the trainee completes the necessary exams and assessments.

Exams

Trainees must complete the Fellowship of the Royal College of Ophthalmologists exam:
- Part 1 FRCOphth completed by end of ST2
- Refraction Module completed by end of ST3
- Part 2 FRCOphth completed after ST4 prior to CCT

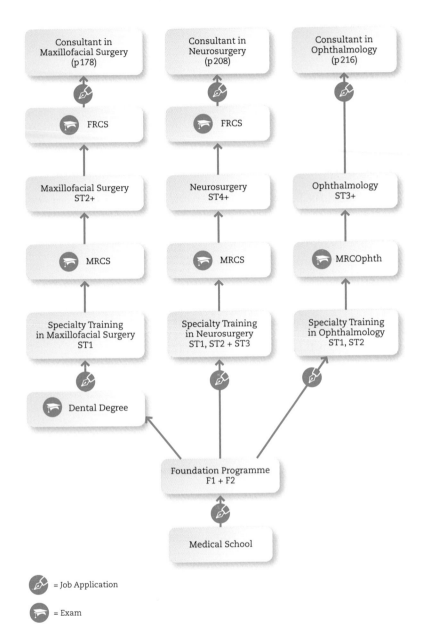

⬤ = Job Application

⬤ = Exam

ℹ️ **For further information:**

British Association of Oral and Maxillofacial Surgeons, 35–43 Lincoln's Inn Fields, London, WC2A 3PE
Tel: 020 7405 8074   Fax: 020 7430 9997   Web: http://www.baoms.org.uk
Society of British Neurological Surgeons, 35–43 Lincoln's Inn Fields, London, WC2A 3PE
Tel: 020 7869 6892   Fax: 020 7869 6890   Web: http://www.sbns.org.uk
Royal College of Ophthalmologists, 17 Cornwall Terrace, London , NW1 4QW
Tel: 020 7935 0702   Fax: 020 7935 9838   Web: http://www.rcophth.ac.uk

How to get a job

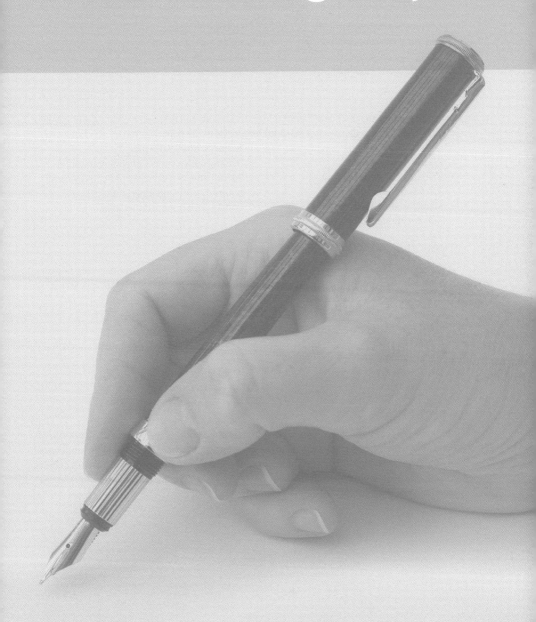

Part 3

How to get a job

Choosing a career

As this book demonstrates, there are many career options available to those with a medical degree. However, the new Modernising Medical Careers system of training forces doctors to pick a career route much sooner after finishing medical school: there is no longer an option to try a variety of jobs until one feels right. Work has a huge impact on day-to-day life and happiness so it is important to think carefully about what really matters when choosing a career.

Priorities

Every medical career offers a different range of working patterns and lifestyles. The career chapters (pp. 90–290) give an impression of how each career compares. Key priorities include:

- Amount/intensity of on-call
- Part-time working options
- Salary and private work
- Living in a city vs village
- Outside interests
- Being part of a team
- Being in control
- Travelling

Skills

Different doctors are good at different things; these skills can determine what type of job suits them. See the career chapters (pp. 90–290) for a guide to the skills required in each career, eg:

- Communication skills
- Practical ability
- Thinking/academic ability
- Attention to detail
- Managerial skills
- Teamwork/leadership skills
- Business/financial skills
- Dealing with a variety of patients/systems
- Specializing in a subset of patients/systems
- Ability to work under pressure
- Coping with responsibility

Type of work

Different aspects of medicine appeal to different people and the opportunities vary between careers. See the sections entitled 'The work' and 'Extras'; in the career chapters (pp. 90–290). Common types of work include:

- Clinics
- Ward rounds
- Procedures
- Operating theatres
- Emergencies
- Laboratory work
- Research
- Teaching
- Presenting at conferences
- Management
- Imaging
- Continuity of care

Competition

Medicine is becoming increasingly competitive and a doctor's experience and achievements determine which careers they are able to pursue. Most doctors have sufficient ability to succeed in any specialty, however they may need to work extremely hard for several years to achieve the necessary qualifications and CV. See pp. 56–59 for MMC competition ratios and the individual career chapters (pp. 90–290) for an estimate of competitiveness by career.

Finding jobs

Foundation programmes

These are advertised via http://www.foundationprogramme.nhs.uk. The application form includes a preference list which entails ranking all the foundation schools (e.g. North West Thames, Oxford) from 1 to 26. The applicant is allocated a foundation school place according to the score of their application form (p 62). Once the doctor is assigned to a foundation school the exact programme of four month placements is chosen; the method of allocating these programmes varies between foundation schools, but is usually based on the application form or CV. Different regions offer different specialties; for less common placements it is worth checking numerous deaneries.

Specialty training and core-training

These jobs are advertised in different places for different specialties; the majority of jobs are shown on deanery websites, however specialties with national application systems may advertise elsewhere. The competition ratios (i.e. how many people applied per place) are published by location and specialty so it is worth considering these when applying. The overall competition ratios per specialty are shown on p 56.

Consultant jobs

Most consultant jobs are advertised on the BMJ Careers website and in the *BMJ Careers* magazine. The website is free and does not require a BMJ subscription. It allows jobs to be searched for by specialty, grade and/or region. There is also a reminder function that can be set up to send emails when specific jobs are available. See also the section on word of mouth below.

Other jobs

There are other options for finding jobs apart from those described above; these include:

Internal jobs Many hospitals will recruit doctors for non-training grades or research-based jobs from those already working in the hospital. This may require a brief interview or simply resubmitting a CV. It is essential to get a written job offer and to sign a contract as soon as possible, otherwise it is difficult to complain if the offer is withdrawn.

Word of mouth While MMC and human resource departments have reduced the old boy network, medicine is a small world and people talk. To get a competitive job, especially consultant jobs, it is essential to be known and liked by those working in the department. Showing interest and visiting departments is still an essential part of getting many jobs.

Locum agencies It is important to sign up with a locum agency well in advance as the process takes two to three months. Choosing the right agency is also important, as some cover different regions and specialties. See p 174 for more on working as a locum.

Contacting organizations Some jobs need to be created rather than found. For specific research interests it is worth contacting research leaders in the field to see if they can offer a suitable research post. Likewise, if pursuing careers outside the NHS (e.g. expedition doctor, journalism) then contacting appropriate organizations directly is often a good way to begin.

Publications Some jobs available to doctors will be advertised outside of *BMJ Careers*, especially those in management or civil service. It is essential to find out where these are being advertised and to subscribe to that publication or a job searching website that covers it.

Competition for ST1/CT1 applications

MMC have published figures on the degree of competition for each specialty. The table below shows the number of applicants per post at ST1/CT1 level. Overall there were 6.4 applicants per post (note that applicants could only apply for four jobs in this round).

	Specialty	Applicants per post[1]
Extremely competitive	Clinical radiology	18.1
	Public health	18.0
	Microbiology and virology, microbiology	18.0
Above average competition	ACCS, acute medicine	9.3
	Oral and maxillofacial surgery (OMFS)	8.8
	Chemical pathology	8.8
	Histopathology	8.7
	ACCS, emergency medicine	8.4
	Ophthalmology	8.2
	Surgery in general, plastic surgery	8.1
	Neurosurgery	7.5
Average competition	Obstetrics and gynaecology	7.0
	Surgery in general, general surgery	6.8
	Surgery in general, trauma and orthopaedic surgery	6.8
	Surgery in general, generic	6.4
	General practice	6.1
	Core medical training	5.8
	ACCS, anaesthesia	5.5
	Microbiology and virology, virology	5.3
	Surgery in general, paediatric surgery	5.2
	Psychiatry	5.1
Below-average competition	Anaesthesia	4.8
	Paediatrics	4.5
	Surgery in general, otolaryngology (ENT)	4.4
Well below average competition	Surgery in general, urology	1.9

---

[1] MMC Competition Ratios Table, ST1 by specialty, March 2007, http://www.mmc.nhs.uk.

Competition in the future

The competition ratios are likely to change year by year; this table acts as a guide. There are slightly more ST1/CT1 posts than there are foundation programme posts (6100 vs 5500), however there is also competition from overseas and senior doctors changing career. MMC estimates that about 75% of F2s will get an ST1/CT1 job (though not necessarily their first choice); most of the rest should get FTSTA jobs (p 14); they are unlikely to be unemployed.

It is possible to apply for ST2 jobs after an FTSTA1 job but the MMC website notes that it is difficult to transfer from an FTSTA to a ST post. An FTSTA is more likely to lead to a staff grade job (p 14).

The key message from these figures is that medicine is competitive and in some specialties only the 'best' will get their first choice of job. To get a first choice job it is necessary to have above average achievements (p 60), a good CV (p 65), a well written application form (p 62) and polished interview skills (p 66).

Competition for ST3/ST4 applications

	Specialty	Applicants per post[2]
Extremely competitive	Cardiothoracic surgery ST3	53.2
	Trauma and orthopaedic surgery ST3	22.6
	General surgery ST3	20.3
	Otolaryngology (ENT) ST3	19.8
	Plastic surgery ST3	18.1
	Urology ST3	17.6
Above average competition	Paediatric surgery ST3	15.9
	Cardiology ST3	15.0
	Neurology ST3	14.4
	Gastroenterology ST3	13.2
	Palliative medicine ST3	12.2
	Sports and exercise medicine ST3	11.8
	Paediatric cardiology ST4	11.8
	Respiratory medicine ST3	10.3
	Neurosurgery ST3	10.2
Average competition	Infectious diseases ST3	9.1
	Dermatology ST3	9.1
	Endocrinology and diabetes ST3	8.9
	Rheumatology ST3	7.8
	Renal medicine ST3	7.7
	Forensic psychiatry ST4	7.2
	Medical oncology ST3	7.1
	Anaesthesia ST3	7.0
Below-average competition	General adult psychiatry ST4	6.9
	Haematology ST3	6.8
	Clinical oncology ST3	5.9
	Child and adolescent psychiatry ST4	5.8
	Old age psychiatry ST4	5.8
	Acute medicine ST3	5.6
	Genitourinary medicine ST3	5.4
	Geriatric medicine ST3	5.3
	Psychiatry of learning disability ST4	4.8
	Clinical genetics ST3	3.9
	Psychotherapy ST4	3.9
	Occupational medicine ST3	3.0
Well below average competition	Clinical neurophysiology ST3	2.3
	Audiological medicine ST3	2.0
	Rehabilitation medicine ST3	1.9
	Medical ophthalmology ST3	1.5
	Emergency medicine ST4	1.4
	Allergy ST3	1.0
	Nuclear medicine ST3	1.0
	Immunology ST3	0.6

For those in run-through specialties (p 8) a job is guaranteed (though competitive application for specific jobs may still occur). However, the majority of hospital-based careers have uncoupled training (p 8), meaning that doctors have to apply for their definitive career at ST3 or ST4 level depending on the specialty. Competition is even more fierce at this level with an average of 8.5 applicants per post (again applicants could only apply for four jobs in this round).

---

[2] MMC Competition Ratios Table, ST3 and ST4 by specialty, March 2007, http://www.mmc.nhs.uk.

Staying competitive

Medicine is a competitive career; getting through medical school is only the start. The competition ratios on pp 56–59 show that many specialties will only take the 'best' candidates. It is important for applicants to be objective about their CVs and experience. What is lacking? What would make for a better application?

Achievements and qualifications

Application forms can be objectively graded based on the applicant's achievements and qualifications. This will often involve ticking boxes if the applicant can demonstrate something relevant to each category. As a result diverse experience is better than a great deal of experience in one category (e.g. a diploma, publication and award may score more than a PhD).

Intercalated degrees Only a small proportion of medical students undertake intercalated degrees (BSc) during medical school. These look very good on the CV as they show a commitment to research and help the student to stand out from the crowd. It is of even greater benefit if it leads to a presentation or publication in a peer-reviewed journal.

Postgraduate qualifications These include diplomas, masters, medical doctorates (MD) and PhDs in order of status from low to high. The time commitment also varies; it is possible to take a diploma alongside a full-time job whilst a PhD is at least three years full time.

Membership exams (p 10) It is essential to pass these to progress through specialty training. Passing these early and first time gives a big advantage. Note that some exams only allow a set number of retakes or time to pass, so it is important to plan when to take each part.

Prizes/awards Any prize looks good; the majority of applicants will leave this section blank. Opportunities to win prizes include research presentations and essay writing. Some of these can be surprisingly uncompetitive so it is worth being proactive.

Courses These include advanced life support (ALS), advanced trauma life support (ATLS), advanced paediatric life support (APLS).

Publications This is a key area. Any form of publication will set an applicant above the crowd. The ideal is as the first author of original research in a peer-reviewed journal. In the early years of training a single publication makes a big difference; to maintain an advantage more are needed in higher-impact journals as careers progress.

Letters/reviews/reports/case reports While original research has the highest status there are lots of other ways to be published in journals.

International presentations Research can also be submitted to international conferences as an abstract; this can be before or after publication. The best abstracts will be selected to present at the conference, an opportunity that is well worth the cost of a plane ticket and hotel.

Presentations Presenting at UK conferences has slightly lower status than international conferences but is still extremely worthwhile.

Posters If an abstract is not accepted for a conference presentation it will often be accepted as a poster. Again international conferences have higher status.

What standard is the competition? It is important to remember that applicants are not only competing against peers; there will also be applicants from overseas, doctors with PhDs or more experienced doctors changing career direction. Such applicants may have had more time to accumulate achievements and qualifications. For the most competitive careers it is necessary to show achievements in most, if not all, of the categories above.

Demonstrating an interest

Achievements and qualifications are not the only measure of an applicant. The phrase 'demonstrate an interest in the specialty' often appears on application forms. Essentially this is asking the applicant to prove that they really want to train in this specialty and have had this desire for a while. This is not an unreasonable request, as many specialties appear very different from outside compared with working in them. If pursuing a career in a specialty consider some of the following:

Medical student special study module Many medical schools offer clinical modules in a specialty of the student's choice. Medical schools often offer students a list of suitable specialties; it is important to see this as a guide rather than a limit. If a specialty is of interest then it may be possible to approach a consultant in that specialty and create a unique module.

Medical student elective This is a great chance to get a feel for a specialty. It is also a great chance to travel the world and have a good time before starting a job with long and antisocial hours. For really competitive specialties you cannot beat working in a quaternary referral centre (i.e. international specialist centre). These are often in the USA.

Attend clinics/surgery While this can be difficult when carrying a bleep it is one of the best ways of showing an interest. Consider using days off after on-calls. Note that many application forms ask specifically what extra-curricular work the applicant has done towards developing an interest in the specialty.

F2 Taster sessions During the F2 year trainees should be offered the chance to spend week-long tasters in specialties of their choice. Be imaginative and look for interesting options by approaching a consultant in an interesting specialty.

Audit projects Audits are required throughout training; in most placements it is possible to choose a topic that fits with the specialty of interest.

Research project This is an excellent way for a trainee to show that they are serious about a specific specialty. It may also result in a publication relevant to the specialty.

Postgraduate qualifications e.g. diploma or masters in the specialty or a subject relevant to the specialty.

Join relevant societies Most specialties have a society, college or association; the contact details for many of these can be found under the career chapters (p 90). Many have options for student/junior doctor membership and this is an excellent way to hear about opportunities.

Conferences Information about conferences can be acquired through trainees in the specialty or relevant societies. Attending conferences shows commitment and also provides a good idea of the current important issues within the specialty.

Getting the balance

Some doctors spend every waking minute furthering their medical career by the means above, while others choose to do their job and nothing more. Neither extreme is wrong and there is a spectrum between them. It is important for trainees to think about where they fit on this spectrum and assess which careers are compatible. An incompatible choice is likely to lead to frustration with colleagues or job applications. There is no right or wrong answer to this, but it is important to think about it objectively, after all, this life is more than just a read through.[3]

---

[3] 'Can't Stop', Red Hot Chili Peppers.

Surviving the application system

The marking scheme for foundation programme and specialist training applications has never been published, but there has been some description of the general process. Furthermore different specialties have different application forms. These pages should act as a guide.

CV points Try to get a wide range of experience and qualifications. The forms ask specifically about publications, posters, presentations, audits, courses, conferences and exams. Diversity is likely to score more highly than excellence in a single category, i.e. it is better to have one example of each category than twenty publications and nothing else.

Experience It helps to spend as much time in the chosen specialty as possible to demonstrate an interest (p 61). Consider taster weeks during the foundation years, clinics, conferences and joining relevant societies/colleges. Talk to people doing the job about the work and their experience.

Choosing jobs The following points are very important:
• Check the essential criteria for the job, e.g. the GP/specialty person specifications on the MMC website. If in doubt speak to a consultant or the deanery.
• When applying for competitive jobs or regions, consider including less competitive back-up choices. The competition ratios are shown on p 56, 59 and the MMC website.[4]
• Apply for as many jobs/regions as possible. This will greatly increase the chance of success.
• Only apply for jobs that are preferable to being unemployed.

Applications Although it sounds obvious, it is important to fill in *all* the sections and answer *all* the questions. If a question is made of two or more components then ensure all of these are covered by the answer. Read and reread each question to make sure the response answers exactly what is being asked. Check that every page and section are complete and go through applications with colleagues to make sure.

Buzz words It is important to emphasize key qualities like communication skills, reflective practice, patient-centred care etc., but this should not distract from answering the questions. Look at the MMC person specification and state which of the selection criteria are fulfilled by the answer, e.g. 'this demonstrates teamwork'. Whenever an experience is described it should be followed by what was learnt and how this will affect future actions.

Reviewing Show application forms to as many people as possible, including peers, educational supervisors, seniors and human resources (who spend lots of time reading them). Applicants who do not speak English as their first language should ask a native English speaker to read their form.

Portfolios Make sure these have all the required information and are well presented. Do not leave this to the last minute as it can take a long time to track down signatures.

Interviews Practice interview technique with senior colleagues; this will improve confidence, style and familiarity with common questions. Check what current/previous candidates were asked at interview and prepare likely questions.

Reapplying If an application is unsuccessful then try to find out why. Contact the assessing institution (e.g. deanery) and ask for feedback. It is also useful to look at the application forms of successful colleagues and compare these to your own.

---

[4] http://www.mmc.nhs.uk, Specialty Training, Specialty Training 2008, Vacancies and competition.

Answering the questions

Many of the application forms developed since Modernising Medical Careers have relied heavily on short answer questions about the candidate's experiences, reflective abilities and commitment to the specialty. While these questions may be tedious to answer it is extremely important to write responses as well as possible—over 50% of available application form marks may be based on these answers.

Preparation

Download a copy of relevant documents, for example *Specialty Training Person Specifications*, *The New Doctor* (GMC), *Good Medical Practice* (GMC), the *Foundation Applicant's Handbook*, *Foundation Curriculum*, or a job description. The qualities, skills and experiences described in these documents will be exactly what are being assessed on the application form so they basically describe what the answer needs to say.

- Start early (for example, the foundation programme application form is published on the website three weeks before applications open).
- Keep a list of interesting clinical cases in the portfolio to use as examples.
- Read all the questions on the form before starting. Jot notes about what qualities each one might be asking about and any suitable examples that spring to mind.

Answering the question (see examples p 64)

- Read and reread the question. Break it into sections that need answering. Check what format the response should be in. Usually this is text in full sentences without bullet points.
- The *Foundation Applicant's Handbook*[5] highlights the following words that often appear on these forms. Be clear about exactly what they are asking:
  - **Analysis** Examining facts/events and making relevant conclusions.
  - **Reflection** Considering an experience and how it affected/changed you.
  - **Learning** How gaining knowledge/experience has changed what you do.
  - **Relevance** (e.g. relevance of learning to training) How gaining knowledge/experience has helped you meet training objectives or change the way you approach training.
- Assume that the person marking each answer can only see that single answer and not the rest of your form. Repeat key qualities, skills or achievements in multiple answers.
- If a question has multiple parts then break the answer into parts too. Clarify which part is being answered, e.g. "This experience made me realize . . . This is relevant to my training because . . . ." This makes the questions much easier to mark.
- Never write the answers on-line; the system is bound to crash and lose all the answers. Copy and paste the questions into a text document which can be backed up, then copy the answers into the form once they are finished.
- Never copy someone else's answers; it is very easy to run all the application forms through a computer and look for similarities. Being caught could result in a GMC disciplinary hearing. While copying is not allowed, comparing application form answers with other applicants to spot mistakes or misunderstood questions is a good idea.
- Be honest. Interviewers may ask about the application form answers in an interview and it is much easier to remember the truth. Being caught lying on the application form could also result in a GMC disciplinary hearing and no job.

---

[5] Foundation Applicant's Handbook, 8 October 2007, http://www.foundationprogramme.nhs.uk.

Application form example question[6] 1

Describe an example relevant to your medical training where you have felt personally under pressure and/or challenged. What did you do to manage this and what did you learn from this experience that will be relevant to your foundation training? (150 words)

Comments Do not be fooled; this question is not about who has dealt with the most challenging situation, but who is best able to 'reflect' upon a difficult experience. Before choosing an example think about which qualities to highlight using relevant documents (p 63), for example: prioritization, teamwork, communication, putting the patient's needs first, asking for help. Think of an example that allows discussion of these qualities and spell them out, e.g. "I contacted my senior and discussed the situation; this taught me the importance of asking for help and communication." Try not to use too many words describing the example and make sure it is an example where your management of the situation was good.

Application form example question 2

Give one example of a non-academic achievement explaining both the significance to you and the relevance to foundation training. (150 words)

Comments The example must be non-academic, but not non-clinical. The marks will not be awarded for the achievement, but for ability to reflect on it. Again, try not to waste too many words on the example but concentrate on describing how the experience affected/changed you (e.g. 'Helped me realize the importance of teamwork') and how the experience helped meet a training objective (e.g. 'Helped me to work more effectively as a member of a team').

Application form example question 3

Describe one example of a recent clinical situation where you demonstrated appropriate professional behaviour. What did you do and what have you learned? How will you apply this to foundation training? (150 words)

Comments The more questions you are asked, the harder it is to give a full answer (the example has three questions plus describing the example). The important qualities for this question include ethical behaviour, probity, integrity, confidentiality, consent and patient-centred care. Make sure that the example allows demonstration of some of these qualities. Many of the marks will be awarded for reflection and describing the training outcomes that were covered.

Other common questions

- Demonstrate your commitment to this specialty. What extra-curricular activities have you undertaken to promote your career (see p 61)?
- Give an example of patient care that was less than ideal. **This does not mean *your* care had to be less than ideal.**
- Describe a time you explained a complex term or procedure to someone.
- Give an example of a complex case and your approach. How did this alter management?
- Describe your experience of clinical audit.
- How will this training programme help you meet your career objectives?
- Describe your commitment to professional development.

---

[6] Example questions adapted from the Foundation Programme Application form available online at http://www.foundationprogramme.nhs.uk/pages/home/how-to-apply/uk-graduates.

Curriculum vitae (CV)

A CV is a document that summarizes a doctor from a professional point of view, including education, qualifications, employment and achievements. They are primarily used to apply for jobs, especially more senior clinical posts (e.g. consultant jobs). Nowadays, CVs are rarely requested for junior doctor jobs, having been largely replaced by application forms, though these forms usually follow a similar format to a CV.

It is important to keep a CV up to date alongside a portfolio. When applying for a job the CV should be revised so that it emphasizes relevant experience to the specific specialty, job or location.

Personal details Full name, date of birth (±age in brackets), contact details (address, telephone numbers, email), GMC number. Consider gender, marital status, career aspiration, current post, job applied for (shows the CV was written specifically for that job).

Qualifications List significant qualifications including doctorates, masters degrees, bachelor degrees, diplomas, medical degrees and A/AS levels. Start with the most recent and include the awarding institution, grade (if relevant) and date, e.g. 2007, BMBS, Nottingham University, upper second class.

Awards, prizes, distinctions These should be listed with the most recent first. Include the name of the award, the reason it was awarded, the awarding institution and the dates. For those with many awards consider listing them in different categories (e.g. international, national, regional, institution).

Education Include secondary school and university. Education is sometimes combined with the employment section. List the most recent first and include the dates and institutions.

Employment Starting with the most recent job list all relevant jobs; early in medical careers this may include non-medical jobs. Include dates, institutions, educational supervisors and important roles (e.g. acute admissions, on-call).

Publications List with the most recent first. Provide information in this order: authors (include all authors but highlight your own name), title, journal title (this can be abbreviated to standard journal abbreviations), year, date, volume and pages. A quick approach to this is to copy the reference from http://www.pubmed.com. Those with numerous publications should either display a selection (most impressive/relevant) or put them into categories in order of status: peer-reviewed original research, peer-reviewed reviews, reports, letters, textbooks, posters.

Presentations These include presentations at conferences, invited lectures, grand rounds, departmental presentations and journal clubs. The more senior the applicant the more selective this list will become. Once again the most recent should be listed first.

Audits List these with the most recent first including a brief description of the aim, methods, results and conclusions. If the audit will be repeated then state this.

Other sections A CV is a very personal document and it should reflect the applicant. Some people choose to include the following: personal statement, other interests, a description of why they are suitable for the job (this may also go in a covering letter submitted with the CV instead), teaching experience, management also experience, research interests.

Referees It is usual practice to include two referees, though many forms require three or four. Referees must be asked if they are willing to write a reference prior to submitting the CV; each referee should be sent a copy of the updated CV. Include the referee's name, position, institution and contact details (address, telephone, fax, email).

Interviews

The application procedure for almost all jobs after the foundation programme includes some form of interview. Different specialties use different interview formats; they may also vary between deaneries. Common interview formats include:

- Discussion of portfolio, experience and/or career intentions
- Discussion of management of a clinical scenario
- Discussion of clinical examples on the application form
- Communication skills assessment
- Simulated patient contact
- Group discussion exercise
- Giving a short presentation

Preparing

Interview preparation does make a difference; knowing what to expect makes it easier to be relaxed and make a favourable impression. There are a number of means to prepare:

- Talk to doctors who went through the application process the year before and ask them specifically about the format and questions they were asked. Seniors may be involved in the application process as assessors and be able to give you an insider's view.
- If there are multiple days of interviews then ask colleagues on the earlier days for details about the format and questions. The specific questions are likely to change each day, but the types of questions may be the same (since they must assess the same qualities).
- Consider what qualities are being assessed. These are actually stated by the Specialty Training Person Specifications. Interviews often use standardized question and mark schemes; the marking is likely to be based around the qualities shown on the person specification.
- Become familiar with the specialty by spending time working in it (outside of normal hours if necessary); this makes it much easier to give the impression of being a suitable trainee. Read through your application form answers and be familiar with any examples given.
- Practice interview skills with colleagues and seniors.

What to take Up-to-date portfolio (including proof of qualifications and completed placements), copy of application form answers, letter confirming the time and place of the interview, directions to the interview locations. The interviewers may ask for: identification (e.g. passport, driver's licence), GMC certificate, signed references, proof of visa/work permit status.

What to wear Appearance has a huge impact at interviews. Aim to appear as a safe, responsible and professional doctor who deserves to be trained in the specialty of the interviewer. The choice is easy for men (suit and tie); women should dress smartly, in either a trouser/skirt suit or a smart top and trousers/skirt. If in doubt dress conservatively, but make sure you are comfortable.

On the day

The interviewers will probably be other doctors and on the whole they are friendly and trying to help maximize interviewees' potential. Try to relax and be yourself. Take time to think about the answers rather than saying the first thought that occurs. If in doubt ask the interviewer to repeat the question (this also allows more thinking time).

What happens if you don't get a job?

The competition for medical jobs means it is relatively common not to get a job after a round of applications. It is, however, a serious situation; without a specialty training job it is very difficult to become a consultant and there is a risk of being stuck in non-training jobs. The first objective is to work out why the application was not successful; consider the following:
• Not meeting the eligibility criteria of the jobs—check the person specifications carefully
• Not listing sufficient jobs on the preferences forms (p 62)
• Applying to competitive specialties/deaneries (p 56, 59)
• CV and experience (p 60)
• Application form answers (pp 63–4)
• Interview performance. Some deaneries offer interview feedback and score; this vital information can be obtained by contacting the deanery to which you applied (p 66)

Improving the CV

Failure to be invited to interviews or to be offered jobs suggests the need to improve the CV and application significantly for the next round. The time between rounds can be used to follow the suggestions on p 60. Getting a job can be a difficult hurdle and one which gets harder with each successive unsuccessful application. It is important to make a big effort early to improve the CV, application form and interview technique as soon as possible.

Apply to other deaneries or specialties

The application date for specific specialties varies between deaneries. Furthermore different specialties will be advertised at different times within the same deanery. This means there may be time to reapply to a different deanery or specialty within the same round of applications.

Further application rounds

Each deanery can run three rounds of applications each year in each specialty; the dates of these rounds should be shown on each deanery's website. The main recruitment round for all deaneries should be between January and May with the view to applicants starting in early August. Check to see if the deanery will be running further application rounds in the chosen specialty and apply to these, using the time in between to improve competitiveness.

Jobs outside of specialist training

There are many doctors' jobs apart from the specialist training posts. Consider the following:
• FTSTA (p 14) These are year-long jobs to gain experience though there is a risk of having to reapply at a more competitive level and they may not look good on the CV.
• Staff and associate specialist grades (p 14) Working as a middle grade or senior doctor without the responsibilities of being a consultant. It is difficult to re-enter the training career track and the pay may be relatively lower.
• Time out (p 68) Use the time to work in different countries or to travel, making sure that there is some clinical experience to justify the time out.
• Research jobs These can offer an amazing insight into a specialty and also look good on the CV. Look in *BMJ Careers* and specialty journals for adverts.
• Locuming (p 174) This pays the rent, but will not count as training and does not look good on a CV unless the time was used to do something else 'worthwhile'.

Taking time out

Taking a break from clinical medicine feels like a risk and will often be a logistical nightmare. It might also be a wonderful and life-defining experience. There are many reasons to take a break:

- Research (p 16)
- Alternative careers (p 20 and p 24)
- Working overseas (p 69)
- Simply having a break and/or travelling
- To enjoy a family

Does a break affect job prospects?

This depends on the nature and duration of the break. The key question is how the break could be justified at an interview or on an application form. Some application forms include questions such as, 'Do you have any gaps in your employment history of more than 4 weeks duration?' Consider observerships, conferences and publications to help show the educational benefit of the time out.

A break can also enhance job prospects through standard routes (research or writing up that case report that's been hanging around) but also by less objective measures (developing a more rounded, interesting or personable doctor). Most consultants entirely understand the desire to take a break from training, and even from medicine itself, of up to a year, providing this had a clear and fulfilled objective. However a year spent doing ad-hoc locums whilst working out what to do next will usually be viewed much more negatively.

Important considerations

Along with career impact there are logistical issues to consider:

- Changes in standard of living due to reduced income.
- What will happen to a house, belongings, car, etc. when travelling?
- Getting a job/place to live after coming back.

When to take a break

There are stages in medical career when it is easier to have time off:

- **Before university** the standard gap year is probably the easiest opportunity
- **After the F2 year** by not applying until the next year, though it may be necessary to be present for ST interviews as deferred entry is very rarely possible
- **After ST training** though career pressure might be high

It is possible to get time off within medical school, foundation or ST programmes with a very good reason, e.g. pregnancy, otherwise this can be an extremely difficult battle. Some ST programmes tolerate breaks of up to a year; this depends on specialty, region and supervisors.

Arranging a break

Short breaks (weeks) The options include taking study leave or unpaid leave. Talk to educational supervisor and consultants. Trainees are usually expected to work out how the on-call rota will be covered in their absence, which may include paying for locums.

Medium breaks (months) These will almost certainly be unpaid. The options include asking for a deferred start to a job or locuming until the next round of applications.

Longer breaks (years) This basically entails leaving a job and reapplying upon return. Breaks from medicine for several years may require a period of retraining.

Working abroad

Many doctors choose to enhance their skills by working abroad and whilst reasons for going differ, many value the experience. Whatever the reason for going (e.g. emergency relief work, learning specialized techniques or research opportunities) it is essential to plan well ahead, speak to relevant people and arrange key aspects before going.

Registration and immigration

Doctors need to be registered with the appropriate regulatory body in the country they are working in, and this can be a very lengthy process. It is necessary to provide various documents (often originals), including certified translations where appropriate. The best sources of information are the regulatory body themselves; some have websites with specific sections for international doctors. The regulations vary according to the country:

European Economic Area (EEA) Under European legislation doctors are entitled to full registration in any EEA member state provided they fulfil two criteria: they are citizens of an EEA member state and they completed primary medical training and gained their primary medical qualification in an EEA member state.

Outside the EEA The type of registration, and whether or not exams will need to be taken, depends on where a doctor wishes to practise, the type of work and the duration. In some countries doctors must prove their linguistic competency. Bear in mind that even if the intention is to work with an English-speaking community, doctors need to liaise with local staff and will need some knowledge of the local language.

Immigration This can be a very complex issue and doctors should investigate their options with the relevant embassy well before going. Usually a simple tourist visa is not sufficient to work in a foreign country. Bear in mind that it can be difficult to change status once in the country, so it is essential to have the right visa before travelling.

Medical indemnity This needs be arranged in advance; some UK defence bodies can offer packages depending on the destination.

Fitting in with training

Doctors in specialty training posts can seek approval from the postgraduate dean to undertake clinical training overseas and, if approved prospectively by the PMETB, this can count towards the CCT or GPCCT. Retention of specialty training places for out of programme training (i.e. training not approved by PMETB) is at the discretion of the postgraduate dean and will not count towards the CCT.

Finding a job

The internet, *BMJ Careers* and other journals are valuable resources, as are people who have already been. Look into local working practices as well as terms and conditions of service before going. If there are any concerns, get the contract checked by the national medical association in the country of interest.

General planning

There are many additional things to consider including accommodation, insurance, schooling and whether partners can work. Furthermore, financial considerations such as UK mortgages, tax, insurance policies and pensions. BMA members can get advice on the latter from the Pensions Department. For other information on working abroad contact the BMA International Department at internationalinfo@bma.org.uk.

Applying from overseas

Requirements

Visa The requirements vary between countries (see http://www.ukvisas.gov.uk). Applicants from many countries outside of the European Economic Area (EEA) will require a work permit, which will only be given if the organization can prove that the job cannot be filled by a member of the EEA or for a training position of a fixed duration.

Immigration To work in the UK permanently from a country outside of the EEA it is necessary to apply through the Tier 1 (General) Scheme, a points-based system for highly skilled workers. See http://www.hsmp-services.co.uk for details including a points calculator. At least 95 points are required to be accepted.

Language All doctors must be able to demonstrate that they can speak English:
- Medical degree taught in English and practicing in an English-speaking country A letter from the university and regulating medical authority is usually sufficient.
- Medical degree not taught in English but practicing in an English-speaking country If an English exam was required to register with the medical regulatory authority in the English-speaking country then this exam can also be used to apply for GMC registration.
- Medical degree not taught in English and practicing in a non-English-speaking country Applicant needs to take the International English Language Testing System (IELTS) exam, see http://www.ielts.org.

GMC To work as a doctor in the UK it is essential to register with the GMC. The means of doing this depends on the country of the applicant's medical degree and nationality:
- Both medical degree and citizenship of EEA or Switzerland (a list of these countries is available on the GMC website) Registration is relatively easy. The applicant must apply online through MyGMC (http://www.gmc-uk.org) then attend an identity check at a GMC office in person with original identity documents, qualifications, references and Certificate of Good Standing from the regulating medical authority. All documents must be translated into English by an official translator (list available on GMC website). Registration takes about five days after identity and documents are checked.
- Either medical degree from, and/or national of any other country Applicants need to demonstrate their medical knowledge and ability. There are four ways of doing this:
  - (i) PLAB exams, these consist of two parts: an MCQ and a clinical exam
  - (ii) Sponsorship by a medical College or Association for further postgraduate training
  - (iii) Membership exams e.g. MRCP (p 10)
  - (iv) Eligibility for entry in the Specialist or GP Register (e.g. Article 14 p 82).

Types of jobs

Foundation programme This is a two-year internship that follows medical school. A place is guaranteed to UK medical graduates and this leaves 5% of jobs available for international medical graduates. Those who have completed an internship in a different country should aim to apply to F2 jobs or get another year of experience and apply for specialty training.

Specialist training This is the stage that most overseas doctors apply to; it is highly competitive, see p 56–9. It is necessary to demonstrate foundation competencies, basically this means two years of supervised work as a doctor and completing a 'Declaration of Foundation Competence Assessment – Document D' with the educational supervisor from the last job.

Consultant/GP It is necessary to join the GP or specialist register to apply for these jobs. This entails demonstrating suitable experience through Articles 14 or 11. See p 82 for more details.

Doctors' pay

Medicine does not offer superstar pay; however it does offer a good, secure wage for life to almost everyone who practices. A very small minority make megabucks from private work or special awards, but this requires extremely hard work and a degree of luck. This page provides a guide to pay at different career stages, but the figures vary every year so are only approximate. See http://www.bmjcareers.com, 'Careers', 'Salary Scales' for most recent figures.

Junior doctors

Pay is split into two sections:
- Basic pay
- Banding supplement

Basic pay is determined by grade (F1 or F2/ST) and duration in that grade. Basic pay should never go down, instead it should go up by about £1700 for every completed year of service.
- Basic pay for F1   £21 700
- Basic pay for F2   £26 500
- Basic pay for ST1/CT1   £28 200

A banding supplement is determined by the number of hours of work (rated as 1 or 2) and the sociability of those hours (rated from A to C). The definitions of these bands are beyond the scope of this book, but the details are available at http://www.bmjcareers.com. Basic pay is multiplied by the number below (e.g. 1.5) to give the full salary. Most junior doctors work band 2B or below.
- Band 2A   1.8
- Band 2B   1.5
- Band 1A   1.5
- Band 1B   1.4
- Band 1C   1.2

Consultants

Consultants get a basic full-time pay of £71 800, which increases by about £2250 per year for the first five years and can reach a maximum of £95 800. Pay is in 4-hour blocks (called programmed activities). 40 hours equals 10 PAs. There is a small supplement (1–8%) for on-call.

Clinical excellence awards (CEAs) Awarded on top of basic pay either locally (Level 1 £2800 to Level 9 £34 200, equivalent to a bronze award) or nationally (bronze £34 200, silver £45 000, gold £56 200, platinum £73 100). Only a few consultants receive the higher-paying awards, for example 1% of consultants receive a bronze award or above.

Private work Opportunities vary dramatically between specialties, location and reputation.

Staff and associate specialists

The basic pay scale varies from £31 500 to £45 000, however this can be extended to £77 000 as a reward from the Trust for good performance. New terms, conditions and rates of pay are under negotiation at the time of writing.

General practitioners (GPs)

There are two main ways to work as a GP:
- Salaried (employed by the practice) full-time pay £52 000 to £78 000
- Partner (own all or part of the practice) full-time pay £80 000 to £120 000

Actual figures are variable depending on location, demand and how well the practice is functioning as a business. Like any business there is also the risk of poor performance which could significantly reduce pay, though this is uncommon.

Flexible training

Flexible training, also called 'less than full-time training' (LTFT) or part-time, allows trainees to fulfil the requirements of foundation programmes and specialist training whilst working reduced numbers of hours. They should still perform the same activities as full-time trainees, but with a proportional decrease in the number of hours of each activity (pro rata). This means that on-calls, night shifts and working on national holidays are still necessary. Flexible training enables a doctor to reduce their working week to 50% of full-time (this is the minimum that can be approved for training) but the actual percentages available vary between deaneries. The national target is for 20% of trainees to be training flexibly by 2010, subject to demand.

Eligibility

Doctors can apply for flexible training if they have a well-founded reason for being unable to work full time. The reason for wishing to work flexibly determines the priority of the request:

Category One	Parents of young children who wish to spend part of the week at home
	Doctors caring for sick or dependent relatives
	Doctors who are unable, for health reasons, to work full time
Category Two	Doctors wishing to train part-time, while in alternative paid employment for the remainder of the week
	Doctors wishing to train part-time in order to pursue non-medical interests

Deaneries usually restrict flexible training to Category One applicants as they do not have sufficient funding for both categories.

Types of flexible training posts

Reduced sessions in a full-time post An unfilled full-time post is filled by a doctor working part-time leaving a gap in hours; no postgraduate deanery funding is required.

Slot share Two doctors working part-time share a full-time job. Each slot sharer can work more than 50% if the relevant postgraduate deanery chooses to fund the additional hours over the normal full-time post. For example if two slot sharers work 80% each (160% in total) the deanery can choose to fund the additional 60%.

Supernumerary posts A doctor working part-time works in addition to the full-time staff so that their hours are extra. The postgraduate deanery has to fund the daytime sessions while the Trust funds the out-of-hours (OOHs) supplement.

The budget for flexible training is limited and the number of doctors requesting flexible training is increasing so reduced sessions in full-time posts or in slot-sharing is preferred.

Out-of-hours (OOH)

A flexible trainee should work the same proportion of on-calls as a full-time trainee (e.g. 60% of daytime shifts and 60% of on-calls). The Trust may put pressure on those in supernumerary posts to do little or no on-call to reduce costs. However, the training programme must be approved for training and if this requires OOHs then OOHs must be included.

European legislation allows exemption from OOHs if an employee is breastfeeding and trainees may be able to obtain OOHs exemption or modification of their working hours if they are pregnant. The rules on exemption from OOHs apply equally to full- and part-time employees but exemption could mean the post is no longer approved for training.

Whole time equivalent training

This table shows the duration of flexible training posts in months compared with full-time training:

Full-time	6 months	12 months	18 months	24 months	30 months	36 months
80%	7.5	15	22.5	30	37.5	45
70%	8.5	17	25.5	34	42.5	51
60%	10	20	30	40	50	60
50%	12	24	36	48	60	72

Educational approval

If flexible trainees are working in a slot share or reduced sessions in a full-time training post then educational approval should already be in place. However, for supernumerary posts educational approval must be obtained from the Postgraduate Medical Education and Training Board (PMETB) before starting in post. If it is possible to obtain experience of emergency work within normal working hours, PMETB may be prepared to accept this but it must be agreed in writing before starting the post. If on-call is not required for training approval there is no compulsion upon the Trust to provide it.

Recruitment

Flexible trainees are appointed through the same competitive application process as full-time colleagues for foundation programmes and specialty training posts. Applicants are not obliged to state that they would like to train flexibly until after they have accepted a training programme, however it is wise to consult the flexible training department in their postgraduate deanery to establish their eligibility for funding and it helps the deanery if doctors indicate their intention on their application form. Those assessing applicants will not be told that the applicant plans to train flexibly as this is protected information at the interview stage.

Once accepted to a training programme deaneries, specialty schools and foundation schools will give guidance on organizing flexible training, however an individual placement is subject to an employer being willing to employ the doctor on a flexible basis. The individual doctor is responsible for organizing their flexible training placement.

Summary

Flexible training is not an easy option and takes time, patience and resilience to organize. Trainees will need to use all their negotiating skills, but there should be plenty of help and advice available. It remains the primary responsibility of the trainee to organize their flexible training. Flexible trainees should no longer be seen as different, but just another way of working, within employment legislation. As the demand for flexible training increases the majority of placements will need to become mainstream with supernumerary posts only used in special circumstances.

i **For further information:**

The following documents can be downloaded from the Internet and are available on numerous NHS and deanery websites (e.g. mmc.kssdeanery.org), though the exact links change frequently.
Doctors in flexible training: equitable pay for flexible medical training. NHS Employers (2005).
Doctors in flexible training: principles underpinning the new arrangements for flexible training. NHS Employers (2005).

The organization of medical careers

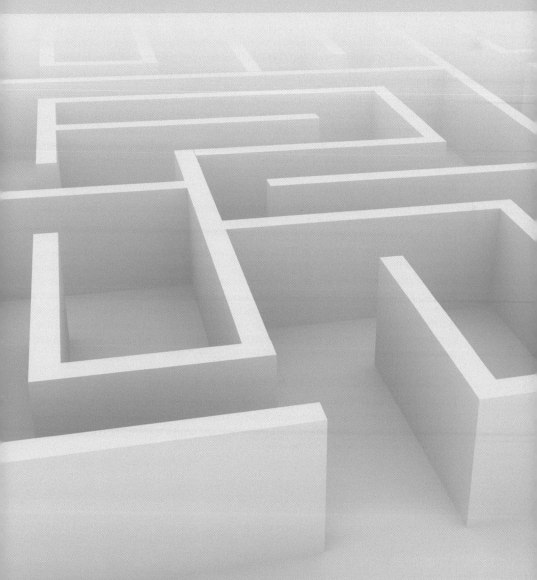

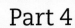

Part 4

The organization of medical careers

Postgraduate training: MMC

The postgraduate training system in the UK has undergone two wholesale changes in living memory and is currently going through a third. Despite this impression of constant flux, many aspects of training remain pretty constant; although the steps on the path may vary, the overall route to becoming a consultant or GP will remain recognizable in the future.

History

It is easy to forget that prior to the Calman reforms of 1996 there was little fixed structure to postgraduate medical training in the UK. There were four training grades (PRHO, SHO, registrar and senior registrar) with the onus on the junior doctor to arrange their next post at six-monthly or yearly intervals. Posts could be anywhere in the country, involving multiple applications and moving long distances in the more competitive fields. There was also no defined end point, with senior registrars staying in posts for up to a decade waiting for the right consultant post to come up.

The then Chief Medical Officer (CMO), Sir Kenneth Calman, decided to structure training. Rotations were standardized and the registrar and senior registrar grades were replaced with a single, time-limited specialist registrar (SpR) grade. Training culminated in a Certificate of Completion of Specialist Training (CCST) with six months' grace to find a consultant post. Once accepted for an SpR rotation, training was secure in one region. The downside was that a lost tribe developed at SHO level, waiting for SpR numbers.

In 2002 the next CMO, Sir Liam Donaldson, published *Unfinished Business* in which he highlighted the plight of the large numbers of young doctors marking time in the SHO grade, half of whom were not in formal training posts. In 2005 Modernising Medical Careers (MMC) was launched with the arrival of the foundation programme (p 6). The CCST was also replaced by the Certificate of Completion of Training (CCT), which was otherwise identical to CCST.

Modernising Medical Careers

The aims of MMC were to streamline training and to ensure that trainees achieved clearly described competencies rather than just training for a set length of time. The introduction of run-through training (p 8) meant that trainees had to make decisions on their final specialty far earlier than many felt ready to. This was compounded by the apparent inflexibility of the training routes, making it difficult for trainees to change career path (p 78). The competencies and their assessments have also been criticized for settling for the minimum rather than allowing and encouraging young doctors to excel.

However, the biggest problem of all was the immediate transition from the old to the new system in August 2007 resulting in very high levels of competition as trainees below the SpR grade competed for a limited number of training posts. This perceived unfairness was hugely compounded by a national electronic application scheme: MTAS.

MTAS (Medical Training Application Service)

Despite the appeal of a national 'matching' application scheme similar to the US model, the development of the UK system was deeply flawed in terms of selection and shortlisting criteria, timescale for development, professional involvement and actual delivery. The system was consequently abandoned, to widespread relief.

Postgraduate training: Tooke and the future

The Tooke Report

In 2007, Patricia Hewitt, the Secretary of State for Health at the time, commissioned an independent inquiry into MMC, chaired by Professor Sir John Tooke. The final report was published in January 2008.

The Tooke Report will form the basis for the shape of medical training in the UK. The principal recommendations are directed towards the governance and structure of postgraduate training. The Report recommends three training grades:

1) a single first foundation year of generic training (this has been rejected);

2) three years of core specialty training giving a broad base of experience; and

3) higher specialist training (varying from approximately three to six years).

The recommendation to merge PMETB with the GMC to govern training has already been adopted and the report recommends the creation of a new body: NHS Medical Education England. This body will coordinate professional involvement in workforce planning, policy development and postgraduate training as the Report highlighted the medical profession's weak involvement in policy-making.

Two further findings were:

1) that the ongoing lack of a clearly defined role for junior doctors needs to be resolved (are they trainees or responsible for service delivery?)

2) doctors in training lacked a sense of belonging to their employing organizations and the mix of ownership by hospital Trusts, deaneries and colleges needs fixing.

The Report firmly states that UK medical training should aim to produce the very best doctors possible and not settle for ensuring basic competence; hence the title—*Aspiring to Excellence*.

Finally, those with an interest in the shape of the future of the medical profession in the UK should pay particular attention to the international comparison in appendix 7 of the Tooke Report. The UK remains an outlier in many respects and still has a relatively low number of doctors and lower health spending than comparator countries.

The future of medical training

Irrespective of how the Tooke Report is implemented and subsequent changes to training, some aspects are likely to remain constant. For example: the three grades of postgraduate trainee (generic, basic specialty and higher specialist); postgraduate exams as the hurdle to get into higher training; the need to provide 'emergency-safe' doctors who can deal with all the common causes of deranged physiology; and the ability to differentiate between the ability level of trainees and to limit progression of weaker doctors.

There are areas which may change from the models of the last ten years. For instance, there is debate over the need to better compare medical graduates across the country. Britain and Australia are unusual in not having a common medical graduate exam allowing nationwide comparisons.

Another major area of change may be in the immediate post-CCT period. It is unclear whether hospitals will start offering jobs which are substantially different from current consultant posts, but this looks likely (e.g. junior consultant posts). Furthermore, the mechanism for obtaining subspecialty training after the acquisition of a CCT is still very unclear.

Finally, the biggest change to face new medical graduates is almost certain to be increased competition for training places at every stage. The number of medical graduates has increased dramatically over the last six years with a slightly smaller increase in the number of training places for all grades, leading to an excess of trainees. The era of 100% of UK doctors being employed may well be at an end.

Switching specialist training pathways

Flexibility in training programmes was one of the underlying principles of the plans for Modernising Medical Careers (MMC). In the document *Modernising Medical Careers—the Next Steps* it was clearly stated that:

> there will be in-Programme opportunities for trainees to move to other preferred or more suitable specialties. The processes for doing this must be clear, explicit and fair—it will be a very important feature of the new training system. They should match the choices of individuals with career advice, assessed potential and, importantly the demands of the NHS for particular specialists and for GPs.

It was widely understood that there would be opportunity to switch specialty training pathways for trainees that decided who they had made the wrong career choice.

There was much discussion about the concept of 'transferable competencies', and while the details of specialty training were being planned it was suggested that there should be broad training bands immediately following foundation where generic skills for the specialties would be enhanced and trainees could take some time to decide on their future, narrower, specialty career path. Unfortunately this was not considered to be achievable, for reasons largely related to workforce planning, and there was reversion to run-through training immediately following foundation training.

Career planning

One of the other pillars on which MMC was based was that there should be a system of 'rigorous counselling and career advice which should be present throughout training'. The document went on to say 'underpinned by practical career advice and coaching, there should be opportunities to change direction later on'. Despite these assurances, there has been significant difficulty in providing even basic career planning advice for all trainees and significant differences have been perceived between deaneries and specialties. Much of the careers advice has been based on limited information and experience; many trainees, particularly those coming out of foundation programmes may have had limited or no experience of the specialty for which they have expressed a preference.

Specialty selection

The timing of the run-up to the selection rounds early in 2007 necessitated a considerable amount of specialty-specific information being available at very short notice. The college curriculum documents had only very recently been approved by PMETB and many were not accessible. The colleges and specialty societies worked hard to get accurate person specifications and specialty profile information available in time for the selection round to begin, but many trainees had very limited time to choose their specialty and many educational supervisors were ill-informed about both the process and content to aid completion of application documentation.

With the subsequent failure of the Medical Training Application Service (MTAS) system and the confusion surrounding the different rounds of the subsequent application process, many trainees felt disadvantaged and pressured into making rapid career decisions and felt too exposed to make career choices that were considered to be too risky.

Changing specialty

Against this background there are, inevitably, going to be some trainees who have made the wrong career choice for themselves and their ability to change career paths at the current time is limited. Much depends on the stage of training at which doctors find themselves and the type of post in which they have been placed.

For those trainees who have taken up the option of a Fixed Term Specialty Training Appointment (FTSTA) the options are easier than for those who were successful in being placed into one of the run-through training grade posts because of the time-limited nature of these posts. The further on in training, the more difficult it is to change career path, although at all stages there is the option to surrender a training programme and compete for a non-training post, including the staff and associate specialist grade (p 14). Although these posts have not been universally popular, they may well suit some individuals who choose to have a less pressured lifestyle and a slower training pathway—with the warning that such posts need to be selected with care as they embrace a wide range of service delivery commitment and have a variable degree of training and career progression opportunity.

At the current time, any trainee who decides that they are in the wrong training programme will need to apply through a competitive process for an alternative specialty training programme unless there are particular circumstances that mean a trainee is unable, for any reason, to pursue their original career path. Such exceptional circumstances should be discussed at an early stage with the specialty tutor and the deanery as special arrangements might need to be made.

Reapplication

The Person Specifications of Specialty Training Programmes state how much experience is required at each ST level and in which specialties this experience must take place. For radical changes of career path, e.g. paediatrics to public health, this will require restarting training at ST1 level. For specialties that are closely related, e.g. cardiology and respiratory medicine, the applicant would need to apply to the point at which these career paths diverge, i.e. ST3. Specific guidance has been given to both applicants and selection panels to take due note of competences that have been gained in posts undertaken prior to the date of application. There are many non-specialty-specific skills which are transferable across specialties and would potentially enhance training within the new specialty. Once again, additional careers advice is beneficial from a more experienced clinician within the new specialty.

Progress in the new specialty

If you are successful in achieving a post in a new specialty then it is likely to have to be at the beginning of the training programme, as the Postgraduate Medical Training and Education Board (PMETB) will only approve training towards a CCT that takes place within prospectively approved training posts within a specialty. However, it has always been a principle of PMETB, and supported by the colleges, that training should be competency and not time-based. It is therefore possible, in theory, to have accelerated progress which may be the result of levels of competence gained within another specialty and demonstrated within the new specialty. Once again, this will be something which will need to be discussed with a specialty tutor and the deanery representative.

Summary

Although there was a clear desire within the concept of MMC to allow flexibility within training programmes and encourage opportunities for trainees to move cross programmes once they had been selected for specialist training, this has not been appropriately facilitated in the current system. However, there has been significant pressure from many bodies through the review of MMC to increase flexibility in the ability of trainees to move across training programmes. It is highly likely that this is one aspect of postgraduate medical training which will be significantly changed in the future.

Overseeing education

From the time of leaving medical school until completion of specialist training there is a network of support designed to ensure that training goes smoothly. This includes a number of important individuals and organizations, all of whom play a role in the wider context of medical education. It is important to understand the function of each, and their role in helping trainees to complete their training without difficulty. They may also offer a point of contact in case of anxiety or concern related to aspects of training and education.

Educational supervisor

Every doctor in training should have a nominated educational supervisor. In the majority of cases these will be consultants with whom the trainees work, who will therefore have an understanding and knowledge of their strengths and weaknesses. Meetings with educational supervisors should take place regularly to discuss progress and offer support and advice when necessary. Trainees should be prepared to discuss their educational needs and use their portfolio as a resource to help identify what they hope to get out of their job (personal development plan), along with additional learning needs and how these can be achieved during the time in the placement. Occasionally educational supervisors might also act as clinical supervisors to the same trainee.

Clinical supervisor

All consultants who supervise a doctor in training act as clinical supervisors. They will be responsible for overseeing clinical work, completing assessments as required and offering support as part of a clinical team. Other health professionals may also fulfil a clinical supervisory role. While not all consultants will wish to take on the role of educational supervisor, most are happy to act as a clinical supervisor offering good training opportunities and ensuring that time spent in post is valuable and productive.

Clinical tutor

The clinical tutor, sometimes also known as the director of medical education, is the individual who has been appointed by the dean and the Trust to manage postgraduate medical education within the Trust. It is their responsibility, on behalf of the dean, to ensure that the learning environment within the Trust supports the provision of high-quality postgraduate medical education and training. They are responsible for all medical education issues, working closely with the postgraduate dean, foundation school and specialty schools to develop the team of consultants and other health professionals who are responsible for supporting elements of the foundation programme as well as the provision of specialty training. As a general rule they are supported by an administrative team from within an education centre.

Deanery

The Postgraduate Deans bear the responsibility for managing postgraduate training programmes which start with foundation programmes and span the whole of specialty training until completion of a Certificate of Completed Training (CCT). At the current time (July 2008) they are responsible for providing the infrastructure to recruit to training programmes and managing the programmes to standards which are agreed by the Royal Colleges, established in curricula and quality assured by the Postgraduate Medical Education and Training Board (PMETB). In order to fulfil this task they have highly experienced teams with expertise in all aspects of medical education and training, and are co-signatories to educational contracts with Trusts and the strategic health authorities that manage the funding streams. They are an important resource for advice and support outside the Trust and generally include individuals with specific interests and roles (e.g. flexible training, refugee doctor programmes).

Royal Colleges

The colleges and faculties are the organizations which have the responsibility for setting the standards of practice for their specialist professional groups. They fulfil this role through a collegiate structure which develops a curriculum for training accompanied by an assessment programme, both of which have to be approved by PMETB as appropriate in structure and content to be able to produce a specialist who is trained to a standard appropriate for the award of a CCT. Many colleges have long histories and traditions which offer the benefit of maintaining standards which span generations. Colleges have also taken responsibility for maintaining standards for trained staff through programmes of continuous professional development (CPD) for career-grade doctors and often have to play an independent role when there have been breaches in acceptable practice.

PMETB

This is the body that was established in 2005 to oversee standards for medical education and training. It was initially accountable to the government but following the Tooke report it will become part of the GMC. PMETB works closely with the deaneries and royal colleges to assure quality in the process of medical training. All training programmes are required to be approved by PMETB prospectively before they can offer training that will be counted towards the issuing of a CCT. PMETB is required to approve all college curricula and assessment programmes and is developing a quality assurance programme that will ensure that all approved training programmes are delivered to an appropriate standard. PMETB also has the responsibility for approving Certificates confirming Eligibility for the Specialist Register (CESR), an alternative route to achieve specialist certification for those who are not in training programmes (p 82).

Foundation schools

The establishment of foundation programmes throughout the UK required the development of foundation schools to manage the programmes. These provide a vital link between the deaneries and the medical schools and undergraduate training courses. They are jointly accountable to the General Medical Council (GMC) and PMETB who are responsible for ensuring the fitness of graduates to join the medical register at the completion of foundation year 1. They are run by foundation school directors who work closely with foundation training programme directors based within Trusts. They are responsible for administering foundation programmes from recruitment to completion of foundation year 2.

Following the Tooke Report there was discussion about reducing the Foundation Programme to one year. This has been rejected so they will remain two-years long for now.

Specialty schools

Most deaneries are establishing specialty schools to manage the training programmes after completion of foundation training. They will be responsible for ensuring that the new training programmes are delivered and meet the curricula that have been approved by PMETB. They will take responsibility for ensuring that assessment programmes are in place and that all trainees have an Annual Review of Competence Progression (ARCP). Their primary role is to ensure that trainees progress through training programmes to completion of their CCT.

Alternative routes (Articles 14 and 11)

The primary objective of medical training is to produce doctors who are capable of fulfilling the role of a specialist or a general practitioner and are therefore allowed to have their names included on the specialist or general practice registers held by the General Medical Council (GMC). The standard route is to complete a full PMETB approved training programme (i.e. specialist training or GP vocational training scheme) and to apply for a Certificate of Completion of Training (CCT) or a General Practice Certificate of Completion of Training (GPCCT). However, there are alternative routes, the most common of which is for a doctor to apply to PMETB for the Certificate of Eligibility for Specialist Registration (CESR) or for General Practice Registration (CEGPR).

Article 14 and Article 11

PMETB was established by *The General and Specialist Medical Practice (Education, Training and Qualifications) Order 2003* to develop a single, unifying framework for postgraduate medical education and training. Article 14(4) applies to the section of the order which describes the means by which a doctor who has not followed a PMETB-approved training programme may apply to PMETB offering evidence of equivalent training, qualifications or experience to have their name added to the specialist register. Separate arrangements exist for those who wish to apply to practice in a specialty for which a CCT is not awarded in the UK and for those who wish to apply for a CCT in research or academic medicine.

Article 11 describes a similar process for applying for recognition of previous training, qualifications and experience to be assessed against the standard required for the award of a CCT in general practice. In all cases applicants have to demonstrate that they have achieved the knowledge and skills consistent with practice as a General Practitioner (11) or a consultant (14) within the NHS.

The process

PMETB offers detailed guidance on how to submit an application and the documentary evidence that must be supplied. All evidence is required to be validated and the evaluation criteria are based on the General Medical Council's document *Good Medical Practice*. In general the evidence required relates to general standards of practice, which are similar between specialties (e.g. working with colleagues, relationships with patients etc.), and evidence specific to the specialty in which the doctor is applying for a CESR.

PMETB aims to process applications within three months of receiving the complete application, however many applications are delayed, either because they contain inadequate evidence or due to the time required by the college or specialist society to review the evidence of specialist practice before agreeing to grant a CESR/CEGPR. If an application is not successful then PMETB will advise on what further training or assessment is required and there is opportunity for resubmission if considered appropriate. There is a right of review or appeal on the judgement made by PMETB.

Curricula and posts

From August 2007 all training programmes will be required to conform to the new curricula for each specialty approved by PMETB. It is a requirement that doctors applying through alternative routes are expected to meet the standards attaining to the equivalence of the CCT/CCGPT at the time of approval. This means that all submissions will now have to demonstrate compliance with the new curricula.

Since August 2007 the only route to a CCT is through a training programme in which all posts have been prospectively approved by PMETB as being suitable for inclusion within a training programme for the new curriculum for that specialty. PMETB have made it clear that they will not give retrospective approval to posts already undertaken. This means that trainees entering a trainee programme at any level above ST1 (first year of specialist training) will have to have undergone training in posts that have previously been approved by PMETB if they are to be awarded a CCT. If they have worked overseas or within the UK in non-approved posts they will not be eligible for the award of a CCT and will have to apply for a CESR or CEGPR.

Staff and associate specialist grade posts (p 14)

Traditionally posts at staff grade and associate specialist grade have been perceived as non-training opportunities. A number of other types of posts have been developed by Trusts, often to meet service needs and the hours required for the European Working Time Directive. These posts are variously labelled Trust doctor or Clinical Fellow and may include some research posts. Because these posts are not necessarily approved by PMETB for training, the time spent in these posts cannot be counted towards the award of a CCT or CCGPT.

It is widely recognized that many of these posts offer excellent training opportunities and many meet exactly the same standards and conditions as training posts within the same department. Incumbents of such posts are encouraged to undertake CPD and through these opportunities may progress towards achieving the standards required by PMETB for the award of a CESR. However, attention should be drawn to the fact that all evidence submitted for consideration for a CESR needs to be validated; therefore it is essential that doctors within SASG posts avail themselves of a mentor or supervisor so that their practice can be validated. All applications to PMETB through this route require six referees to provide structured reports offering a range of views to allow a fair judgement to be made.

Summary

The conventional route for a doctor to get their name on the specialist register within the UK is to complete a PMETB-approved training programme leading to the award of a CCT. Doctors wishing to have their names added to the register who have not completed a full training programme within the UK or who are applying from abroad need to demonstrate that they have achieved the standards required of a consultant or GP practicing within the UK. Article 14 and Article 11 of the Order (2003) allows doctors to supply validated evidence to PMETB for approval for the award of a CESR or CEGPR enabling them to have their name added to the specialist or GP Register.

Discrimination

Discrimination in medical careers is choosing between doctors on the basis of a quality that they possess. Some forms of discrimination are allowed and even encouraged, for example choosing a doctor on the basis of merit (i.e. how good they are at the job). Many other forms of discrimination are illegal under British law (particularly discrimination by gender, race, disability, religion, sexual orientation, age or political opinion) unless there is justification (e.g. a disability that prevented the person from performing the job despite reasonable support).

Discrimination can take two forms:
- Direct e.g. not giving someone a job because they are female
- Indirect e.g. an unjustified job requirement that makes it harder for women to apply.

Since medicine is a competitive career with numerous job applications between entering medical school and reaching a final career, there is ample opportunity for unfair discrimination. In the past discrimination within medicine has been widespread, e.g. the old boys network and prejudices of interviewers. With time, attitudes and application procedures have changed so that discrimination has been drastically reduced. NHS Trusts have to prove that their application process does not discriminate unfairly and any allegations of foul play are taken very seriously.

It would be unrealistic to think that discrimination has been eradicated entirely though; for example overseas and female doctors are still under-represented in senior jobs (see p 86).

What to do if you have experienced unfair discrimination

Advice If you believe you have been subject to unfair discrimination it is a good idea to talk the matter over with someone you trust before you act. This may be a colleague your educational supervisor or the BMA (members can phone 0870 6060828).

Informal complaint You can complain directly to the person or institution who you believe has been unfairly discriminatory. It is best to complain in writing so that you have a record of the issue: note that this is a serious accusation and should not be made lightly.

Formal complaint Making a formal complaint will begin a legal process to determine if you have been subject to unfair discrimination. It is essential that you act promptly since complaints must be made in writing or online to an employment tribunal within three months minus one day of the alleged discrimination. Details of employment tribunals can be found at http://www.employmenttribunals.gov.uk including an online claim form.

Harassment and bullying

Harassment is threatening or disturbing behaviour based on a specific characteristic of the victim (e.g. race, gender, sexual orientation) whilst bullying is similar behaviour without a discriminating cause. Either behaviour may be vocal, physical or psychological. Acknowledging harassment or bullying can be difficult and it takes courage to raise the issue. The main options for dealing with this behaviour are:
- Talk to a colleague, senior, educational supervisor or BMA
- Confront the person and ask them to stop behaving in this manner
- Make a written complaint to the member of staff's immediate manager

Women in medicine

Why include a chapter about a non-marginalized majority?

Over 50% of medical students have been female for over a decade, yet in 2006 only 10% of consultant surgeons were female and only 11% of medical professors were female.

Historical angle In the 1970s there were fewer women at medical school, so many of the professors and senior consultants of today are males in their fifties. The application process has also changed; until the 1990s every 6–12 months required a new fight for the next junior doctor post alongside working 104 hour weeks and operating most nights during the critical childbearing years (age 25–35).

What has changed? There have been a number of beneficial changes in medical practice, UK law and application procedures, mostly affecting those who wish to have families and children: The European Working Time Directive only allows 48 hours of work per week.

- The CEPOD (Confidential Enquiry into Postoperative Outcome and Death) reports stopped night-time operating, except for life- or limb-threatening cases.
- National Training Numbers (NTNs) were introduced in the 1990s and gave 4–8 years of almost-guaranteed training until the Certificate of Completion of Training (CCT, p 13). This means that it is possible to take 6 months out for childbirth and still have a training job to go back to. These have been replaced with specialist training posts.
- Working less than full-time (LTFT) also called flexible training or part-time working. It can take some time to set this up, but it has become much more acceptable (see p 72).
- New consultant contract: a full-time contract amounts to 3½ or 4 days of direct clinical care per week, some hospitals allow a degree of flexibility about management/teaching/admin at other times (e.g. permitting some of this work to be done at home). It may also be possible to work flexi-time.
- New general practice (GP) contract. This removed the necessity to do any on-call work.
- More team-working (lots of protocols, nurse-led care, physiotherapy-led discharge, etc.) so that one doctor does not have to work single-handed.
- New curriculum: all specialties are now transparent in what is required for training.
- Advances in surgical equipment and technique mean even very physical surgery (e.g. ortho-paedics) is a matter of finesse, not brute strength.
- Academic posts: there is clearer path for these now, see p 16.

Is there still a gender imbalance?

Yes. So few women apply to surgical specialties (10%) that the ones who do actually stand a better chance of being selected. The critical career-defining moment is obtaining a specialist training post in your chosen specialty. This is decided by a selection panel, which has to be fair. Once you have a specialty training post it is quite difficult to lose it as long as you pass the necessary exams and assessments.

Everyone needs to be aware that some specialties are highly competitive: some special-ties have rejected 90% of all applicants for many years, as there are not enough posts and these specialties are very popular (p 56–9). All candidates need to work on their CVs (p 65), especially audit experience, prizes, posters, presentations, teaching experience, management experience, sporting, team-work, etc. Some specialties with a heavy out-of-hours burden have 40–50% of women in ST posts (e.g. emergency medicine, anaesthetics, obstetrics and gynaecology, paediatrics).

Does sexist behaviour still exist?

Yes. There are some male consultants who can't seem to help mentioning physical attributes of their trainees and medical students. These are often the ones who paradoxically demand a female trainee 'because girls work harder'. There is some, often inadvertent, discrimination from other NHS staff: 'Sorry, love, I thought you were the dietician', 'Oh, I assumed the [male] doctor was the consultant', 'Oh, I didn't realize *you* would be doing the operation'. This may change when a critical mass of female doctors is reached in each specialty and as society's assumptions change.

The practicalities for women in medicine

Working while pregnant A risk assessment need to be arranged through occupational health. The manager should consider any risks and means to reduce them. There are papers suggesting that the risk of using X-rays is low. Morning sickness may be helped by regular snacks and often settles after the first trimester. Some tasks undoubtedly get harder in the third trimester.

Maternity leave NHS employees are entitled to up to 8 weeks (~2 months) full-pay, 18 weeks (~4 months) half-pay and 29 weeks (~7 months) unpaid leave. Jobs should be held open for a year. It is best to announce the date of expected departure and return well in advance, though avoid announcements before 13 weeks gestation since 20% of pregnancies miscarry in the first trimester. Doctors must be employed at least 11 weeks before the due date to receive these benefits.

Breastfeeding and work Doctors are entitled to take breaks to feed their child. In practice, most babies will mix-and-match bottle and breast. There is also the option to express breast milk whilst on-call and freeze it to take home.

Childcare Looking after a small child is a full-time job; doctors are just fortunate to earn enough to pay someone else to do it for some of the time. Care needs to be arranged well in advance since nurseries have long waiting lists; some people choose a nanny. Both options are expensive. Also consider whether parents or a partner's parents may be handy for weekend or evening on-calls.

Working less than full-time (LTFT) This must be organized far in advance; deaneries arrange LTFT for specialist training posts (see p 72).

Some useful websites

* Royal College of Surgeons of England http://www.rcseng.ac.uk (look for 'Women In Surgery')
* Medical Women's Federation http://www.medicalwomensfederation.org.uk
* BMA http://www.bma.org (look for 'Maternity Leave')
* Intercollegiate Surgical Curriculum Programme http://www.iscp.ac.uk (look for 'Curriculum Project in Surgery')
* London Deanery http://www.londondeanery.ac.uk (look for 'Less Than Full-time working')
* National Confidential Enquiry into Postoperative Outcome and Death http://www.ncepod.org.uk
* National Patient Safety Agency http://www.npsa.nhs.uk
* Association of Surgeons in Training http://www.asit.org

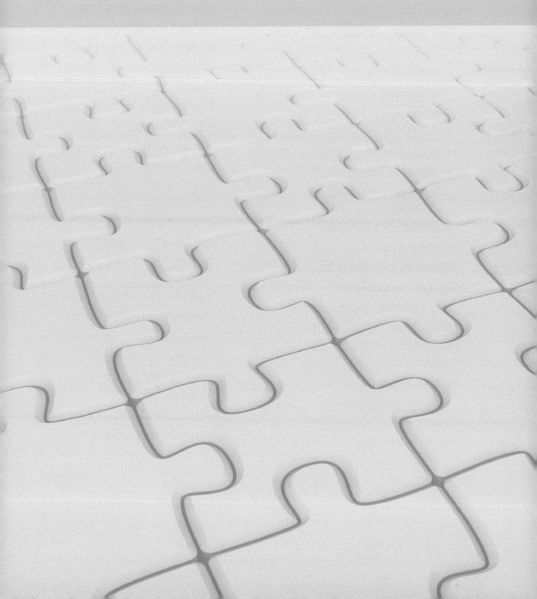

Part 5

Career chapters

Career chapters

Academic GP

Academic GPs have the best of both worlds: they have the challenge and diversity of clinical care along with dedicated time for research to improve general practice. Their role includes providing the research evidence to improve clinical care, teaching medical students and offering general leadership to the profession. Every medical school has a core of GPs who teach and a smaller number of Academic GPs.

the patients are important. Almost all academic GPs still do surgeries, maybe one or two days a week. It's the reality of patient care that keeps them grounded and provides the most interesting research ideas on which to reflect. Some work as salaried GPs, but many are partners (p 71). As with any GP job the patients can come from any demographic (babies to the elderly, rich to poor, etc.) and present with any problem. Their clinical role is equivalent to a GP working part-time.

the work is not for the faint-hearted. Universities are demanding employers who allocate funding and promotions based on academic success. Research can be frustrating, difficult and tortuous, but when it all works out it can be terrifically rewarding; there is also the excitement of working on a chosen research interest from conception to answer. Many find the teaching aspects to be a genuine pleasure. Research is usually about the organization of GP services (e.g. methods to prevent teenage pregnancy) or best practice in specific diseases (e.g. ideal management of hypertension). The GP role is covered on p 144.

the job cannot be pinned down easily. Every academic GP carves out their own niche with unique activities, workload and responsibilities. Most jobs are a combination of research, teaching, committees (local and national), conferences (often overseas) and university administration. Most academic GPs work in a team, though each has a different research interest; there are also research assistants and research fellows to help with the research.

extras Part-time working is easily arranged and on-call is optional. Pay is a mixture of the consultant contract (including clinical excellence awards) and the GP contract (salaried or partnership p 71). Academic GPs are in a good position to pursue leadership or management interests in health care.

ⓘ *For further information:*

Royal College of General Practitioners, 14 Princes Gate, Hyde Park, London, SW7 1PU
Tel: 020 7581 3232;   Fax: 020 7225 3047; Web: http://www.rcgp.org.uk
GP Recruitment: http://www.gprecruitment.org.uk
Academic clinical fellowships: National Co-ordinating Centre for Research Capacity Development (NCC RCD), Leeds Innovation Centre, 103 Clarendon Road, Leeds, LS2 9DF
Tel: 0113 346 6260;   Fax: 0113 346 3272;   Web: http://www.nccrcd.nhs.uk

08:30	Surgery in the practice: 20 patients in 8-minute slots, some are familiar faces with ongoing health issues, others visiting for the first time
11:30	Home visits: one requires acute admission for exacerbation of chronic obstructive pulmonary disease (COPD)
13:00	Research team meeting in the university
14:00	Teaching session with medical students; seminar based in small groups
16:00	Working on the draft of a paper for the BMJ about access to healthcare services for refugees
17:00	Telephone conference for a national collaborative research project
19:30	Seminar with local general practitioners

myth	Lives in an ivory tower divorced from reality
reality	A weekly dose of clinical reality with time to pursue research ideas that make a big difference
personality	Obsessive, good at seeing projects through to completion, hard working, leadership skills, good at teaching and writing
best aspects	The joy of a good seminar; having ideas be taken up by the profession; seeing a paper published
worst aspects	Competitive, so success is hard won; profession can be reluctant to accept change despite good evidence
route	A combination of an Academic Clinical Fellowship (p 16) and GP Vocational Training (p 32); requires nMRCGP and a higher degree (e.g. PhD)
Numbers	185
Locations	Teaching hospitals and surrounding GP surgeries

life					work
quiet on-call					busy on-call
boredom			☺		burnout
uncompetitive					competitive
low salary					high salary

Academic medicine

In terms of scope, saying 'I want to be an academic' is not far off the same as saying 'I want to be a doctor'. The world is your oyster, as academia can relate to any specialty you care to think of and a huge range of types of research. Medical academia is now primarily about research rather than teaching and the balance between clinical work and research varies widely. MMC has resulted in structured career paths into many academic specialties though many people move into academia from full-time clinical practice.

the patients Clinical practice can be in any specialty that forms a chapter of this book. The extent ranges from one outpatient clinic (or equivalent) a week to nearly full-time clinical with a bit of protected research time (a solution close to hell!). 50:50 is the most common arrangement. The clinical contact is essential to supply research ideas and practical applications of the research so that the patients ultimately benefit.

the work It is all about creating new knowledge in a disciplined manner to produce reliable results that stand up to critical scrutiny. It all starts with an interesting idea, then framing it as a question, working out how to find the answer and who will pay for doing so, then conducting the experiment to find an answer. While running research projects and analysing the results is the heart of it, the work is a balance between indulging the enquiring mind and the hard and competitive world of getting research grants, submitting publications, smooth project organization and dealing with the regulations that ensure researchers don't cheat or hurt their patients.

the job It can be anything from gene sequencing in a laboratory to talking to patients about their illness or to staff about their working practices. The job entails a lot of talking and a lot of writing, including the obligatory grant proposals and scientific papers. The job path starts easily with learning the trade of conducting research and writing up the findings. Then come presentations at conferences, trying to answer impossible questions about what was done or not done and publishing papers in peer-reviewed scientific journals. A researcher has 'made it' when they write their first research grant proposal, receive funding and can employ researchers themselves.

extras Teaching (always rewarding), conferences in nice places meeting people who are fascinated by the same issues. A rewarding academic career is about having the time to pursue passionate research interests in the manner that seems best. Contrary to popular belief this is not a route for high income or extensive private practice.

For further information:

Academic Clinical Fellowships: National Co-ordinating Centre for Research Capacity Development (NCC RCD), Leeds Innovation Centre, 103 Clarendon Road, Leeds, LS2 9DF Tel: 0113 346 6260   Fax: 0113 346 3272   Web: http://www.nccrcd.nhs.uk

A day in the life ...

08:30	Catch up on e-mails and plan the day – every day is different
09:00	Ward round or outpatient clinic
11:30	Deal with clinical paperwork and letters, call colleagues for advice and answer questions about specific patients
13:00	Read latest journals and some papers from a literature review
14:00	Meet with research team, review progress and talk about ways round problems in a current project
16:00	Start writing the results section of the first paper on a completed project
19:00	Clear head on the way home to reengage with reality and family

myth	Academics spend their lives in ivory towers and aeroplanes and have difficulty finding their way home
reality	Being paid to pursue your own interests and ideas. It is hard work and competitive though.
personality	Self-disciplined, persistent, eternally optimistic
best aspects	The world really is your oyster. You can research almost anything you if you can find someone to fund it.
worst aspects	It is like riding a bicycle. Once you start you have to keep pedalling, i.e. getting the research grants, or you fall off.
route	Academic Foundation Programme followed by Academic Clinical Fellowship (p 16); Membership Exam and higher degree (MD/PhD); it is possible to transfer to an academic career path at any stage in a medical career
numbers	3000 of which 25% are women
locations	Universities or hospitals and laboratories linked to a university to a greater or lesser extent

life		work
quiet on-call		busy on-call
boredom		burnout
uncompetitive		competitive
low salary		high salary

Acupuncture

Almost any doctor can include acupuncture within their clinical practice. Patients are increasingly seeking drug-free alternatives and acupuncture research is showing how useful the therapy can be. Acupuncture is best known for treating pain and musculoskeletal conditions, however its use is not confined to anaesthetists and GPs as it can be used in many other situations. The last decade has seen a great increase in opportunities for training, research and work, something of a renaissance for a specialty that began about 5000 years ago!

the patients The Chinese say that the very old and the very young do very well with acupuncture. In reality all ages and both sexes can benefit from acupuncture whether or not they believe in it. Acupuncture works best with an intact nervous system, which can limit its use in some conditions (e.g. diabetic neuropathy). Treatment often requires multiple sessions so be prepared to see your patients over a period of time.

the work Acupuncture is a hands-on treatment. It requires knowledge of anatomy, clinical awareness, diagnostic skills and an ability to communicate well with patients and colleagues. It can be used in any aspect of medicine where there are painful conditions; it often forms part of pain clinic treatments. Where the problems are musculoskeletal acupuncture may be used by physiotherapists, osteopaths and chiropractors. There is also a role outside of pain and musculoskeletal conditions, for example in psychiatry for anxiety and depression, oncology and gynaecology for nausea and vomiting and gastroenterology for irritable bowel syndrome.

the job Acupuncture skills can supplement a specialty or GP career; alternatively it can be a full-time role in a pain clinic, GP setting or private practice. For private practice there is also the need to run a small business alongside therapeutic sessions; this includes the risk of the business not performing well. Treatment can take place in almost any setting including hospitals, GP surgeries, private clinics or the patient's home.

extras Private practice is well established. There are some academic opportunities including a teaching clinic at the Royal London Homeopathic Hospital in central London, conferences and the journal *Acupuncture in Medicine*.

ⓘ *For further information:*

British Medical Acupuncture Society, BMAS House, 3 Winnington Court, Northwich, Cheshire, CW8 1AQ
Tel: 01606 786782   Fax: 01606 786783   Web: http://www.medical-acupuncture.co.uk
British Acupuncture Council, BAcC 63 Jeddo Road, London W12 9HQ
Tel: 020 8735 0400   Fax: 020 8735 0404   Web: http://www.acupuncture.org.uk

A day in the life ...

09:00	Clinic in private rooms at home; 45-min appointments: first patient has multiple problems despite seeing six professors and seven consultants and she hopes acupuncture will improve her well-being and reduce her pain
10:00	Grab a coffee and continue clinic with common cases: hay fever, primary subfertility, low back pain and a frozen shoulder
13:00	Speedy lunch and travel to chiropractic clinic; contact with chiropractors, aroma-therapists and homoeopaths
14:00	Clinic with 20-min appointments including cases of IBS, stress, sinusitis, endometriosis, osteoarthritic knee and many sciaticas
19:00	Back home to do the accounts, mail, check equipment supplies and sort out the bookings for tomorrow; reply to messages from GPs, colleagues and patients; may have clinical or GP meeting
20:30	End of a varied, interesting and often entertaining day in private practice

myth	Patients looking like porcupines with boosted energy levels
reality	Uses a few fine disposable needles; medical acupuncture rejects the traditional 'energy-based' methodology; the evidence base for use in specific diseases is developing
personality	Compassion, patience, listening skills, good business sense
best aspects	Flexible training, enormous variety, independent practice
worst aspects	Constantly having to prove the beneficial effects of the therapy, competing in the open market, being ranked alongside lay practitioners
route	BMAS training programme and Diploma, other training colleges are also available
numbers	About 5000 registered practitioners (both doctors and non-doctors); number of unregistered acupuncturists is unknown
location	Anywhere, from hospitals to private practice at home

life						work
quiet on-call						busy on-call
boredom						burnout
uncompetitive						competitive
low salary						high salary

Acute medicine

Acute medicine is a new and evolving specialty that concentrates on 'front door' medicine and the first 24–72 hours of care. It is an exciting mix of being a generalist in a specialist setting where making the right decision is essential. Patient presentation is wide-ranging, with anything from cerebral malaria to a suspected pulmonary embolus to musculoskeletal chest pain. Many hospitals are now developing their own medical assessment units (MAU) and/or short stay wards that focus on rapid investigation and management of acute medical problems.

the patients Adult patients aged 16 to 115 from all backgrounds and walks of life. Most MAUs look after medical patients only, although a minority take all comers, e.g. surgery, orthopaedics etc. About 40% of emergency medical admissions can be discharged within 24 hours, with rapid follow-up if necessary. Short stay patients (<72 hours) may remain under the care of the acute physicians while the rest are triaged to specialist care wards. Over one third of admissions are cardiovascular in nature with respiratory problems coming a close second.

the work Every day is different and is defined by the diversity of clinic problems that present. Everything from acutely septic patients requiring liaison with ITU to discussing the (un)likelihood of a deep vein thrombosis in somebody who has experimented with wearing stilettos for the first time. Consultants still clerk patients alongside their juniors, but also lead the ward rounds and offer advice for the more challenging patients. Practical skills are important as procedures are common (from cannulation to endoscopy) and often need to be done immediately.

the job Often based on a medical assessment unit (MAU) and/or emergency department (ED). Many centres also run rapid assessment/rapid follow-up clinics. Multidisciplinary care and good relationships with specialist colleagues are essential. Acute physicians often work closely with fast response nursing teams and other clinical nurse specialists.

extras The Society of Acute Medicine is the young, lively 'trade union' of the specialty and has been actively promoting itself over the last few years. Compared with others, it is very multidisciplinary and this is reflected in its membership and the contents of its conferences. There are academic opportunities (e.g. testing new care pathways) and frequent opportunities to teach enthusiastic medical students and junior doctors. The scope for private practice is limited. Acute medical skills are useful in a range of settings around the world (p 22).

ⓘ *For further information:*

The Society for Acute Medicine, Combined Assessment, Royal Infirmary of Edinburgh, 51 Little Frances Crescent, Edinburgh, EH16 4SA
Web: http://www.acutemedicine.org.uk

00:00	Acute physician on-call; rapid assessment of medical patients in emergency department then sleep in on-call room; called at 03:00 to assess a patient with acute liver failure, back in bed by 04:15
08:30	Post-take ward round of 22 acute medical patients; 7 discharged; 6 others triaged to specialist teams
10:00	Team cup of tea to review patient list and allocate jobs
10:30	Mini ward round of patients who have been in for over 24 hours
12:30	Medical grand round or acute medicine journal club (with sandwich!)
14:00	Follow-up clinic or specialist skills session e.g. bronchoscopy
16:00	Review of patient list and mini ward round
18:00	Home to watch *Scrubs* and cope with any acute DIY emergencies

myth	Medicine for fast runners with a short attention span
reality	The exciting bit of being a physician!
personality	Friendly, dynamic, unflappable, team player, practical
best aspects	Enormous variety of cases; spotting patients who need to be in hospital and discharging those who don't
worst aspects	High intensity; some consultant posts involve sole responsibility over a large MAU; on-calls often in hospital rather than over the phone from home
route	ST1 Acute care common stem, acute medicine (p 28) followed by ST3 acute medicine; MRCP exam
locations	Teaching hospitals and larger DGHs; normally on an MAU

life						work
quiet on-call						busy on-call
boredom						burnout
uncompetitive						competitive
low salary						high salary

Anaesthetics

Anaesthesia is an exciting and varied specialty, allowing doctors to work with patients at critical points in their treatment. Ever since the first demonstration of ether (Morton 1846) was greeted with the phrase, 'Gentlemen, this is no Humbug', anaesthetic agents have enabled the advances in surgical practice that have occurred over the last 150 years.

the patients Anaesthetists are involved in the treatment of two-thirds of all patients admitted to acute hospitals. The patients can be of any age and from any background, though most children are managed by specialist paediatric anaesthetists. Contact with conscious patients is usually limited to pre- and postoperative assessment, but communication skills are important to allay anxiety. During anaesthesia the patient is entirely dependent on the anaesthetist's skill to maintain cardio–respiratory function. In many respects anaesthesia is like flying a plane: a smooth take off, flight and landing result in a satisfied passenger.

the work Modern anaesthetic practice requires a functional knowledge of anatomy, physiology, pathology and pharmacology with particular focus on the cardio–respiratory and central nervous systems. The work requires a mix of clinical analysis (e.g. how the patient's current physiological state will respond under anaesthesia), and practical skills (e.g. central or regional nerve blocks, arterial lines, intubation). All anaesthetized patients can deteriorate rapidly and the anaesthetist needs to be able to respond immediately since interventions can have immediate life-saving results. Anaesthetists are key to acute services, forming a vital part of cardiac arrest teams and critical care 'outreach' services.

the job Most of the work is carried out in the operating theatre or on the intensive care ward and is multidisciplinary, involving interactions with surgeons, obstetricians, radiologists, physicians and non-medical clinical staff. The out of hours work is usually a full or partial shift rota. There is a broad variety of work including chronic pain clinic, emergency theatre, cardiac work, day surgery lists and ophthalmic and obstetric anaesthesia.

extras The work is sessional, allowing other activities to form part of the normal working week including teaching, research (clinical or basic science), management, private practice or subspecialty interests including intensive care and managements. Overseas training opportunities occur in the USA, Canada and Australia.

For further information:

Royal College Of Anaesthetists, Churchill House, 35 Red Lion Square, London, WC1R 4SG
Tel: 020 7092 1500   Fax: 020 7092 1730   Web: http://www.rcoa.ac.uk
Association of Anaesthetists, 21 Portland Place, London, W1B 1PY
Tel: 020 7631 1650   Fax: 020 7631 4352   Web: http://www.aagbi.org

A day in the life ...

08:00 Intensive care unit (ICU) ward round; 8 patients with a mixture of post-operative recovery, severe trauma and reversible medical conditions

10:30 After a civilized cup of coffee carry out ICU procedures

13:00 Lunch

13:01 Pre-operative assessment for patients on the afternoon operating list

14:00 Anaesthetize the first patient on the afternoon list; prepare for an afternoon of banter with theatre team and life-saving interventions

18:00 Predicted finish time for afternoon list

18:30 Actual finish time of afternoon list

19:00 Put up feet and think of new jokes to tell during tomorrow's sessions

myth	Anaesthesia is delivered by the half-asleep to the half-dead to allow the half-witted to half-kill them
reality	A dynamic specialty where physiology and pharmacology knowledge is applied to patients to sustain them through some of of the most traumatic moments of their life
personality	Dynamic, obsessive, good practical skills, team player
best aspects	Every patient is different, and understanding physiology and pharmacology enable adjusting your technique to the patient
worst aspects	Other specialists who think anaesthesia is easy; jokes about crosswords and Sudoku
route	CT1 Anaesthetics (p 30) or CT1 Acute care common stem anaesthetics (p 28) then ST3 Anaesthetics; FRCA exam
numbers	8700 of which 30% are women
locations	Almost invariably hospital-based, though this can be anywhere from a small DGH to a large teaching hospital to overseas

life					work
quiet on-call					busy on-call
boredom					burnout
uncompetitive					competitive
low salary					high salary

Army medicine

Army medicine is a fascinating, diverse world encompassing primary and secondary care, with an overall emphasis on occupational medicine—keeping soldiers fit to do their job. With a high operational tempo and consequently a packed training cycle, today's army doctor requires a broad skills base and high level of commitment.

the patients The Army's patient population is predominantly young and healthy; the patients tend to be male though there are increasing numbers of female soldiers and also the families of soldiers in overseas bases. Many of the patients are highly motivated and keen to regain their health.

the work Much of the workload of civilian medicine can be found in the forces and it is split into secondary and primary care in the same way. Those choosing secondary care (e.g. surgery) will work for the military in a partly NHS environment for much of their time, whilst primary care (e.g. General Duties Medical Officer (GDMO) or Regimental Medical Officer (RMO) – usually a military GP) is a more 'green' role (i.e. army-based, catering for the unique needs of soldiers in a military setting). All military doctors share a common goal, however, which is maintenance of an effective fighting force. The primary care role covers the common diseases in younger adults including trauma, infections and mental health issues.

the job As a GDMO or RMO, the job is split between many roles. The primary care role includes the occupational health role of ensuring that soldiers are fit for their employment and that the chain of command is appropriately advised on such matters. The close proximity of the doctor to their patients inevitably leads to a much more cohesive relationship, requiring considerable interpersonal, managerial and administrative skills.

extras The responsibility of medical training of the unit's soldiers falls to its doctor, who also needs to manage the junior medical staff. This involves career management, report writing and a pastoral role extending well beyond what may be experienced in the NHS. Later in training there is access to many world-class courses and training secondments to ensure maximum standard of care on operations.

ⓘ *For further information:*

SO1 AMS Recruiting, HQ Army Medical Services, Slim Road, Camberley, Surrey, GU15 4NP
Tel: 01276 412730   E-mail: so1recruiting@ramc.mod.uk   Web: http://www.army.mod.uk

08:00	Sick parade – all soldiers requiring non-routine appointments will be seen
09:00	Routine appointments or continuation of non-routine appointments
11:00	Write referrals, catch up with military medical documentation
12:00	Sport with members of medical centre team
13:00	Lunch in officers' mess, often asked for advice with certain soldiers of concern
14:00	Training battalion's medics or soldiers in basic medical care
16:30	Check in with medical centre; every few weeks this includes sitting on the Unit Health Committee to review soldiers with longer-term problems
17:30	Back to officers' mess, get ready for dinner, often receive more informal referrals

myth	A life spent marching and being shouted at
reality	High calibre clinical care is essential: this may be in the calm of a UK medical centre or the life-threatening environment of modern warfare
personality	Stable extrovert, leadership skills, team player, good at decision-making, calm under pressure, able to communicate to non-medics
best aspects	The camaraderie of military life, access to world-class training, travel, diversity of work, chance to bring care to where it is needed most
worst aspects	Exposure to conflict; demands placed on the family by Army life: partners will need to be understanding and mobile
route	Military cadetship during, or immediately after, medical school (p 18)
numbers	170 in primary care and 65 in secondary care; 7.5% are women
locations	**Primary care** Military bases in the UK and overseas (Canada, Germany, Belize, Brunei) **Secondary care** seven Ministry of Defence Hospital Units in UK **Both** current deployments e.g. Afghanistan

life						work
quiet on-call						busy on-call
boredom						burnout
uncompetitive						competitive
low salary						high salary

Audiovestibular medicine

Audiovestibular medicine (AVM) is a specialty that deals with diagnosis, medical treatment and rehabilitation of children and adults with hearing and balance disorders. It develops the interface between neurology and ENT in adults and children with a mixture of psychology, paediatrics, geriatrics, genetics, phoniatrics, acoustic science, etc. thrown in. Being an audiovestibular physician (AVP) requires a holistic approach to managing patients with hearing and balance problems. Most AVPs work in teaching or regional centres within multidisciplinary teams; they also become members of a small but supportive network of like-minded physicians globally—anonymity is not an option with so few!

the patients From birth to the grave, often following patients throughout their life. Patients come from all walks of life and from all ethnic backgrounds. Audiovestibular problems can affect anyone from the 'normal' population to those with very complex medical problems. Hearing problems affect 4% of children and up to 80% of the elderly, while balance problems will have affected a third of the population by the age of 65 years; there is never a shortage of patients.

the work Intellectually challenging without too much drama. This is a rehabilitative specialty where a doctor can make a real difference to a person's quality of life. Correct management can help a dizzy adult return to work or a deaf child to develop speech and have access to normal education. In addition, diagnostic puzzles will keep even the best clinicians on their toes.

the job is predominantly outpatient-based although patients may occasionally be admitted for specific investigations. On the good side this means there is no on-call and weekends are free. AVPs work as a part of a multidisciplinary team that include audiologists, speech and language therapists, psychologists, teachers of the deaf, hearing therapists. In addition there are close links with clinicians in other specialties, e.g. ENT, paediatrics, care of the elderly, clinical genetics.

extras Progress in this specialty is rapid and exciting; significant advances are being made in every aspect, from cochlear implants that enable the profoundly deaf to hear, to prevention and cures for deafness. There is ample opportunity to contribute to the advancement of the specialty through national and international research, teaching, training and service development. Flexible training is relatively easy to arrange and there is some scope for private practice.

🛈 *For further information:*

British Association of Audiovestibular Physicians: http://www.baap.org.uk

myth	You just fit hearing aids
reality	Hearing aids are fitted by audiologists; audiovestibular physicians diagnose and manage deafness, dizziness, imbalance and tinnitus
personality	Good communication and listening skills, academic, practical
best aspects	Making a real difference for the patients and improving their quality of life; unravelling aetiological mysteries through clinical detective work
worse aspects	The lack of life-or-death situations means there is no glory or on-call payment; lots of paperwork
route	CT1 Core medical training (p 34) then ST3 Audiovestibular medicine; MRCP exam; alternative route via paediatrics
numbers	60 of which 45% are women
locations	Wide range including teaching hospitals, DGHs or sometimes community clinics

life						work
quiet on-call						busy on-call
boredom						burnout
uncompetitive						competitive
low salary						high salary

Breast and oncoplastic surgery

This is a relatively new and rapidly developing specialty that can offer an immensely rewarding career. Oncoplastic breast surgeons diagnose and manage disorders of the breast along with performing plastic and reconstructive breast surgery. The primary focus is to optimize the surgical treatment of breast cancer, by far the most common cancer to affect women. There is an increasingly diverse range of techniques and procedures and the job involves close liaison with several other specialties.

the patients The vast majority are female, though not exclusively since men can have breast problems too. A range of age groups is seen, from young women with benign or cosmetic breast problems, to older women with breast cancer (average age mid-50s but a spectrum from the young, right up to the very elderly). Continuity of care allows a close relationship with patients to be built up, which can continue for many years.

the work Diagnosing and treating breast cancer forms the mainstay of the work. Operations vary from lumpectomies to mastectomy and total breast reconstruction with cosmetic techniques, including breast lifts or nipple reconstructions. Outcomes are improving; approximately 80% of women with breast cancer will survive beyond 10 years. As survival improves, attention focuses more on the cosmetic outcomes of breast surgery. Identifying and managing women at high risk of breast cancer (e.g. BRCA mutations) is also becoming a more common activity.

the job is a mixture of operating theatre sessions, outpatient clinics and ward management; compared with other surgical specialties there is more clinic work than ward-based work. The surgeon works with a large multidisciplinary team including radiologists, pathologists, oncologists, plastic surgeons and specialist nurses. Despite guidelines, treatment decisions often require detailed discussion on an individual basis. On-call is variable, often covering general surgery or plastic surgery, both of which are frequently busy; those who only cover breast surgery will rarely be called in.

Extras Teaching of medical students or junior doctors is a significant part of practice in a large centre. Flexible training is possible but surgical specialties are, on the whole, less suited for this. There is reasonable demand for private work especially if providing a cosmetic breast service. Research opportunities abound due to plentiful charitable funding. Many oncoplastic breast surgeons in smaller centres will also practice some general surgery.

ⓘ *For further information:*

Association of Breast Surgery, The Royal College of Surgeons, 35–43 Lincoln's Inn Fields, London, WC2A 3PE
Tel: 020 7405 5612   Fax: 020 7404 6574   Web: http://www.baso.org.uk

A day in the life ...

07:30   Ward round (2–3 days per week)

08:30   Theatre (2–3 full days per week); mastectomy with node dissections followed by two lumpectomies

13:50   Lunch 'break' (sandwich eaten on the hoof on the way to clinic)

14:00   Outpatient clinic (3–4 half days per week): mixture of new referrals, post-op reviews, result disclosure and specialist cases (e.g. reconstruction)

17:30   Paperwork, checking emails, checking patient results

18:30   Home time, unless doing private work which is often in the evenings

myth	Surgeons who just do private boob jobs
reality	90% of time is spent diagnosing breast disease, particularly breast cancer; the majority of 'boob jobs' are reconstructing a breast due to a mastectomy
personality	Practical skills with an artistic flair, perfectionism, communication skills, empathy, patient, decisive
best aspects	Helping women go through a very negative experience (breast cancer) and providing the best possible management
worst aspects	Disclosing a result of metastatic disease to a patient after years of follow-up; providing a service with limited resources
route	CT1 Surgery in general, general surgery (p 48) followed by ST3 General surgery; MRCS exam; alternative route via plastic surgery
numbers	850 of which 12% are women
locations	Hospital-based

life						**work**
quiet on-call						**busy on-call**
boredom						**burnout**
uncompetitive						**competitive**
low salary						**high salary**

Cardiology

Cardiology is perceived as one of the more glamorous specialties. It is a fascinating career which has something for everyone. Perhaps one of the main attractions is that it allows a doctor to do something that really helps the patients; for those who like instant gratification it is hard to beat. There is a large evidence base that is constantly evolving, resulting in new technologies and medications.

the patients Cardiovascular disease affects people from any age group and any background. Those under 16 years, often with congenital problems, are seen by paediatric cardiologists and adult cardiologists see everyone else. Many patients have chronic problems so may require regular follow-up for many years, while others require one-off interventions or reassurance followed by discharge from the clinic.

the work Cardiology is divided into the following subspecialties: intervention, heart failure, electrophysiology, imaging and grown-up congenital heart disease. Although it is important to have a general knowledge of cardiology, trainees are subspecialising ever earlier; the era of the general cardiologist who does a little of everything is disappearing. Common cases include ischaemic heart disease, post-MI, cardiac failure and arrhythmias. There is a wide range of medical treatments available so it is possible to improve the standard of living for most patients and sometimes relieve symptoms completely through interventions.

the job is highly varied. Most cardiologists split their time between the coronary care unit, ward, outpatient clinic and the catheter lab. This offers a great mixture of acute medicine, practical procedures and more cerebral activity. As more district general hospitals acquire catheter labs, and more procedures are performed without cardiothoracic surgical backup, the difference in roles at a DGH and teaching hospital is narrowing. Cardiology is becoming increasingly consultant-led which entails a large degree of responsibility.

extras There is a heavy bias towards research in cardiology and until recently a period of research was considered mandatory. Carefully chosen overseas fellowships are also looked upon favourably. Opportunities for private practice are generally good and, for a minority, can be extremely lucrative. There are few opportunities for flexible training and the training hours tend to be long with active on-calls.

🛈 *For further information:*

British Cardiovascular Society, 9 Fitzroy Square, London, W1T 5HW
Tel: 020 7383 3887   Fax: 020 7388 0903   Web: http://www.bcs.com

A day in the life ...

08:00	Joint cardiac/cardiothoracic meeting to discuss potential surgical patients
09:00	Cath lab: two angioplasties and a stent placement; supervise a trainee performing the second angioplasty
13:00	Troubleshoot cases in pacing clinic
13:30	Eat lunch whilst walking to the ward to review the cases from the morning cath lab list and review patients for tomorrow's list
14:00	Outpatient clinic; 40 patients split between consultant and trainee. Complete range of cardiac symptoms and diseases
18:00	Home to catch up with paperwork unless on-call or doing a private clinic

myth	Arrogant, Porsche-driving, divorced, wannabe surgeons
reality	A pleasant surprise; some drive Porsches and are still married!
personality	Hardworking, committed, confident, academic, good practical skills, calm in an emergency
best aspects	Procedures going well; successful results from treating life-threatening cardiac disease
worst aspects	Procedures going badly; the long and arduous training
route	CT1 Core-medical training (p 34) followed by ST3 Cardiology; MRCP exam
numbers	1450 of which 10% are women
locations	District general and teaching hospitals

life		work
quiet on-call		busy on-call
boredom		burnout
uncompetitive		competitive
low salary		high salary

Cardiothoracic surgery

If you are the sort of person who enjoys working under intense pressure and making snap life or death decisions then this is the job for you. Cardiothoracic surgery has the dubious honour of being the most competitive specialty in medicine. It requires dedication and long hours but it is hard to imagine a more fulfilling job. Cardiothoracic surgery is a relatively young specialty (the first coronary artery bypass graft was performed in the 1960s) and is still evolving.

the patients For cardiac surgery the patients are usually in the 60–80 years age group, predominantly with coronary artery disease and/or degenerative valve disease, often with multiple other comorbidities. They are mostly referred from other specialties rather than by GPs. The thoracic patients are usually referred via the multidisciplinary team and the majority of the work deals with lung cancer diagnosis, treatment or palliation. These patients also have a high incidence of vascular and coronary disease but tend to be slightly younger (50–70 years). All these patients are unique and require a good deal of preparation so that they will survive an operation. However, this individual preparation is one of the most enjoyable aspects of the job.

the work Cardiothoracic surgeons are only really happy when they are in theatre and away from the other distractions of hospital life (management, dictation, audit etc.). The range of diseases is varied and complex but the majority of work is coronary artery surgery, valve surgery and intrathoracic malignancy. There is tremendous autonomy due to the responsibility for the patients whilst they are in the hospital. Alongside the theatre there are ward rounds and outpatient clinics. On-calls can be demanding and may be frequent depending on the size of the unit; common problems include post-operative complications, trauma and dissecting aneurysms.

The job Cardiothoracic surgeons work as part of a large multidisciplinary team including cardiologists, intensivists, anaesthetists, respiratory physicians, general surgeons, vascular surgeons, radiologists, oncologists and trauma teams. There is extremely high pressure as the mortality is relatively high due to the nature of the surgery and patient population; added to this there is the spotlight of individual mortality rates being publicized.

Extra Alongside standard clinical work there are many opportunities for research and overseas training. Surgeons can choose to subspecialize in paediatric, transplant or thoracic surgery, though this is not necessary. There are small amounts of private practice, though less than some other surgical specialties. Flexible training opportunities are very limited.

For further information:

The Society for Cardiothoracic Surgery in Great Britain and Ireland, The Royal College of Surgeons of England, 35–43 Lincoln's Inn Fields, London, WC2A 3PE
Tel: 020 7869 6893   Fax: 020 7869 6890   Web: http://www.scts.org

A day in the life ...

07:30	Ward round on cardiac intensive care
08:00	Theatre. First case is a 78-year-old man with type 2 diabetes and aortic stenosis requiring an aortic valve replacement
11:30	Leave registrar to close case and inhale some lunch whilst writing up
12:00	Start next case, a CABG for a 63-year-old lady with angina
16:30	Finish in theatre
17:00	Ward round on CICU
17:30	Catch up with phone calls, clinic letters, etc.; chat with colleagues
18:00	Sneaky CICU ward round to check juniors have made correct decisions
19:00	Arrive home; pray that patients survive 30 days or leave hospital alive
19:03	Stop worrying; bask in the glory of a marvellous and technically skilled job that brings respect from colleagues and admiration from patients
19:04	Start worrying about the next day in theatre

myth	Boys with toys; cracking chests and flying blood
reality	Mostly boys with toys; challenging and involved surgery that can produce life-saving results
personality	Hard working, extrovert, competitive, very good practical skills, degree of OCD, dedicated
best aspects	Theatre; working against the clock and getting sick patients through difficult operations never ceases to produce a warm glow of satisfaction
worst aspects	High mortality; government targets
route	CT1 Surgery in general (General surgery or generic p 48) then ST3 Cardiothoracic surgery; FRCS exam
number	460 of which 4% are women
locations	Mostly teaching hospitals with a few district general hospitals

life		**work**
quiet on-call		**busy on-call**
boredom		**burnout**
uncompetitive		**competitive**
low salary		**high salary**

Chemical pathology

Chemical pathology (also known as clinical biochemistry) is a specialty with great variety. A chemical pathologist has two main roles in the hospital: managing the biochemistry laboratory and giving clinical advice on biochemical dilemmas, either to clinicians or directly to patients in clinic. There is the potential for considerable flexibility within the specialty, which is very advantageous. A new subspecialty of metabolic medicine, with a greater clinical emphasis, is developing and is described separately on p 202.

the patients The biochemistry laboratory performs vital diagnostic tests on samples from patients throughout the hospital and community. Alongside this there are patients seen in clinics who are usually adults, unless the doctor is specifically paediatric trained. They can be of either sex, any ethnicity and range from young to old. There is good continuity of care through outpatient follow-ups.

the work The majority of biochemical tests (e.g. U+Es, LFTs, CRP) are automated and the samples are processed and run by a team of clinical and biomedical scientists. The role of the chemical pathologist is to oversee this process, e.g. choosing which tests and machines to purchase and assuring the quality of the tests. Alongside this role is interpreting the results for GPs and other specialists: this is especially challenging for the rare and esoteric tests in endocrine conditions and inborn errors of metabolism. The skill is in combining the test results with the clinical information and underlying biochemistry to formulate a diagnosis. Chemical pathologists also see patients directly in clinic (e.g. diabetes or lipid clinics) either alone or with other specialists such as endocrinologists.

the job The majority of time is spent in the laboratory on clinical work or research, but there are also clinics (1–3 per week), ward rounds with other specialists (e.g. nutrition rounds assessing patients on parental nutrition) and the inevitable management meetings. The laboratory is usually a relaxed environment with a strong multidisciplinary ethos. There are also close connections with the diabetic and endocrinology teams. On-calls tend to be quiet and most problems can be managed from home. Overall the job offers great autonomy, a major advantage over many other specialties.

extras Research opportunities are excellent and a research project is an integral part of training. Flexible training is relatively simple to arrange and the quiet on-calls and predictable working pattern are excellent for family life. Teaching opportunities are also common, e.g. juniors, laboratory staff and other specialists. Private work tends to be limited.

ⓘ *For further information:*

The Royal College of Pathologists, 2 Carlton House Terrace, London, SW1Y 5AF
Tel: 020 7451 6700   Fax: 020 7451 6701   Web: http://www.rcpath.org

09:00   Outpatient diabetes clinic: 15-minute appointments (4 new patients and 11 follow-ups and reviews)

13:00   Lunchtime meeting: journal club with presentation from a trainee

14:00   Laboratory work: mostly assessing/interpreting biochemistry test results; phone discussions with hospital doctors and GPs about interpretation and further investigations

16:00   Meeting to discuss which new diagnostic tests should be offered by the laboratory

17:00   Final check of latest results and some paperwork

18:00   Home after another satisfying and varied day at work!

myth	Lab-based boffin who can recite Kreb's cycle
reality	Metabolic specialist with regular patient contact
personality	Academic, thorough, leadership skills, team player, communication skills are important
best aspects	Great variety of job; interesting case mix
worst aspects	Increasing and persistent bureaucracy
route	ST1 Chemical pathology (p 40); FRCPath exam, for metabolic medicine the MRCP is also essential
numbers	320 of which 20% are women
locations	Any hospital with diagnostic laboratories, though some are run by clinical scientists

life						work
quiet on-call						busy on-call
uncompetitive						competitive
boredom						burnout
low salary						high salary

Civil Service medicine

Moving from a medical specialty to work in the Department of Health is often perceived as having crossed an important divide or even going over 'to the dark side'. In reality, delivering health care which is fit for purpose for a population needs policy development and strategic planning from the Department of Health and Government. This should be informed by the medical profession. The involvement of doctors within the Department of Health is well established, but there is no formal career structure or typical route of entry. Most doctors who undertake this work have had significant managerial experience at clinical or divisional director level or as a medical director in an acute hospital. From a primary care background this may be after managing a big general practice or working in a Primary Care Trust (PCT). Other routes involve public health medicine, work with Strategic Health Authorities or in primary care organizational structure.

Managerial roles are enormously rewarding and give doctors with a broad range of clinical and non-clinical skills the opportunity to represent their specialty at a national level. Doctors working in the Department of Health use their broad medical experience as well as specialist expertise at a senior level in medicine to influence health care in a wider setting than that of an individual's clinical practice.

Working in this environment involves working with committees and contributing to publications and presentations for the Department of Health. Building teams and involving key stakeholders from the delivery end of health care services are vital components. Leadership skills and an ability to manage complicated political situations are essential. The work requires effective communication with medical colleagues, Department of Health officials, politicians, the press and the public.

Jobs vary in their time commitment, with some being full-time and others being secondments from NHS work. Most of these roles cannot be fulfilled without negotiating time formally set aside from clinical work. The vast majority continue medical practice to some degree to maintain their skills and interest. This specialty of medicine is not readily available to those lower down the medical hierarchical ladder and usually is the preserve of senior medical professionals only. There are plentiful opportunities for travelling around the UK and further afield. The job involves working with a very wide variety of other professionals which can be both challenging and very interesting. This kind of lifestyle can limit private practice and also tilt the work–life balance firmly in favour of work.

For further information:

Civil Service recruitment website: http://www.careers.civil-service.gov.uk
Department of Health website: http://www.dh.gov.uk

A day in the life ...

06:00	Travel to London, processing emails en route
09:00	Meeting to discuss policy documents at the Department of Health
10:00	Chairing a national committee
13:00	Meeting with other clinical leads at the Department of Health
14:00	Strategy planning meeting with own Department of Health team
16:00	Travel home
20:00	Emails, reading and editing policy documents

myth	Doctors who are no good at medicine playing at being politicians and medical managers
reality	Doctors wishing to extend their interest in medicine beyond their own field by using managerial and communication skills
personality	Communication and public speaking skills are essential; pragmatic, good time management, thick-skinned
best aspects	Variety of working environments and colleagues; ability to influence strategic planning of health care and national policy
worst aspects	Usually working in an advisory role which can be ignored; job can fill every waking (and sleeping) hour
route	Completed training in any clinical specialty followed by managerial experience
locations	Work often involves travelling; the Department of Health is based in London and Leeds

life						work
quiet on-call						busy on-call
boredom						burnout
uncompetitive						competitive
low salary						high salary

Clinical genetics

Clinical genetics is a rapidly developing specialty which is becoming increasingly important in clinical practice. The conditions are an exciting mixture of the fascinating and the challenging and, since genetic disorders can be found in all age groups, backgrounds and bodily systems, the job includes interaction with virtually every medical specialty. The job is extremely diverse; even experienced practitioners still see genetic conditions that they have not encountered before. Knowledge of genetics is expanding rapidly so that new diagnostic services can be offered to patients every month.

the patients Clinical geneticists see patients of all ages, though they tend to see predominantly either children or adults (according to training). This can include pregnant women, preterm neonates on NICU and the elderly (e.g. discussing carrier testing for disorders in their family). Along with the patient in front of them, clinical geneticists need to think about the implications for the wider family. It is the doctor's responsibility to ensure that all the family members at risk are given the opportunity to understand that risk and to discuss options for managing it. This can raise complex ethical dilemmas.

the work Clinical geneticists have three main roles: to diagnose conditions, to confirm diagnoses with genetic tests and to counsel the family about the implications. The remit includes any disease with a genetic basis. Adults are usually seen because a strong family history (e.g. cancer, neurological disorders, learning difficulties or congenital malformation) suggests that they or their future children may be at risk, or because of multiple abnormalities seen on an antenatal ultrasound. Paediatric consultations include children with severe or multiple congenital anomalies or a strong family history. The work is very focused on patients and clinical skills as this guides the decision as to which of the ~20 000 human genes to ask the laboratory to test.

the job Clinical genetics is an outpatient-based specialty, though there are some inpatient referrals. The consultation times are long (e.g. 45 min) to allow a thorough history, family history, examination and counselling. Many cases require literature searches to gather information and there are a wide range of tools to facilitate this. Clinical geneticists work as part of a close-knit team with other clinical geneticists, genetic counsellors and trainees. They are based in large teaching hospitals. There is usually no out of hours on-call.

extras Clinical genetics is a small specialty and retains a sense of community. While the scope for private practice is minimal, the research opportunities are unparalleled. Flexible training is well established.

ⓘ *For further information:*

The British Society for Human Genetics, Clinical Genetics Unit, Birmingham Women's Hospital, Birmingham, B15 2TG
Tel: 0121 627 2634   Fax: 0121 623 6971   Web: http://www.bshg.org.uk

08:30 Check diary, emails and letters and prepare for clinic

09:30 Genetics clinic with trainee and genetic counsellor; three cases: child with dysmorphic features and learning difficulties, child with potential Ehlers–Danlos Syndrome and an infant with congenital deafness

13:15 Grab a sandwich and touch base with secretary

14:15 De-brief to discuss cases from morning clinic and plan for next week's clinic including likely differential diagnosis and genetic advice

15:15 Touch base with on-call team and discuss queries

16:00 Visit paediatric ward to see an infant admitted for cleft palate surgery

17:00 Dictate urgent letters from morning clinic

17:45 Check e-mail and then head for home after a busy but fascinating day

myth	Doctors who work in labs all day trying to clone mini armies
reality	Direct patient contact with emphasis on communication and clinical skills; genetics laboratories are usually run by clinical scientists
personality	Thoughtful, excellent communications skills, generalist, happy away from acute medicine, good memory
best aspects	Helping to make a difficult diagnosis and communicating it sensitively to the family; helping families deal with challenging situations
worst aspects	Sharing 'bad news' from predictive genetic testing; inability to treat the vast majority of disorders; restricted funding for genetic testing.
route	CT1 in core medical training (p 34) or ST1 in paediatrics (p 38) then ST3 clinical genetics; MRCP or MRCPCH exam
numbers	200 of which 60% are women
locations	Larger teaching hospitals

life						work
quiet on-call						busy on-call
boredom						burnout
uncompetitive						competitive
low salary						high salary

Clinical oncologists

Clinical oncologists are doctors trained to use radiotherapy and radioisotopes alongside other treatments to manage cancer, as opposed to Medical oncologists (p 196) who specialize in non-radiological treatment. The specialty provides a wide variety of opportunities from fascinating scientific research to treating patients with the full range of anticancer treatments. Alongside the clinical interest it is important to remember that most patients are facing an uncertain future and benefit from a caring, empathic doctor.

the patients Anyone can get cancer, however the majority of patients are over 60 years old. All patients have a diagnosis of cancer, but this can be of any histological subtype and any body part. Children receive chemotherapy from paediatric oncologists (usually trained in paediatrics initially) and will only see a clinical oncologist if they need radiotherapy. Cancer is a life-changing diagnosis, so families are usually closely involved. Continuity of care is very good as patients are seen regularly during their treatment and are encouraged to report changes or side-effects directly to the oncology team; this can result in a close relationship during an intensely traumatic experience. Oncology treatments can be physiologically demanding and will not be suitable for all patients, however palliative treatments can be tailored to the patients' capabilities.

the work Patients are usually referred to the department having been diagnosed by another specialty, but the appointment with the oncologist is often their first opportunity to ask questions and start to come to terms with 'life with cancer'. Clinical oncologists may use all the modalities of treatment (i.e. radiotherapy, radioisotopes, chemotherapy, hormone therapy and targeted therapies such as monoclonal antibodies and tyrosine kinase inhibitors) except surgery to attempt to achieve a cure or palliation in each patient.

the job The majority of work is outpatient-based, although patients may need to be admitted as their disease progresses or due to the side effects of treatment. Admission in both cases is usually for symptom management. Multidisciplinary team working (especially with surgeons, radiologists, radiographers, specialist nurses, research nurses and pathologists) is integral to the daily work in an oncology department. Most on-calls can be carried out from home, with regular phone calls for advice.

extras Involvement in research is becoming more integral to the training and daily work of clinical oncologists, and as a result there are regular national and international oncology conferences. Subspecialization, usually by cancer site (e.g. chest), is possible in larger centres. There are significant opportunities for private practice. Flexible training is well established.

ℹ️ *For further information:*

The Royal College of Radiologists, 38 Portland Place, London W1B 1JQ
Tel: 020 7636 4432   Fax: 020 7323 3100   Web: http://www.rcr.ac.uk

A day in the life ...

09:00   Ward round: review patient admitted with neutropenic sepsis

09:30   Clinic: some good responses and cures, some poor responses and recurrences; discuss palliative options with a new patient, enrol another into a Phase III trial, discharge one women after five cancer-free years

13:00   Multidisciplinary team meeting: discussing new referrals and difficult cases with surgeons, radiologists, pathologists and specialist nurses

14:00   Radiotherapy planning using a computer planning system to mark out palliative radiotherapy to control haemoptysis from lung cancer

16:00   Contacted about patient with spinal cord compression; arrange immediate admission and palliative radiotherapy to prevent paraplegia

17:30   Home to enjoy a box of chocolates from a grateful patient

myth	Doctors who just do radiotherapy
reality	Manage full range of treatments for cancer; a chance to really help patients and families in extremely stressful times
personality	Caring, empathic, good communicator, team player
best aspects	Fascinating variety; patient gratitude (often expressed with chocolate); giving hope and restoring quality of life
worst aspects	Restrictions on drugs proven to be effective (NICE); clinics often run late; can be emotionally draining
route	CT1 Core medical training (p 34) then ST3 Clinical oncology; MRCP and FRCR exams
numbers	820 of which 40% are women
locations	Hospital-based specialty, only larger hospitals have radiotherapy facilities but chemotherapy in most district general hospitals

life					work
quiet on-call					busy on-call
boredom					burnout
uncompetitive					competitive
low salary					high salary

Clinical pharmacology and theraputics

Clinical pharmacology and theraputics (CPT) is a medical-based specialty usually working in the NHS, as opposed to Pharmaceutical medicine (p 230), which is an industry- or regulatory authority-based job without the patient contact. CPT specialists are usually doctors who have initially trained in a particular medical specialty (e.g. oncology, psychiatry, paediatrics) then developed a particular interest in the pharmacology of that specialty. Their role becomes split between their initial specialty and CPT in a similar manner to subspecialty academia (in fact the majority are also academics, see p 94).

the patients depend on the training of the consultant. The majority of consultants have trained in a medical specialty (e.g. cardiology, neurology, gastroenterology) and continue to work as a physician, including acute on-take medicine. The clinical pharmacology patients are usually referred by colleagues due to complicated pharmacological issues (e.g. a specific allergy).

the work is hugely varied. It includes patient care in the initial specialty, advising colleagues on the management of their patients, teaching (medical students, junior doctors, GPs, pharmacists nurses, etc. about practical drug therapy), formulating drug policy both locally and nationally, editing and writing important texts (e.g. the BNF) and research (bench work, clinical research or theory). While all doctors are able to prescribe, many are unfamiliar with the intricacies of the drugs they use. CPT doctors have an important role to play in educating their colleagues and helping them with troubleshooting.

the job varies widely between each individual CPT specialist, their specialty and their Trust. Most clinical pharmacologists are also academics working in a teaching hospital with their time split between the CPT/academic role and clinical medicine. The unique role of a CPT doctor gives considerable autonomy and the choice of many job options. A few are not academics, but are employed directly by the NHS and can treat CPT as a subspecialty interest. There is no on-call specific to CPT, though standard on-calls are often expected. There is considerable liaison with pharmacists and other specialties, usually involving the CPT doctor giving advice.

Extras Consultancies with pharmaceutical companies can be very educative, interesting and offer good remuneration. Research opportunities abound and meetings of the British Pharmacological Society, the Clinical Pharmacology Colloquium and other local groups are among the best around. There is little scope for private practice but a high proportion of clinical pharmacologists have clinical excellence awards (p 71). The pharmacy industry is desperate for clinical pharmacologists, providing an easy escape from NHS life.

ℹ️ *For further information:*

British Pharmacological Society, 16 Angel Gate, City Road, London, EC1V 2SG
Tel: 0207 417 0111   Fax: 0207 417 0114   Web: http://www.bps.ac.uk

myth	Doctors who prefer the BNF to patients
reality	Very clinical and diverse job; constantly surprising and challenging
personality	Eclectic interests, academic, decisive, sensitive when advising colleagues (they may have made a mistake)
best aspects	Enormous variety, no two days alike; travel opportunities; chances to influence national/international policy
worst aspects	Research bureaucracy; NHS bureaucracy
route	CT1 Core medical training (p 34) or academic route (p 16) then ST3 Clinical pharmacology and therapeutics; MRCP exam
numbers	200 of which 12% are women
locations	Teaching hospitals

life						**work**
quiet on-call						**busy on-call**
boredom						**burnout**
uncompetitive						**competitive**
low salary						**high salary**

Community paediatrics

Community paediatrics is a diverse, interesting and challenging career pathway. In the mid-1970s it was recognized that children with complex disorders needed ongoing care, but did not need the acute services of a hospital, and community paediatrics was born. With advances in neonatology and acute paediatrics, the survival and life-expectancy of very premature babies and children with multiple disabilities has increased. As a consequence there are many more children with complicated health needs and it is the role of the community paediatrician to support these children through all that life throws at them.

the patients Community paediatrics covers the whole of childhood from birth to school-leaving age. The majority of patients will have significant physical and/or mental disabilities or challenging behavioural problems; they are almost always seen with their families, who are essential to the clinical process. An expertise in communication with both children and their families is required and highly rewarding professional relationships can become established over the years.

the work is extremely clinical with long clinic-based consultations allowing time to cope with complex and multiple problems. Common cases include developmental delay (e.g. late speech, difficulty walking), disabilities (e.g. cerebral palsy), chronic illness (e.g. epilepsy) and challenging behaviours (e.g. autism and ADHD). Many of these problems rely on clinical skills for diagnosis and assessment, so the absence of immediate hospital investigations is not a problem. Interventions consist of medications, empowering parents through advice and arranging suitable services (e.g. specialist schooling, respite care); though few are 'cured' it is possible to make a big difference for the majority. The other important roles are identifying children at risk of harm and supporting those in care.

the job This is a career without the limitations and restrictions of a hospital base, allowing a good deal of flexibility; there is complete control over the day without fear of being bleeped away to an emergency. A high proportion of the working week is spent in, or travelling to, community-based clinics. An ability to work as part of a multidisciplinary team is essential and there is frequent need to liaise with colleagues. Many jobs have the benefit of no on-call; others involve covering referrals for child protection, but even then calls in the middle of the night for such purposes are extremely rare.

extras There are a few academic centres of community paediatrics offering research options. Flexible training is readily available and actively encouraged; there are few medical careers that offer a more family-friendly working environment. Private practice opportunities are very limited.

ℹ️ *For further information:*

Royal College of Paediatrics and Child Health, 50 Hallum Street, London, W1N 6DE
Tel: 020 7307 5600   Fax: 020 7307 5601   Web: http://www.rcpch.ac.uk

09:00	Child development centre multi-professional discussions about the children attending over the next week
11:00	Phone a concerned parent whose child has had a further seizure
11:15	Call a head teacher to discuss a child with challenging behaviour
11:30	Speak to physiotherapists about concerns over a child with cerebral palsy
12:00	Meeting with educational colleagues over lunch to identify pre-school children who will require additional support on admission to school
14:00	Community clinic: six families seen without any interruptions and adequate time allowed for the complexities of the conditions seen
16:30	Return to the office to answer queries from parents taken whilst in clinic
17:00	Return home, safe in the knowledge that without any on-call I can spend the evening with my family

myth	Spend every day examining children for head lice
reality	Ensuring children with significant disabilities, who are often at the bottom of the list of political priorities, are provided with appropriate support and ongoing management
personality	Approachable, relaxed, easy to work with, team player
best aspects	Making a difference in a child's life; enormous variety; the support of a team; the lack of on-call
worst aspects	Frustrations of inadequate funding for children with clear needs
route	ST1 Paediatrics (p 38) with subspecialty training in community paediatrics later in training; MRCPCH exam
numbers	500 of which 75% are women (the highest of any specialty)
locations	All community-based settings, both urban and rural

life		work
quiet on-call		busy on-call
boredom		burnout
uncompetitive		competitive
low salary		high salary

Dermatology

While skin is the primary focus of dermatology, it is essential to see the bigger picture both in terms of the effect on a patient's life and the large number of multisystem diseases that can cause skin lesions. The specialty is made exciting by frequent diagnostic challenges, the dramatic and obvious effects of treatment and the wide variety of patients encountered. It attracts a broad range of clinicians, from those with an interest in molecules to those handy with a knife.

the patients Most dermatologists are trained in both adult and paediatric skin diseases, although additional specialty training is often necessary for paediatric dermatology in teaching hospitals. Skin diseases are common throughout life so dermatologists regularly see patients of all ages. Since skin diseases have such a huge effect on appearance (and therefore a patient's social, family and professional life) the patients are often highly motivated. There is a good mixture of quick interventions to cure diseases and chronic care allowing long-term relationships to evolve.

the work In adult dermatology there is a roughly even split between patients with inflammatory skin diseases (eczema, psoriasis, etc.) and patients worried about lumps and lesions that may be skin cancer. Widespread skin diseases can be life-altering whilst seldom being life-threatening; while GPs often manage simple cases, patients with severe diseases receive systemic treatments that require dermatologist supervision. The increase in skin cancer in a population of increasing age and sun exposure has fostered the development of a subspecialty interested in skin surgery, which requires additional training.

the job The vast majority of the workload is in outpatients, though there is some inpatient work and a high number of referrals from other specialties with diagnostic puzzles or multisystem diseases. Dermatology departments typically comprise 2–5 pleasant and easygoing dermatologists and a number of invaluable specialist nurses. Community services are also important and consultants often support GPs with a special interest in dermatology. On-call is busy, but rarely extends into the night. There are close links with other specialists, especially histopathologists, who are essential for making diagnoses from skin biopsies.

extras Teaching is a large part of dermatology, whether it is to GPs, junior doctors, nurses, trainees or patient groups. Research is important in order to develop the critical skills needed in medicine, but an MD is not needed for many posts. Private practice is flexible, well-paid and common though there is some overlap with other specialties (e.g. plastics) for cosmetic services not provided in the NHS. Flexible training and part-time work is well established and common.

🛈 *For further information:*

British Association of Dermatologists, Willan House, 4 Fitzroy Square, London, W1T 5HQ
Tel: 020 7383 0266   Fax: 020 7388 5263   Web: http://www.bad.org.uk

08:30   Make sure desk and secretary still visible beneath paper work before starting clinic

08.45   Outpatient clinic: some urgent '2-week-wait' possible cancers; see patients of all ages and social backgrounds

12:00   Day case surgery under local anaesthetic: lesions removed from two patients with skin cancer

14:00   Clinic letters, emails, teledermatology referrals and eat sandwich

16:00   Go to wards to see two dermatology patients and referrals from other specialties including a child with an unusual rash and an elderly patient with possible skin cancer

17:30   Work on Trust audit and guidelines and talk with trainee about project

18:45   On the bike to head home unless doing a private clinic

myth	Nobody gets better but nobody dies—'dermaholiday'
reality	Days are busy and long, but many doctors wish they had chosen dermatology; dramatic improvements are common
personality	Academic inclination, attention to detail, generalist, good communicator, calm, practical skills can help
best aspects	Immense diversity; tremendously visual; able to make a big difference to patients' lives
worst aspects	Efforts to suck out the interesting and complex so that it can be left to GPs and nurses
route	CT1 Core medical training (p 34) then ST3 Dermatology; MRCP exam
numbers	770 of which 45% are women
locations	Hospital-based in most areas

life		work
quiet on-call		busy on-call
boredom		burnout
uncompetitive		competitive
low salary		high salary

Ear, nose and throat

Ear, nose and throat (ENT) surgeons have incredibly interesting and diverse jobs. An ENT surgeon treats disorders of the senses (smell, taste and hearing), restores special senses (balance), improves cosmesis (facial appearance) and improves function (voice, breathing and swallowing). Although ENT surgeons deal with some life-threatening illness, ENT is mostly about improving rather than saving life, for example, restoring hearing to the deaf with cochlear implants.

the patients ENT patients are of all ages and both sexes. In fact, 30% of the work is paediatric, making ENT the second largest paediatric surgical specialty (after paediatric surgery). Many of the patients can be treated medically, so the ENT surgeon is also a physican; less than 20% of patients require an operation. Some patients have difficult problems such as cancer or dizziness, for whom the treatment is complex, whereas some are seemingly straightforward, e.g. removing a pea from a lively 3-year-old's nose.

the work covers many different diseases in each area: *ear* includes balance, tinnitus and hearing loss; *nose* covers sinuses, cosmetic repair and sleep apnoea whilst *throat* includes voice problems and tonsils. There are a multitude of other conditions that require diagnosis and treatment; head and neck cancer also makes up a large amount of the workload. The surgery is also diverse varying from 16-hour cancer resections to a 5-minute insertion of grommets to improve children's hearing. ENT is at the forefront of utilizing new technology including microscopes and endoscopes to visualize the lesion or operating field. Good outcomes are common and many patients are treated as day case visits.

the job ENT is both a surgical and medical specialty, so the work is split between theatre, ward rounds and outpatient clinics. Compared with other surgical specialties there are more clinics, but slightly less ward work. An ENT doctor works with audiologists, speech therapists and radiologists, as well as with plastic surgeons, neurosurgeons, general surgeons and maxillofacial surgeons. While ENT is busy during the day, the out of hours is generally quiet; it is uncommon for consultants to be called in at night but when they are the cases are often very urgent (e.g. acute stridor).

extras There are lots of opportunities to make life interesting, from fellowships in overseas units to 'ear camps' in Africa. There is also medicolegal work and healthy amounts of private practice for those who want it. In larger centres sub-specialization is encouraged (e.g. otologists, rhinologists, head and neck cancer). Flexible training is more acceptable than in many surgical specialties but still relatively uncommon.

ℹ️ *For further information:*

ENT UK C/o Royal College of Surgeons, 35–43 Lincoln's Inn Fields, London WC2A 3PE
Tel: 020 7404 8373 or 020 7430 0693 Web: http://www.entuk.org

A day in the life ...

07:30	Take informed consent from five patients with trainee and anaesthetist
08:20	Send for first patient, no bed available so time to chat about cricket
09:00	'Knife to skin'; good mix of cases: paediatric tonsillectomy, repair of a traumatic skull base CSF leak, endoscopic sinus surgery and a rhinoplasty; take turns with the trainee and plenty of time for teaching
13:00	Clinic: hit the ground running and clear 15 patients (mixture of young and old); four operations booked, including a patient for endoscopic orbital decompression to treat severe thyroid eye disease
18:00	Cycle home for family supper followed by circuit training
23:00	Called because 7-year-old has inhaled a macadamia nut shell; trainee removes nut from right main bronchus using new fibre optic telescope under supervision
01:00	Return home to bed and sleep soundly

myth	ENT = Early Nights and Tennis; a minor surgical specialty dealing with snot and wax
reality	Challenging and diverse surgery with the latest technology
personality	Decisive, calm, excellent fine coordination, perfectionist
best aspects	Great patients, mostly sane; varied and challenging work; access to the best surgical 'toys'; a life outside the hospital
worst aspects	Heavy demand for services with some departments severely understaffed; extremely competitive
route	CT1 Surgery in general, otolaryngology (p 48) then ST3 Otolaryngology; MRCS exam
numbers	1100 of which 10% are women
locations	Hospital-based specialty available in most hospitals

life					work
quiet on-call					busy on-call
boredom					burnout
uncompetitive					competitive
low salary					high salary

Elderly medicine

The role of the geriatrician is to optimize the care and well-being of older people; it is a role that can be extremely challenging but rewarding. Because of distaste for the name 'geriatrics', many euphemisms have been coined to try to accommodate people's sensibilities, e.g. 'health care of the older person', 'medicine for the elderly', 'geratology' or even 'medicine for the chronologically challenged'. It's not the name, however, but the quality of service which is important.

the patients By definition the patients are elderly; some hospitals run an age-related model, e.g. allocating patients over 80 years, while others prefer needs-related definitions, e.g. multiple pathology, frailty or specific problems such as stroke, falls and acute confusion. Women outnumber men due to their natural longevity. Like all patient groups there is a spectrum of personality and demeanour, but some have fascinating stories and a high 'loveability factor'. The relatives of patients are often the key to their future. Some are heroic and devoted, others wrestle with guilt and yet others are pre-occupied with inheritance. Geriatricians commonly follow patients up, often until they die.

the work The geriatrician is also a general physician and is a member of the team covering acute take, where the whole spectrum of acute medicine is met. While some older people will die in hospital (usually in the acute phase of their illness), the majority return home with varying degrees of support. A small proportion go to care homes. Ethical dilemmas relating to feeding patients are common. These are challenging and need wide consultation, but can be rewarding problems to deal with. The work is a mixture of optimizing the treatment of multi-system pathology and empowering the patient to have the highest quality of life possible through services and the multidisciplinary team.

the job Inpatients predominate with the resulting ward rounds and multidisciplinary (MD) meetings (physiotherapy, occupational therapy, social worker, nurses, amongst others). Patients often progress from acute to rehabilitation wards and elderly people often need time to rehabilitate. Outpatient clinics are either general or special interest (e.g. incontinence, osteoporosis, movement disorders). The acute takes are busy but most situations can be handled over the phone. There are close links with other specialties including orthopaedics, psychiatry and general medical specialties.

extras The evidence base in geriatrics is relatively small, so the opportunities for research are great; there is also plenty of teaching to be done at all levels. While there is very little private practice, flexible training and working is relatively easy. Some geriatric trainees are moving across to acute medicine or stroke medicine.

For further information:

British Geriatrics Society, Marjory Warren House, 31 St John's Square, London, EC1M 4DN
Tel: 020 7608 1369   Fax: 020 7608 1041   Web: http://www.bgs.org.uk

A day in the life ...

07:30	Check emails
08:00	Ward round of 28 patients on the rehabilitation ward
11:00	Rehabilitation review with the physiotherapist in the gymnasium seeing five patients (from rehab ward) and their relations
12:00	Administration and paperwork
12:30	Medical meeting with lunch
13:45	Continence clinic: two new patients, three follow-ups
16:15	Relatives clinic: discussions regarding six patients from rehab ward
17:30	Home
21:00	On-call for acute unselected general medical admissions
07:00	Post-take ward round

myth	Jack of all trades, master of none. Second-rate physician trying to fight the inevitable 'crumble' at the end of life.
reality	Doctors trained in holistic care managing many complex patients (often with multiple pathology)
personality	Hard working, excellent communication skills, team worker, thorough, energetic, patient, slightly obsessional, thick-skinned, sense of humour; watch out for inferiority complex
best aspects	Being an advocate of fairness for the aged patient; gratitude of patients/relatives; teamwork; successful rehabilitation of complex cases; ethical dilemmas
worst aspects	High death rate; difficult relatives; ethical dilemmas!
route	CT1 Core medical training (p 34) then ST3 Geriatric medicine; MRCP exam
numbers	1600 of which 25% are women
locations	Hospital-based from small district general hospital to teaching hospitals; community-based 'intermediate care' is growing

life					work
quiet on-call					busy on-call
boredom					burnout
uncompetitive					competitive
low salary					high salary

Emergency medicine

Emergency medicine (previously accident and emergency and, for those who can remember even further back, casualty) has evolved into a vibrant specialty with its own college. The name might have changed, but the work remains as exciting as ever! Why else would dramas about working in the emergency department (ED) occupy pole position in prime time television?

the patients A typical ED treats patients of all ages with a diversity of problems unrivalled in hospital practice. Most patients are vulnerable, distressed, in pain and, from their point of view, seen at their worst. Children comprise 20% of the average workload, although there are some well-established paediatric EDs in larger urban centres.

the work Inevitably, the focus is on emergency patient management, particularly in the resuscitation room. The incredible variety of patient presentations is more than enough to maintain interest. Being able to prioritize (juggle) several different tasks at the same time and cope with interruptions is a distinct advantage. In addition to emergency clinical work, most units are responsible for some short stay beds (typically managing minor head injury, soft tissue infections and poisoning) and run follow-up clinics (for patients with soft tissue injuries).

the job There is no time to get bored! An inherently sociable activity, working in the ED is very much a team affair. The team support is especially important at busy and stressful times. Nights on-call can be busy with telephone advice or coming in to lead complex resuscitations, though the frequency of this depends on local arrangements. The specialty is moving towards senior presence around the clock, but consultant numbers are increasing to help offset the effect of this. Alongside clinical work there are teaching, management and administration roles.

extras Teaching is integral, with high demand from various quarters, including resuscitation courses, for example advanced life support (ALS), advanced paediatric life support (APLS), and advanced trauma life support (ATLS). Research has been slow to develop, but there is now a solid academic base and opportunities are amazing due to the diverse patients and presentations. Private practice has not (yet) developed though there is scope to write medicolegal expert reports. Special interests are encouraged and cover a range of areas, including pre-hospital care, major incident planning, injury prevention and management of poisoning.

Paediatric emergency medicine is also a recognized subspecialty. Currently there are fairly few emergency specialists who focus solely on paediatric work, however most departments have (or aspire to have) a paediatric lead with additional training. Registrars can acquire this training by spending an extra year in a children's hospital at the end of their standard training programme.

ⓘ *For further information:*

College of Emergency Medicine, Churchill House, 35 Red Lion Square, London, WC1R 4SG
Tel: 020 7404 1999   Fax: 020 7067 1267   Web: http://www.emergencymed.org.uk

A day in the life ...

08:00	Perform appraisal with junior doctor
08:30	Meeting to discuss new protocol to manage suspected pulmonary embolism (PE)
09:00	Assess patients on short stay ward, refer one for CT scan
10:30	Timetabled teaching of medical students
11:30	Admin and management (punctuated by coffee and lunch): emails, reference requests and a statement for the police
13:00	Clinical 'shop floor' work, mostly supervising junior doctors and nurses
15:00	Review of X-ray reports over coffee whilst the department is quiet
16:00	Lead a resuscitation team and organize patient transfer to ICU
17:30	Brief phone conversation with the Press Officer, then home for tea; not on-call, so it's down to the local cricket club for evening net practice...

myth	Watch ER, a glamorous job with beautiful staff, personal intrigue and a life saved every two minutes
reality	Predictably unpredictable, but always interesting and frequently rewarding; heavy focus on team work and camaraderie
personality	Generalist, calm in emergencies, common sense, practical, leadership and teamwork, unshockable, thick skin
best aspects	Arguably the most varied hospital job and certainly one of the most interesting; occasionally you really do 'save a life'
worst aspects	Hours (and some patients) are antisocial; limited opportunities for patient follow-up; conflict with management/other specialists
route	CT1 Acute care common stem, emergency medicine (p 28) then ST4 Emergency medicine; MCEM exam
numbers	1200 of which 25% are women
locations	Hospital-based in virtually all hospitals providing acute services

life						work
quiet on-call						busy on-call
boredom						burnout
uncompetitive						competitive
low salary						high salary

Endocrinology and diabetes

Clinical work in endocrinology and diabetes offers immense variety. Treatment is available for many conditions and this can dramatically change the course of patients' lives. The majority of specialists cover both endocrine and diabetic conditions though a few subspecialize. The specialty tends to attract doctors who enjoy dealing with the ebb and flow of people's lives but are excited by the diagnostic challenge of eliciting clear information from patients and pursuing investigations in a logical manner.

the patients *Endocrine* The patients come in all shapes and sizes from all ethnic groups; many are young. There is a pleasant mix of straightforward and complex cases. *Diabetes* There is a great spread in age from young people with type 1 diabetes, through to patients with either type 1 or type 2 diabetes in later life; diabetic patients have to live with treatment that interferes with their habits and lifestyle and sometimes have to contend with disabling complications. Both specialties offer great continuity of care often over many years.

the work *Endocrine* Thyroid disorders, thyroid lumps (and therefore possible malignancies) and prolactinomas form much of the workload. Patients with adrenal disorders, sex hormone disorders and pituitary disease add variety and interest. Clinical outcomes are often very good. *Diabetes* Supporting and educating people at the diagnosis of their type 1 or type 2 diabetes is very important. Many people with diabetes need regular assistance to make the lifestyle changes that are needed to maximize their chance of a long healthy life. Part of the challenge is finding ways to help people grasp the need for change in their lives.

the job A large proportion of the work is in outpatient clinics. There are also inpatients under the endocrine team with acute deteriorations or complications of their condition, while others are admitted for investigation. Endocrinologists work with large multidisciplinary teams (specialist nurses, dieticians, specialist midwifes, chiropodists and eye screening technicians). They also collaborate with a range of specialists, e.g. ophthalmologists, nephrologists and neurosurgeons. Many endocrinologists cover acute general medicine on-calls, which adds even more variety to the job. The hours tend to be slightly more predictable than other medical specialties due to the higher proportion of outpatient work.

extras Endocrinology and diabetes has a strong research emphasis and most consultants will have spent some time in research; there are also many chances for teaching. There are some opportunities for private practice in both endocrinology and diabetes. Flexible training is more acceptable than in other general medical specialties.

ℹ️ *For further information:*

Society for Endocrinology: http://www.endocrinology.org
Association of British Clinical Diabetologists: http://www.diabetologists-abcd.org.uk

A day in the life ...

08:00	Mark medical students' special study module submissions
08:30	Emails: 30% clinical, 30% managerial, 40% wide miscellany
09:00	Endocrine clinic: 16 patients of which about 25% are new
12:30	Lunch time at the medical grand round
13:30	Sandwich lunch with IT team
14:00	Ante-natal/endocrine clinic
16:30	Case discussion meeting with obstetricians
17:30	Check recently returned results
18:30	Paperwork: a solid 7 inches stack
20:00	Put 3½ inches of paper back in 'in tray' and head home

myth	Academics chasing hormones but only finding diabetes
reality	Diagnostic challenges in a wide range of patients with the excitement of acute general medicine too
personality	Thinkers, good communication and diagnostic skills, attention to detail, good team work, leadership skills
best aspects	Great spread of patient ages; diagnostic problem-solving; continuity of care
worst aspects	Paperwork; patient complaints; patients refusing to engage with treatment or lifestyle changes and getting progressively worse
route	CT1 Core medical training (p 34) then ST3 Endocrinology and diabetes; MRCP exam
numbers	1050 of which 25% are women
locations	Hospital-based, from district general hospitals to teaching hospitals

life						work
quiet on-call						busy on-call
boredom						burnout
uncompetitive						competitive
low salary						high salary

Expedition medicine

Most expedition doctors have regular careers and take time off to use their hard-earned medical skills as a passport to adventure. A few work for groups such as the British Antarctic Survey for up to 18 months at a time. The expedition doctor can combine a love of mountaineering, diving or sailing with medicine.

the patients People of all ages and backgrounds go on overseas expeditions. Many are fit, highly motivated individuals (but not always!). Participants could come from any country and the doctor may end up treating expeditioners, other team members (guides, muleteers, porters) or local villagers encountered en route. It is wise to treat only those who are seriously ill or injured to avoid depleting the medical kit or administering health checks to entire villages. As well as the potential communication problems, there are ethical issues when treating local people, for instance the risk of undermining local services, while follow-up is usually impossible unless the expedition returns via the same route.

the work Some say expedition medicine is the last bastion of clinical medicine because conditions must be diagnosed and treated clinically. Much of the work occurs before the expedition leaves: advising on suitable jabs, anti-malarials, medical training and medical kits. The commonest problems are minor injuries (e.g. blisters, sprains, cuts), diarrhoea and, on climbing trips, high-altitude symptoms (e.g. headache). Almost everyone will recover in the field with simple treatments such as dressings, antibiotics and analgesia. Rarely, evacuation and repatriation may be required. Caring for patients in remote environments often requires specialist adventure sport skills—diving, climbing, sailing, etc.

the job Work can be in any environment: on or under the sea, in the desert, in the jungle or on high mountains. Most doctors act independently but on larger expeditions there may be nurses or other health professionals operating in different locations and communicating by radio. There may be recourse to senior advice via satellite phone, email, etc. The group should be informed when 'clinics' will be held otherwise the doctor may face a never-ending barrage of requests whilst the medical kit heads over a distant sand dune on a camel! There are opportunities to teach the team medical skills and some doctors will undertake studies in the field as part of research projects. On-call is 24/7 unless another doctor accompanies the group. That said, it is rare to be kept very busy although one seriously ill or injured person will keep a doctor fully occupied.

extras Expedition medicine does not provide a career for most, but can rejuvenate flagging morale and adds spice to a CV. A few doctors use their experience to advise expedition companies on a professional basis, briefing staff and advising on risk assessments and appropriate medical kits.

🛈 *For further information:*

Diploma in mountain medicine: http://www.medex.org.uk
Training courses: http://www.wildernessmedicaltraining.co.uk; http://www.expeditionmedicine.co.uk

A day in the life during a Himalayan trek ...

06:00	Wake and start to melt snow for morning cuppa; help prepare breakfast
07:00	Check team for illness including altitude sickness; redress a porter's leg wound and dispense antibiotics for persistent diarrhoea in a team member
08:30	Pack the medical kit (to be carried on a yak); brief team on dangers of sun, dehydration and altitude; walk for three hours carrying all personal kit (18 kg)
11:30	Stop for lunch on the trail and examine a swollen, twisted knee
13:00	Ascend 800 m slope; stay at the back to encourage the slower team members
17:00	Put up tents and advise two people with diarrhoea and sickness
18:00	Reiterate altitude advice and inform the group leader that a rest day may be necessary tomorrow as many are suffering from altitude-related illness
21:00	Turn in with a book after supper and hot chocolate
00:00	Get up to inject an anti-emetic and give antibiotics for vigorous vomiting
04:00	Wake feeling nauseated
06:00	Get up and melt snow for morning cuppa, despite nausea; another day ...

myth	Indiana Jones-like characters dealing with snakebite and lion attacks
reality	Most work is preparing and maintaining the team's health; while most problems are minor there is great responsibility if things go wrong
personality	Good team player, ability to improvise and work independently, sound outdoor skills (important not to be a liability to the team)
best aspects	Opportunity to work in challenging environments and to use your medical skills to look after a team of like-minded adventurers
worst aspects	Being ill oneself; often unpaid (though may get a free/subsidized trip)
route	No established route (p 20); broad experience particularly in emergency medicine or general practice, training courses are available (see opposite)
locations	Anywhere on earth

life						**work**
quiet on-call				●		**busy on-call**
boredom			☺			**burnout**
uncompetitive		●				**competitive**
low salary	●					**high salary**

Forensic medical examiner (police surgeon)

Forensic medicine is a rapidly developing and fascinating field where clinical medicine meets the criminal justice system. It includes numerous specialties including forensic medical examiner (FME, also known as a forensic physician or police surgeon), coroner (who may be medically and/or legally qualified), forensic pathologist (p 138) and medicolegal adviser to the medical defence organizations (p 180). The FME's role is to offer therapeutic services to detainees and perform examinations and investigations in a manner that could be used in court; this requires an understanding of law, negligence and consent.

the patients include detainees in police stations, police officers with injuries, victims of physical or sexual assaults (both child and adult), torture victims, prisoners, drug packers/mules and even terrorist suspects. Many detainees have drug, alcohol and/or mental health problems. Occasionally FMEs may be asked to confirm whether a death is suspicious. Patients are referred by judges, lawyers, policemen and other medical specialists.

the work necessitates an excellent general medical background to provide the experience to deal with the broad presentations of patients. Work with detainees includes attending police stations to manage drug and alcohol intoxication or withdrawal or to examine detainees for their fitness to be detained, interviewed, transported or charged. The forensic role entails the collection of specimens (e.g. blood, urine, intimate and non-intimate swabs), detailing injuries where present and commenting on their nature. Examining children following sexual assaults is usually performed alongside a suitably trained paediatrician. Writing reports or giving evidence in court as a professional witness or expert becomes common as a specialist's reputation, knowledge and credibility develops.

the job is on a call-out basis so it is paid per case or per session on-call. Many FMEs work through locum agencies (e.g. Medacs, p 174). The workload varies between shifts and region (large cities being much busier); like emergency departments there is usually a rush of work after pubs and nightclubs close. It is essential to be able to drive to get between police stations, though mileage is usually paid. Due to the legal nature of the work a previous criminal conviction may prevent employment as an FME. There is interaction with other specialists including forensic odontologists (bite mark specialists), scene of crime officers, forensic pathologists, serious fraud officers and forensic scientists.

extras There is plenty of extra work, including acting as an expert witness or writing reports, once sufficient expertise is developed. The work is inherently flexible, but a large proportion takes place at night. Training opportunities are developing and there are a number of diplomas, courses and conferences.

ⓘ *For further information:*

Faculty of Forensic and Legal Medicine, 3rd Floor, 116 Great Portland Street, London, W1W 6PJ
Tel: 020 7580 8490   Web: http://www.fflm.ac.uk

A day in the life ...

06:00	Shift starts: take blood from those with borderline breath alcohol tests
07:00	Review drug addict prior to transfer to court
09:00	Review drunk for fitness to be interviewed
10:00	Mental health assessment for detainee arrested for assault
11:00	Examination of detainee (drug addict) for fitness to be interviewed and examination of the injuries of the assaulted police officer
12:00	Detainee sectioned under Mental Health Act
14:00	Review withdrawing drug addict (managed with dihydrocodeine) and alcoholic (managed with diazepam)
15:00	Assess a diabetic and epileptic detainee for fitness to detain, prescription for insulin and carbamazepine written for police to obtain
17:00	Return to administer insulin
18:00	Review of alcoholic and drug addict being kept in overnight, then home

myth	Somewhere between *Quincy* and *CSI*
reality	Clinicians who are independent of the police and responsible to the criminal justice system
personality	Strong and independent nature, open-minded, generalist
best aspects	The independent nature of work, respect shown by police officers and having a view of the other side of life
worst aspects	The disruptive last-minute call to attend court
route	Initial training varies, e.g.: GP, emergency medicine, general medicine, psychiatry; membership exam likely to start in 2009, until then Diploma of forensic medicine among others
locations	Police stations, sexual assault centres

life		**work**
quiet on-call		**busy on-call**
boredom		**burnout**
uncompetitive		**competitive**
low salary		**high salary**

Forensic pathology

Forensic pathology is a subspecialty of pathology and a part of forensic medicine, along with forensic medical examiners (p 136), coroners and medicolegal advisers to the medical defence organizations (p 180). Forensic pathology is in the public eye through television dramas such as *CSI*; this has raised unrealistic expectations from juries about what the specialty can, and cannot, do. The role of the forensic pathologist is to look for evidence in cases of suspicious death alongside forensic scientists (usually non-medical scientists) who perform DNA analysis, fire investigation, ballistics, etc.

the patients are mostly, but not exclusively, dead. A forensic pathologist may be involved if the death was suspicious, related to toxins, drugs or alcohol or due to trauma. Occasionally they may be asked to assess an injury in a living patient.

the work Forensic pathology is an interesting and varied career requiring energetic, resilient practitioners who have a thorough approach to their work, integrity in their opinions and the ability to present complex evidence to a lay jury. Whilst conducting autopsies remains the core skill of the forensic pathologist, it is not all about murder as there are many other causes of unexplained death. The other key aspect of the work is presenting evidence in court, which can be a nerve-racking experience. The work has become more specialized and pathologists often have specific areas of interest including paediatric forensic pathology, drug-related deaths, forensic neuropathology and human rights abuses.

the job Forensic pathology was initially practiced in university departments. This is still the case in Scotland, Wales and Northern Ireland but in England the majority are now self-employed. This leads to a fragmented service and not all jobs are advertised, so obtaining a post is not always straightforward. The day-to-day work varies between individual practices but will involve travelling to mortuaries to perform autopsies, reviewing histology, studying documentary evidence and giving evidence in court. A lot of suspicious deaths are examined out of normal hours and travelling to courts and hanging around waiting to give evidence remains a bugbear for many forensic pathologists.

extras Forensic pathologists are popular teachers and lecturers. Forensic medicine in general needs a stronger evidence base and more research is needed, but tissue retention laws hamper research. There are opportunities for international travel, though many of the places are not in holiday brochures. Being a small specialty it is easy to become acquainted with both national and international colleagues.

🛈 *For further information:*

The Royal College of Pathologists, 2 Carlton House Terrace, London, SW1Y 5AF
Tel: 020 7451 6700   Fax: 020 7451 6701   Web: http://www.rcpath.org

A day in the life ...

06:00	Phone call from Coroner's office asking when an autopsy on a suspicious death can be performed
10:00	Attend inquest – give 5 minutes of evidence with no questions
11:00	Go to Crown Court; sit outside reading book
12:05	Start giving evidence but break for lunch at 13:00
14:05	Return and complete giving evidence
16:00	Commence autopsy on suspicious death
19:00	Leave for home
20:00	Spend evening completing report required by lawyers for the next day

myth	TV detective who autopsies the victim, interviews the suspect, traces the path of the bullet and solves the crime
reality	Skilled medical practitioner who performs autopsies as part of a team investigating a suspicious death
personality	Strong, resilient, often extrovert, attention to detail, systematic
best aspects	Not knowing what will happen next; assisting in the administration of justice
worst aspects	Poor facilities; waiting around courts; lack of proper national structure; unpredictable working day
route	ST1 Histopathology (p 40) then forensic pathology training from ST3; FRCPath (forensic pathology) exam
numbers	70 of which 15% are women
locations	Independent practice, mortuaries, courts, hospitals, universities

life						work
quiet on-call						busy on-call
boredom						burnout
uncompetitive						competitive
low salary						high salary

Forensic psychiatry

Forensic psychiatrists diagnose and treat psychiatric conditions in patients who have been imprisoned. The work is often challenging and coping with risk-related anxieties is part of the job. Separating professional and personal life is vital: while stepping into the mind of a killer is fascinating it is essential to step out again after the interview! Gratitude from patients is less common compared to other medical disciplines, but there are numerous other rewards.

the patients are mostly mentally disordered offenders. They may display the full range of psychiatric disorders including psychotic illnesses (e.g. schizophrenia) and personality disorders. Many also abuse substances and may have physical health problems, so generic doctor skills remain important. The patients may have committed a range of offences, such as violence (including homicide), arson and sexual offences (including rape).

the work Forensic psychiatrists offer psychiatric management for patients in secure hospitals and assessment of psychiatric illness for those in prison. The work focuses on exploring the mental state of individuals who have carried out offences. This can be challenging but intellectually stimulating as one tries to understand why they committed their offence. This understanding is crucial both to plan treatment and to give an accurate estimate of future risk or prognosis. The other important role is as an expert witness in court where one faces cross-examination on issues such as diagnosis, criminal responsibility, risk and whether a patient should go to prison or a secure hospital. Infrequently hospital psychiatrists may ask for help in dealing with dangerous non-offenders.

the job Most forensic psychiatrists are employed by the NHS to work in secure hospitals; these are usually medium-secure units (double-locked doors, high fences and nursing supervision in a structured, safe environment) but a few are high-secure units. There are also some outpatient clinics for ex-offenders. Liaison with the police, Home Office and lawyers is interesting and forces the forensic psychiatrist to balance an individual patient's welfare with the welfare of others.

extras Forensic psychiatry is an expanding specialty with much scope for teaching and personal professional development; there are also a few academic posts. There are opportunities for subspecialization, e.g. forensic psychotherapy and forensic child and adolescent psychiatry.

ℹ️ *For further information:*

Royal College of Psychiatrists, 17 Belgrave Square, London SW1X 8PG
Tel: 020 7235 2351   Fax: 020 7235 1231   Website: http://www.rcpsych.ac.uk

A day in the life ...

09:00	Check emails, make telephone calls
09:30	Ward round; detailed multidisciplinary discussion and interviews with 4–5 patients, coffee break halfway through
12:00	Supervise trainee
13:00	Lunch
13:30	Tutorial with medical students discussing arson and possible motivations
14:30	Joint assessment at local prison with trainee and medical student of remand prisoner with history of schizophrenia and charged with murder
16:30	Check messages with PA, make final telephone calls then head home
19:00	Read papers of a Crown Court referral for tomorrow (witness statements, police interview); watch late-night repeat episode of *Cracker* on UK Gold

myth	A medical *Cracker*-type character giving profiles to police on serial killers and caring for Hannibal Lecter
reality	Fascinating work on the interface of medicine and the law with complex, challenging patients
personality	Inquisitive, decisive, obsessional, thrive on analysing and overcoming complexity, realistic, able to defend opinions
best aspects	Time to explore and understand the darker recesses of the human mind; contact with interesting colleagues; potential for good and varied professional development
worst aspects	Patients who seriously harm others, resulting in distress and inquiries into your work; lots of paperwork
route	CT1 Psychiatry (p 42) then ST4 Forensic psychiatry; MRCPsych (forensic psychiatry) exam
numbers	480 of which 30% are women
locations	Secure hospitals

life					work
quiet on-call					busy on-call
boredom					burnout
uncompetitive					competitive
low salary					high salary

Gastroenterology

Gastroenterology is a branch of internal medicine and gastroenterologists are physicians who investigate and treat patients with gastrointestinal (GI) disorders, including diseases of the bowel, liver, pancreas and biliary tree. The advent of fibre-optic endoscopy has had a huge impact; it is now complemented by capsule endoscopy, endoscopic ultrasound and positron emission tomography (PET) scanning, allowing greater visualization of the GI tract. The gastroenterologist needs a holistic approach but requires a surgical temperament because they will perform diagnostic and therapeutic procedures which can go wrong. Gastrointestinal diseases are very common, accounting for one in six of all hospital admissions.

the patients Many gastrointestinal diseases start in the young (e.g. inflammatory bowel disease) whilst others present later in life (e.g. colon cancer). Consequently gastroenterologists treat patients from a wide age range. A proportion of patients are alcoholics and present a significant medical and ethical challenge. Many conditions are chronic so patients are managed for many years through the vagaries of their condition, resulting in long-term working relationships with patients and their families, which can be rewarding.

the work A tremendous variety of cases are seen and the gastroenterologist often needs to be a detective, searching for causes of anaemia or weight loss, for example. Other common presentations include abdominal pain, PR bleeding and diarrhoea. Endoscopy is an important part of the work load and may be for diagnosis (e.g. colon cancer), for treatment (e.g. strictures) or acute and life-saving (e.g. endoscopic banding of oesophageal varices).

the job The majority of patients are managed as outpatients with several clinics and endoscopy lists each week. There is also significant inpatient work in disorders such as GI bleeding, jaundice, liver failure, severe diarrhoea and cancer. These patients can be very unwell and their management requires an ability to cope well with the rigours of high-dependency medicine. Gastroenterologists work closely with general surgeons, radiologists and pathologists and there are regular multidisciplinary meetings. Most gastroenterologists in the UK take part in the acute general medical on-call, alongside a 24-hour emergency endoscopy on-call for acute GI haemorrhage.

extras Having a 'procedure' leads to good opportunities for private practice and ensures a very busy NHS practice, with emergency and elective work. There are excellent opportunities for teaching and research. Subspecialization is becoming important (e.g. GI oncology, nutrition), whilst hepatology is becoming a separate specialty with 'pure' hepatologists focusing on hepatobiliary disease and transplantation. Flexible training is difficult with the long hours and busy on-calls.

🛈 *For further information:*

British Society of Gastroenterology, 3 St Andrews Place, Regent's Park, London, NW1 4LB
Tel: 020 7935 3150   Fax: 020 7487 3734   Web: http://www.bsg.org.uk

08:00 MDT meeting for GI cancer, involving discussion with radiologists, pathologists, surgeons, oncologists and specialist nurses

09:00 Outpatient clinic, an interesting case mix including an 18-year-old with malabsorption, a 35-year-old with alcoholic liver disease and a 51-year-old with an inherited risk of colon cancer

13:00 Meet with trainee to catch up on inpatients; discuss whether a patient needs to have his ascites drained

14:00 Endoscopy list, perform banding of oesophageal varices and use diathermy snare to remove colonic polyps

17:00 Nutrition round, discuss starting total parenteral nutrition (TPN) in a patient on the intensive care unit (ICU)

18:00 Home to spend evening improving own nutritional intake and drink alcohol (in moderation of course!)

myth	Frustrated surgeons who see patients through an endoscope
reality	An enjoyable specialty which combines clinical medicine with sophisticated investigative and therapeutic techniques
personality	Academic, excellent practical abilities, able to communicate with patients and colleagues (especially surgeons)
best aspects	Technical aspects (e.g. endoscopy); application of science to disease; great variety of conditions
worst aspects	Acute medical on-call as well as emergency endoscopy on-call
route	CT1 Core medical training (p 34) then ST3 Gastroenterology; MRCP exam
numbers	1300 of which 15% are women
locations	Hospital-based specialty present in most hospitals

life					**work**
quiet on-call					**busy on-call**
boredom					**burnout**
uncompetitive					**competitive**
low salary					**high salary**

General practice

General practice is a challenging, ever-changing career offering the chance to develop and use diverse skills. In a health care system that is producing more and more specialists, general practice offers the opportunity to be a true all-round doctor. Generalism is a specialty in its own right. The job requires a vast breadth of knowledge along with the skill to know when to seek further advice via referral. In this way General practitioners (GPs) act as the gatekeepers to the rest of the health service for the patients.

the patients General practice cares for patients and their families from birth until death (and sometimes beyond)! Patient mix can include the homeless, refugees, commuters, the very young and the very old, as well as the worried well. Looking after several members of the same family can raise confidentiality issues but also offers valuable insight. Patients often form strong bonds with their family doctor which can be both rewarding and frustrating.

the work Includes clinical medicine/surgery, psychiatry, social problems and health promotion. One of the major challenges is having no idea what the patient is going to present with and getting into the correct gear within 7–10 minutes, then doing that again and again up to 40–50 times a day. One minute you might be dealing with a child with eczema (paediatrics and dermatology) and the next you may be called upon to resuscitate a diabetic with a myocardial infarction (MI) (endocrinology, cardiology, emergency medicine). The diversity is endless.

the job Many GPs become partners within a practice and are jointly responsible for running the practice as a business (usually partly delegated to a practice manager). Other options are to work as a salaried GP without the management responsibilities but with a similar clinical workload (p 71). GPs mainly work alone during surgery times, but with support from other practice team members (partners, nurses, etc.). They form part of a wider multidisciplinary team including district nurses, health visitors and other community professionals. It is also possible to carry out minor operations and procedures in the GP surgery.

extras Good opportunities for part-time/flexible hours. Option to subspecialize and become a GP with a special interest or 'GPwSI', pronounced 'gypsy', (p 152). Opportunities to work in private sector are expanding. Becoming a partner offers chance to 'buy-in' to the business and premises which remains a good long-term investment. Multiple research opportunities for the interested but there is no obligation for those who are not. There is also the chance to train future doctors and GPs by becoming an F2 supervisor or a GP trainer.

🛈 *For further information:*

Royal College of General Practitioners, 14 Princes Gate, Hyde Park, London, SW7 1PU
Tel: 020 7581 3232   Fax: 020 7225 3047   Web: http://www.rcgp.org.uk

A day in the life ...

08:00	Paperwork: checking/actioning results, reading letters, insurance reports
08:50	Surgery: 7–10-minute consultations with 25 patients, cups of tea appear at regular intervals from the receptionist; consultations include earache, depression, urinary frequency, antenatal check and diabetic review
13:00	Home visits: agree to post letter for one housebound old lady who just needed a chat; negotiate bed for another with confusion related to a urinary tract infection (UTI)
14:00	Lunchtime meeting with partners discussing cases, practice and gossip
15:00	Dictate referral letters and sign repeat prescriptions
15:30	Surgery: 22 patients, runs late after admitting child with appendicitis
18:30	Surgery closes, hand over responsibility to out-of-hours service; quick chat with practice manager about waiting room which needs repainting
19:00	Home to relax with family

myth	Failed hospital doctors who stay in one job until they retire
reality	Becoming a GP is an active choice for most; a GP is jack-of-all-trades and master of many; many start as salaried doctors and move around until they find a practice that suits them
personality	Calm, open, logical, good listening skills, non-confrontational, able to deal with uncertainty, business mind helps
best aspects	Seeing the same patients over and over again; getting to know patients as people and seeing their homes and families; wide diversity of presentations; optional out-of-hours
worst aspects	Seeing the same patients over and over again! Not enough time to deal with multiple problems (e.g. the patient with a list)
route	GP vocational training scheme (p 32) with nMRCGP exam
numbers	38 300 of which 45% are women
locations	Anywhere from city to countryside; practice-based with home visits and possible to do some hospital sessions

life					work
quiet on-call					busy on-call
boredom					burnout
uncompetitive					competitive
low salary					high salary

General surgery (colorectal surgery)

This branch of surgery focuses principally on abdominal surgery, but spans from itchy bottoms to resecting liver cancers. The variety of cases is amazing; emergency cases are particularly diverse, though seat belt legislation has significantly reduced abdominal trauma. The specialty is being slowly divided into upper GI surgery (oesophagus, stomach, hepatobiliary and pancreas) and lower GI surgery (colon, rectum and anus) with the lower GI surgeons being seen as the 'on-call abdominal surgeons'. Further subspecialization occurs according to a technique or organ (e.g. laparoscopy, pancreas).

the patients range from teenagers upwards as those under 16 years are seen by paediatric surgeons (p 222). Many are elderly because the conditions treated are more common with advancing years. Informed discussions with both patients and relatives (or carers) are increasingly important, as there is the potential for significant complications from all major operations in this age group. Contact with patients ranges from one-off (e.g. day case operations) to regular meetings throughout a career (e.g. malignancy and inflammatory bowel disease).

the work The work encompasses the complete spectrum of pathology from the concerned hypochondriac to the life-threateningly acute. Many operations are carried out as day case/overnight stay procedures (e.g. cholecystectomies, hernia repairs) with laparoscopic techniques becoming increasingly common. The bulk of major resections for cancer are still done as open operations and these form the vast majority of the inpatient work. Emergency admissions include 'acute abdomens', appendicitis, pancreatitis and bowel obstruction.

the job The work is split nearly equally between clinics, wards and theatre. The size of the team varies between hospitals, but is commonly made up of about four surgeons along with numerous junior doctors. Increasingly major upper GI resections are restricted to larger hospitals, though lower GI surgery takes place in most hospitals. Multidisciplinary teams are important including specialist stoma nurses, cancer nurses and close links with radiology, oncology and pathology. On-calls can be busy, but modern practice prevents all but the most urgent operations being performed outside office hours.

extras The wide range of patients provides good options for research and the competitive nature of the specialty makes publications almost essential. Teaching is important as surgery is an integral part of training for medical students and junior doctors. Private practice is common and can be lucrative. Flexible training remains uncommon, making it difficult to arrange.

🛈 *For further information:*

The Royal College of Surgeons of England, 35–43 Lincoln's Inn Fields, London, WC2A 3PE
Tel: 020 7405 3474   Web: http://www.rcseng.ac.uk

A day in the life ...

08:00 Ward review of acute admissions and sick patients, ending on intensive care unit (ITU); give instructions to junior staff

08:30 Outpatient clinic: a mix of 22 patients of which 14 are new and 8 are follow-ups; four operations booked including a hemicolectomy

12:30 Lower GI cancer multidisciplinary team meeting with lunch

13:30 Operating list: one total colectomy followed by a hernia repair, haemorrhoidectomy and diagnostic laparoscopy

17:30 Review of post-op patients, assess if any can go home tonight

18:00 Liaise with junior staff about inpatients and post-op patients

18:30 Home unless doing a private clinic

myth	Giblet doctors, the butchers of the hospital
reality	Fascinating, rewarding area of practice with increasing opportunities for specialization
personality	Calm, team worker, leadership skills, decisive, good practical skills, resilient, good time management
best aspects	Personal satisfaction of curing by operation alone
worst aspects	Serious complications with serious outcomes inevitable
route	CT1 Surgery in general, general surgery (p 48) then ST3 General surgery; MRCS exam
numbers	1600 of which 12% are women
locations	Hospital-based, present in most hospitals

life						work
quiet on-call						busy on-call
boredom						burnout
uncompetitive						competitive
low salary						high salary

Genitourinary medicine

Good communication skills and a non-judgemental attitude are essential for a career in genitourinary medicine (GUM). The specialty offers a fascinating insight into a very private world and the ability to offer essential treatment or reassurance. Sexual health issues are varied and along with general GUM clinics there are services for HIV, psychosexual issues, contraception, syphilis, herpes and sexual assault.

the patients Most patients attending GUM clinics are young and otherwise fit and well. Specialists see patients of both genders, though men and women are usually physically separated in the waiting room and clinic. Specific services are often provided for those who are homosexual or bisexual, commercial sex workers and prisoners. HIV patient demographics reflect the risk factors for HIV acquisition (e.g. multiple partners, IV drug use). General GUM provides little opportunity for continuity of care, however a few patients with chronic problems, e.g. HIV, may require years of follow-up.

the work focuses on the management of individuals with sexually transmitted infections or genital disorders along with health promotion, screening, contact tracing and outreach services. Diagnosis is very hands on, including a general and sexual history, thorough examination and microbiological investigations (some of which are analysed immediately by the doctor); patients are often seen and treated on the same day, usually with good outcomes. The job can raise challenging ethical dilemmas, due to the sensitive nature of the information shared against the need for contact tracing.

the job GUM is almost entirely outpatient based. In larger centres a few GUM specialists also provide inpatient HIV care including ward rounds, MDT meetings and on-call duties; alternatively HIV care may be managed by infectious diseases (p 168). Both GUM and HIV care are multidisciplinary with doctors, nurses, health advisors and administration staff working closely together to ensure good-quality services. The specialty has strong links with microbiology, virology, dermatology, women's health and public health. HIV care often interacts with many other specialties and a good all-round general medical knowledge is essential. GUM usually has no on-call and HIV on-call is not onerous, generally consisting of telephone advice and a weekend ward round.

extras There are good opportunities for teaching; research interests and attendance at national and international conferences are encouraged. Flexible training is well established and part-time working is common, making the specialty very family-friendly. Private practice opportunities are limited.

For further information:

British Association of Sexual Health and HIV (BASHH), Royal Society of Medicine, 1 Wimpole Street, London, W1G 0AE
Tel: 020 7290 2968   Web: http://www.bashh.org.uk

08:30	Check emails and post
09:00	General GUM clinic, 15 patients seen, some jointly with junior doctor; treated with a mixture of reassurance and medicines
13:00	Lunch and patient-related admin
14:00	HIV clinic: nine patients seen with medical student sitting in
17:00	Discuss management of complex patient with trainee
17:30	Head home or for quick drink with work colleagues
19:00	Evening out with friends hoping not to meet grateful patients

myth	Doctors who can't cut the mustard dealing with drippy willies
reality	Rapid developments in HIV treatment and care make this a complex and challenging specialty; many opportunities to develop services in innovative ways to manage an increasing patient demand
personality	An eclectic bunch, often a bit alternative, very accepting of diversity, excellent communication skills, non-judgemental
best aspects	Friendly working environment; good support from colleagues
worst aspects	Dealing with stigma and discrimination particularly as regards HIV; little scope for private practice
route	CT1 Core medical training (p 34) then ST3 Genitourinary medicine; MRCP exam
numbers	470 of which 45% are women
locations	Hospital and (increasingly) community-based clinics

life						work
quiet on-call						busy on-call
boredom						burnout
uncompetitive						competitive
low salary						high salary

GP in a rural setting

Rural general practice brings holistic general medical skills to a new level beyond the urban settings to which so many specialties are bound. Some say it remains the only true form of traditional general practice, but it requires commitment and an independent mind.

the patients are fantastic and that's the point! The doctor is central to the community, whose members respect and care for the doctor who cares for them. Likewise, the doctor must consider the needs of the whole community as well as the individual patients within it. Patients may become friends and friends may become patients. The range of patients is diverse, including, perhaps, the Lord in his castle, the traveller in his caravan, tourists and eccentric characters with stories to tell. Medical practice can seem much calmer among people who live by the rhythm of the land and seasons.

the work All the variety of general practice but potentially in a beautiful location: perhaps a Scottish island, the Peak District or rural Wales. Many rural GP practices also function as the community pharmacy and liaise with a community hospital for rehabilitation medicine and care of the elderly. The teams are small so good working relationships are essential. In the absence of typical hospital hierarchies, all aspects of the work are inevitably shared. The GP is the leader of a small business, and some of the team may be their employees, but they will still have to take their turn at washing up!

the job Single-handed practice, though unusual elsewhere, is common in rural or remote settings. The job requires independence and self-reliance and it is important to build up peer networks for support and advice to avoid professional isolation. Emergency drills, regular skills courses and keeping up to date are now made much easier by video conferencing and e-learning. GP care continues in community hospitals which can provide a very satisfying balance.

extras In addition to the professional advantages of working in rural settings, living in the country can offer a very different lifestyle. Some locations may provide a safer environment with good schools for families, and some may offer eco-friendly living. Sailing, diving, canoeing, mountaineering, fishing, horse-riding, camping, ornithology and even smallholding can be a regular part of life, although time off can be a problem in remote practices. Undergraduate teaching and clinical research add academic interest. Doctors' spouses and families may be highly esteemed in remote communities.

ℹ **For further information:**

Royal College of General Practitioners, 14 Princes Gate, Hyde Park, London, SW7 1PU
Tel: 020 7581 3232   Fax: 020 7225 3047   Web: http://www.rcgp.org.uk

A day in the life ...

09:00	Check email and latest patient's results/letters
09:30	Booked GP consultations every 15 minutes
11:30	Coffee with community nursing team to discuss a palliative care patient
12:00	Ward round in community hospital. Talk to a city cardiologist about the management of a patient admitted with a MI at the weekend
13:00	Nip home for a quick lunch with the new medical student
13:45	Video conference to update management of paediatric emergencies with colleagues at the other end of the country
14:30	Booked GP consultations and emergency slots in parallel with the medical student. Plan to reassess a febrile child later.
16:00	Home visit to a farmer's wife who is dying at home from terminal cancer
17:00	Dictate referral letters. Plan the first aid course for the lifeboat crew.
18:00	Drop in to check febrile child on way home

myth	*Peak Practice!*
reality	Clinical generalist; key member of a self-contained community
personality	Independent, self-reliant and pragmatic
best aspects	True generalism and variety; sincere appreciation from individuals and the community; life in a beautiful, safe area
worst aspects	Living in a goldfish bowl where everyone knows the gossip
route	GP vocational training (p 32) and nMRCGP then a rural fellowship for the extra bits city GPs don't do
locations	England, Wales and Scotland all have some remote and rural general practice, but mostly Highlands and Islands of Scotland

life						work
quiet on-call						busy on-call
boredom						burnout
uncompetitive						competitive
low salary						high salary

GP with a special interest

A GP with a special interest (GPwSI, pronounced 'gypsy') is first and foremost a GP. The majority of their clinical time is spent doing the same types of clinics as other GPs, however some of their time is dedicated to specialist clinics. The specialist role is supported by hospital-based consultant colleagues. GPwSIs evolved to treat patients more quickly and conveniently and to save consultants time, enabling them to focus on the more complex cases. The GP can also bring a new dimension to the specialist role because they are an expert in community medicine and services. It is an opportunity to develop and use a special skill for increased job satisfaction.

the patients vary according to the chosen specialist interest. Many referrals come from other GPs who require specialist services to diagnose and manage the patient. Consultant colleagues will also refer patients; these tend to be patients with complex conditions who need a community-based specialist.

the work Likewise the nature of the work depends on the chosen specialty, but there is a wide range available. Specialist clinics (e.g. dermatology, gynaecology, substance misuse) often form the core of the work and the GP may be given direct access to operating lists or special investigations. In some specialties GPs perform diagnostic procedures, e.g. sigmoidoscopy, 24-hour blood pressure monitoring or minor surgery (e.g. hernia repairs, vasectomy, carpal tunnel release). With their community-based practice GPwSIs are also in an excellent position to work with multidisciplinary teams to manage chronic disorders (e.g. diabetes, palliative care, HIV).

the job Most GPwSIs spend one or two sessions a week in their specialist role as it is essential to maintain skills in traditional general practice. Like their general session, a GPwSI has full clinical responsibility for their specialist service. The location also varies; many work from their own surgery while others work in the hospital, especially if surgery or invasive procedures are required. The relationship with the hospital consultants is often built up over years, resulting in effective working relationships and good clinical support.

extras GPwSIs usually specialize in clinical specialties, but other possibilities include management, academic medicine or public health. A GPwSI's role also involves training, teaching and being a bridge between primary and secondary care.

ℹ️ *For further information:*

Royal College of General Practitioners, 14 Princes Gate, Hyde Park, London, SW7 1PU
Tel: 020 7581 3232   Fax: 020 7225 3047   Web: http://www.rcgp.org.uk
Association of Practitioners with Special Interests (APWSI), Rila Publications Ltd, 73 Newman Street, London, W1A 4PG
Tel: 020 7631 1299   Web: http://www.apwsi.co.uk
Search Department of Health website (http://www.dh.gov.uk) for 'Practitioners with special interests'

A day in the life ...

08:30	Meet with specialist nurse and supporting consultant to allocate patients attending hospital clinic to the most suitable professional
09:00	Clinic: seven patients with 20–30-minute appointments; mainly new patients with a couple of follow-ups; consultant on hand for problems
10:30	15-minute coffee break; discuss difficult cases, review results, sign letters
12:30	Finish seeing patients; review outcomes and triage new referrals
13:00	Rush back to practice to do home visits, lunch in the car on the way
15:00	Afternoon GP clinic: 20 patients with 8-minute appointments
18:00	Dictate letters and finish paperwork
18:30	Head home

myth	Frustrated consultant or GP with an inflated ego
reality	GP by name, GP by nature; all the fun/trials of GP life but with the interest of being a 'super GP' in a very narrow field
personality	Same qualities as a standard GP but with a passion for a specialty
best aspects	Doing that little bit more for the patient in primary care; empowering other GPs to have the confidence to do the same
worst aspects	Initial scepticism from GP and consultant colleagues; fear of failing so that other GPs and consultants will say 'I told you so'
route	GP vocational training (p 32) and nMRCGP to become an established GP; special interest accreditation route is defined by the Department of Health; specialties available vary between PCTs
locations	Depends on specialty and facilities needed; includes GP surgery, community hospital, private intermediate care centre and hospital

life		work
quiet on-call		busy on-call
boredom		burnout
uncompetitive		competitive
low salary		high salary

Gynaecological oncology

Gynaecological oncologists manage cancers of the female reproductive tract; this does not include breast cancer which is managed by breast surgeons (p 106). An attractive feature of the specialty is that it combines the hands-on practical skills of a surgical specialty with close collaboration with medical oncologists (p 196) and clinical oncologists (p 118), all working towards a common goal. It is the mixture of surgery, medicine and psychology which makes for high levels of satisfaction amongst practitioners, particularly since more than 50% of all cases are cured.

the patients are exclusively female. Like most cancers the incidence rises with age so a large number of the patients are elderly, though by no means all of them. They are usually referred by gynaecologists with the diagnosis of cancer having already been made. Prolonged continuity of care and intensive pre-op and post-op counselling lead to close clinical relationships.

the work The majority of the cancers are of the ovary, endometrium or cervix; less commonly the vagina, vulva and placenta may be involved. Even though they are often discussed as one group, they differ significantly in causes, detection, treatment and likelihood of cure. Diagnosis of cancer has serious psychological implications for the patient and her family and this presents challenges for the specialist. The primary role of a gynaecological oncologist is to perform complicated surgery to excise the cancers whilst limiting the damage to other pelvic organs. The surgery is often long (e.g. 3–4 hours) and difficult. In younger patients the issue of fertility can introduce complications.

the job Gynaecological oncologists practice in cancer centres, mostly based in teaching hospitals. The job is split between the operating theatre, outpatient clinics and the post-op patients on the ward. Patients benefit from management by highly experienced interdisciplinary treatment teams composed of gynaecological oncologists, therapeutic radiologists, medical oncologists, clinical oncologists, pathologists and nurse specialists. On-call is relatively mild since most problems are elective rather than acute.

extras The work is highly specialized in nature and most gynaecological oncologists are involved in research, ranging from studies in molecular genetics to clinical trials or surgical research. Consultants are expected to participate in the teaching of juniors and medical students. Private practice is available, but is less common than for general gynaecologists.

ⓘ *For further information:*

Royal College of Obstetricians and Gynaecologists, 27 Sussex Place, Regents Park, London, NW1 4RG
Tel: 020 7772 6200   Fax: 020 7723 0575   Web: http://www.rcog.org.uk

A day in the life ...

07:45	Ward round; most patients are recovering from major pelvic surgery
08:30	Theatre session: single case—a complicated total abdominal hysterectomy and salpingo-oophorectomy
13:00	Lunch, catch up with paperwork and emails
14:00	Multidisciplinary team meeting: each case is discussed in detail with input from oncologists, pathologists and radiologists
17:00	Ward round including a review of the patient from the morning list
18:00	Home to read latest research on treatments

myth	Extensive and mutilating surgery to delay the death sentence of a cancer diagnosis
reality	Individually tailored therapies give good chances for cure and many women retain their fertility; even those with incurable disease often have good quality of life for several years
personality	Ability to listen, sympathize and communicate effectively, excellent practical skills, boldness in surgery combined with compassion in the clinic
best aspects	Specialized field with great variety of skills and knowledge to acquire; enjoyment of working in a team
worst aspects	Physically and emotionally draining
route	ST1 Obstetrics and gynaecology (p 36) then subspecialty training in gynaecological oncology at ST6; MRCOG exam
numbers	200 of which 33% are women
locations	Hospital-based in teaching hospitals

life						work
quiet on-call						busy on-call
boredom						burnout
uncompetitive						competitive
low salary						high salary

Gynaecology

Gynaecology is an exciting career option for both men and women. The majority of consultant posts include a mixture of obstetrics (p 212) and gynaecology, however a small number of exclusive gynaecology jobs are available in tertiary centres. There are a number of subspecialties such as urogynaecology (p 282) and gynaecological oncology (p 154) that can be developed as special interests or full-time subspecialty posts in larger hospitals.

the patients include the complete age range of women, from children to teenagers to adults of reproductive age to postmenopausal and elderly women. Delivery of care must be modified according to each woman's individual needs, including religious beliefs and social attitudes. The job includes discussing sexual and reproductive problems; these can have relevance to male partners, so the job includes more frequent contact with men than many expect. Gynaecological conditions are diverse so a patient may be successfully treated in a single visit or may need long-term follow-up for years.

the work is a mixture of medical and surgical work. Common presentations include menstrual disorders, vaginal bleeding, pelvic pain, infections and urinary incontinence. Each of these can be caused by a number of conditions, however a careful history and examination can often yield the diagnosis and there are a wide range of treatments available. Gynaecologists also manage cancer of the reproductive tract, spontaneous miscarriages and sexual and reproductive difficulties, all of which require empathetic counselling skills. The majority of surgical work is elective, with a range of operations from the quick diagnostic laparoscopy to intricate and long cancer resections. On-call emergencies include vaginal bleeding and suspected ectopic pregnancies, both of which can be serious. Overall most of the patients are relatively well so the mortality rate is low.

the job is split roughly three ways between outpatient clinics (general and specialist), ward-based inpatient management and surgery (both elective and emergency). Outpatient clinics tend to be busy, however trainees can usually manage emergencies so on-call is relatively quiet. Consultants have regular contact with other health professionals including trainees, specialist nurses, anaesthetists and pathologists.

extras There are many opportunities to teach medical students and junior doctors. Subspecialty interests and research are encouraged and numerous training courses and conferences take place. Opportunities for private practice are ample and pay well. The specialty accommodates both flexible trainees and part-time consultants well.

ℹ️ For further information:

Royal College of Obstetricians and Gynaecologists, 27 Sussex Place, Regents Park, London, NW1 4RG
Tel: 020 7772 6200   Fax: 020 7723 0575   Web: http://www.rcog.org.uk

08:00 Ward round of post-op and sick patients followed by coffee with team

09:00 Outpatient clinic: mixture of new patients and follow-ups; two patients booked for theatre (prolapse repair and hysterectomy), one couple requiring investigation for subfertility and a range of common presentations

13:00 Called to emergency department to review a woman with a suspected ectopic pregnancy and moderate blood loss; advise on resuscitation

13:30 Surgical removal of Fallopian tube of woman with ectopic pregnancy followed by several elective cases

16:30 Teaching session with trainees

17:30 Review post-op patients

18:30 Home, on-call but should be able to manage with phone advice

myth	Endless hysterectomies and complaints about the menopause
reality	A combination of medicine and surgery that can make a real difference to the lives of women
personality	Good practical skills, empathetic, good communication skills, open-minded, calm in an emergency
best aspects	Rarity of mortality and morbidity in most of gynaecology
worst aspects	Ethical concerns with terminations of pregnancy
route	ST1 Obstetrics and gynaecology (p 36); MRCOG exam
numbers	3100 (combined with obstetrics) of which 33% are women
locations	Hospital-based in most hospitals

life					work
quiet on-call					busy on-call
boredom					burnout
uncompetitive					competitive
low salary					high salary

Haematology

Haematology is all about blood; since you can't live without blood, it is a vital specialty! Historically the specialty was purely laboratory-based but over the last 20 years the role has become fully clinical, although haematologists still supervise the laboratory and give advice about lab tests and blood transfusion (see Transfusion medicine, p 276). The outcomes for most haematological conditions are improving, with treatments being developed through greater understanding of the underlying disease processes. The specialty is highly innovative, with rapid translation from research to clinical use of many new drugs.

the patients Haematologists cover patients of all ages, including children. In areas with large African or Asian populations, the haemoglobinopathies (e.g. sickle cell, thalassaemia) can form a significant part of the workload. Many of the conditions are chronic so long-term clinical relationships can develop. Since haematological problems are commonly inherited the care often extends to the entire family.

the work The clinical work is split between malignant (haemato-oncology) and non-malignant haematology. Malignant conditions include leukaemia, lymphoma and myeloma along with stem-cell transplants (previously called bone marrow transplants). Non-malignant conditions are extremely varied ranging from clotting disorders (e.g. haemophilia, idiopathic thrombocytopaenia [ITP], thrombosis) to red cell disorders (anaemia, polycythaemia), haemoglobinopathies and white cell disorders. Haematologists also supervise the haematology and transfusion laboratories using clinical experience to interpret test results and advise on treatment. The routine laboratory work is done by biomedical scientists.

the job The job is split between inpatients, day treatment units, outpatient clinics and the laboratory, making for highly varied day-to-day work. Multidisciplinary team-working is important, particularly with biomedical scientists, nurse specialists, physios and social workers. Close liaison is also important with other specialties including joint clinics (e.g. obstetric haematology), radiology (diagnostic imaging and vascular access) and histopathology and cytogenetics (interpretation of bone marrow samples and accurate classification of leukaemias and lymphomas). On-call can be busy but is mostly handled over the phone.

extras There are many opportunities for research during training and most larger departments have academic haematologists. Much of the research is translational, i.e. converting research into clinical applications. Alongside the research there are numerous conferences and many chances for teaching. Subspecialization is common in larger centres. Private practice is virtually non-existent outside London.

🛈 *For further information:*

British Society for Haematology, 100 White Lion Street, London, N1 9PF
Tel: 020 7713 0990   Web: http://www.b-s-h.org.uk

08:30	Arrive at work; check there were no disasters in the lab or on the ward overnight
09:00	Ward round: review inpatients
11:00	Laboratory: looking at blood films or reporting other tests; phone call from a surgeon about a patient bleeding in theatre: give advice on haemostatic support
12:00	Go to day unit to review patients or examine a bone marrow sample
13:00	Grab lunch and attend a multidisciplinary team meeting
14:00	Outpatient clinic
16:00	Dictate letters, answer emails and check all is ok on the ward and in the lab
18:00	Back home, though can be later on busy days or if on-call

myth	Vampires who prefer microscopes, blood films and coagulation cascades to patients
reality	Highly varied clinical work with regular direct patient contact and the added dimension of supervising a laboratory; the coagulation cascade can actually be quite interesting once it becomes clinically relevant
personality	Good communicator, team player, calm in an emergency (e.g. severe bleeding requiring rapid haemostatic support), academic
best aspects	Being at the centre of hospital life with regular interaction with most specialties; great variety so that most find a niche that suits them
worst aspects	Some patients go through a lot of intensive treatments but ultimately don't survive, though overall survival rates are improving
route	CT1 Core medical training (p 34) followed by ST3 Haematology; MRCP and FRCPath exams; alternative route via paediatrics
numbers	1200 of which 40% are women
locations	Hospital-based specialty, found in all hospitals

life						work
quiet on-call						busy on-call
boredom						burnout
uncompetitive						competitive
low salary						high salary

Hand surgery

Hand surgery covers the hand, wrist and elbow, without which we can't work, play or gesticulate. So many things can happen including birth defects, injury, arthritis, nerve compression, tumours and work-related pain. Disorders are common: over 20% of trauma in the emergency department includes a hand injury, 1 in 500 babies are born with a hand defect and 1 in 30 people get a nerve compression syndrome during their lives. Anyone from a goalkeeper to a violinist can have their work or hobbies curtailed by a hand problem; hand surgeons do their best to give people their lives back.

the patients are referred from a wide mixture of sources including paediatricians, emergency departments, GPs and sports clubs. Some patients enter the hand surgeon's realm only briefly (e.g. a simple injury that is promptly fixed); others require a year or two of treatment and follow up (e.g. a complex injury or widespread arthritis); yet others are patients for ever (e.g. those with rheumatoid arthritis).

the work Despite its small size, the complexity of the hand makes the surgery extremely diverse. On a daily basis injuries are repaired, arthritic joints (fingers, wrist and elbow) are replaced, tight nerves are released, the inside of the wrist or elbow is inspected endoscopically and tight tendons or joints are freed. Most patients do very well and the gratitude of a patient who can get back to their work or hobby is priceless.

the job A hand surgeon's time is distributed roughly equally between clinic, theatre and administration/research. The intensity of on-call varies greatly between working practices in different Trusts: it is usually light if the service only covers hand surgery but much more onerous if participating in the general orthopaedic or plastic surgery rotas. Hand surgeons interact with many other specialties (e.g. orthopaedics, rheumatology, paediatrics and neurology). The most important relationship is with the hand therapist, a physiotherapist dedicated to disorders of the hand; many patients improve with therapy alone and it is essential after an operation to restore function.

extras Hand surgery has a thriving academic base; there are regular scientific meetings and instructional courses along with two dedicated research journals. Flexible training is available and many hand surgery trainees are female. There are also good opportunities for making money in private practice because people treasure their hands and will pay for the best advice. Furthermore people with injuries will need a medicolegal report to support their claim for compensation.

ⓘ *For further information:*

The BSSH awards two £760 bursaries to medical students doing an elective in hand surgery units

British Society for Surgery of the Hand, Royal College of Surgeons, 35–43 Lincoln's Inn Fields, London, WC2A 3PN

Tel: 0207 831 5162   Fax: 0207 831 4041   Web: http://www.bssh.ac.uk

A day in the life ...

07:45	Pre-operative assessment and consent of patients due for surgery today
08:30	Start operating list: diverse range of patients and operations
13:00	Finish operating list: review post-op patients and let them know how well it went
13:30	Travel to clinic in community setting
14:00	Hand clinic, alongside hand therapy team and trainees
17:00	Finish clinic
18:00	Private practice or a well-deserved night off with the kids
21:00	Finish private practice or send kids to bed; have a well-deserved (rest of) night off with the spouse

myth	The cream of orthopaedic and plastic surgeons
reality	The cream of orthopaedic and plastic surgeons
personality	Calm, organized, meticulous, thoughtful, excellent fine manipulative skills, perfectionist
best aspects	A broad spectrum of work; usually able to make big differences to patients; good opportunities for private practice
worst aspects	Poor initial treatment causing problems later; on-calls can be very busy if covering orthopaedics; extremely competitive
route	CT1 Surgery in general, trauma and orthopaedic surgery or plastic surgery then ST3 Trauma and orthopaedic surgery or plastic surgery (p 48); MRCS exam
numbers	300 (far fewer are 'pure' hand surgeons)
locations	Hospital-based from district general hospitals to regional plastic surgery centres

life		work
quiet on-call		busy on-call
boredom		burnout
uncompetitive		competitive
low salary		high salary

Histopathology

Histopathology is one of the most varied and intellectually challenging branches of medicine. A pathological investigation plays a part in over 70% of health care decisions including making a diagnosis or choosing a treatment, so there is huge scope for influencing patient management. The role of a histopathologist is to diagnose disease processes through the examination of tissues (from biopsies or surgical resections). The specialty is intimately associated with almost all specialties from surgery to paediatrics to primary care, often providing the definitive diagnosis in a huge variety of diseases.

the patients For most histopathologists there is no direct patient contact, however the samples that are processed come from patients of all ages, genders and backgrounds. Furthermore the sample can come from any site in the body. Sound clinical knowledge is essential since it is the combination of the tissue appearance with the clinical details that enables an accurate diagnosis to be made. Some histopathologists also practice cytopathology (analysis of the cells rather than tissues, often used to diagnose cancer) which may involve performing the fine needle aspiration (FNA) to obtain the cell sample themselves.

the work The majority of the workload is examining surgical specimens and medical biopsies to help make a diagnosis. The variety of cases is wide-ranging from simple diagnostic biopsies to complex cancer resection specimens; like any specialty the variety is greater in teaching hospitals where complex cases are more likely to be managed. The provision of rapid intra-operative diagnosis is often requested for unexpected findings during surgery, essentially emergency pathology. Post-mortems are also performed by histopathologists, usually for the Coroner in order to determine a cause of death, however, this is a minor component of the job for many.

the job Histopathologists spend most of their time working in a pathology laboratory (though this often looks like an office with microscopes). Many are specialists in certain areas, such as dermatopathology, or gastrointestinal pathology. Histopathology is key to many diagnoses, especially cancer, so histopathologists work closely with all types of surgeons and many other clinicians throughout the hospital and in primary care. They routinely participate in, or lead, multidisciplinary team meetings in surgery and oncology.

extras There is ample opportunity for research and teaching alongside the diagnostic work. Subspecialization is possible in larger centres (e.g. paediatric pathology and neuropathology). Flexible training is well-established. Private practice is widely available and it is possible to do this on a flexible basis, even at home!

🛈 *For further information:*

The Royal College of Pathologists, 2 Carlton House Terrace, London, SW1Y 5AF
Tel: 020 7451 6700 Fax: 020 7451 6701 Web: http://www.rcpath.org

08:30	MDT meeting of recent cases with surgeons, radiologists and oncologists
10:00	Surgical cut-up; examination and tissue sampling from the surgical specimens sent from theatre including a colectomy specimen from a patient with carcinoma, skin excision biopsies and a kidney from a patient with an undiagnosed tumour
13:00	Grand round; presentation of the histopathology findings in a liver biopsy from a patient with previously undiagnosed Wilson's disease
15:30	Reporting of slides from the previous day's cut-up and biopsies
16:30	Call from theatre asking for a frozen section diagnosis on an unexpected liver nodule in a patient undergoing a colectomy; accurate diagnosis is essential as the interpretation may result in the operation being aborted due to metastases
16:45	Good news, not a metastasis; phone theatre then back to reporting
17:45	Home to enjoy the freedom of life without on-call

myth	Histopathologists live in the mortuary, only let out in the dead of night to visit the recently deceased with the police
reality	Autopsy is usually a minor part of the job and the police work with forensic pathologists (p 138); the key job of the histopathologist is in diagnosing the living—a vital and interesting role
personality	Academic, good visual skills, excellent general medical knowledge, communication skills are still important for liaising with other clinicians
best aspects	Variety of work and diagnostic challenges; 9–5 working week with limited on-call allowing an excellent work–life balance
worst aspects	Low pay as a trainee (no on-call); lack of direct patient contact
route	ST1 Histopathology (p 40); FRCPath exam
numbers	1900 of which 40% are women
locations	Hospital-based, present in majority of hospitals

life					work
quiet on-call					busy on-call
boredom					burnout
uncompetitive					competitive
low salary					high salary

Homeopathic medicine

Homeopathic medicine is a job for generalists who are prepared to be a bit different. There are two basic premises to homeopathy: first that illness should be treated with a substance that replicates the symptoms, secondly that these substances should be extremely diluted. Across the board about two-thirds of those treated claim a benefit to an extent that it makes a difference to their daily lives. As a holistic form of practice, homeopathy makes no clear distinction between physical and mental health problems. This is a job which involves a lot of empathic listening; those who love listening to people's stories will love this job.

the patients Patients of all ages come for homeopathic treatment. All of them have chronic problems and most of them have already tried conventional treatments without success so the homeopath is their last resort. Some patients come for homeopathic treatment because they believe in 'alternative medicine' and may be taking a wide range of 'natural' medicines with which they will expect the homeopath to be intimately familiar. Others may be trying a complementary therapy for the first time.

the work Homeopaths deal with a great range of conditions including children with asthma, elderly patients with arthritis, women with PMT and people of all ages with illnesses which are hard to categorize. Consultations follow a similar format to other areas of medicine including history and examination followed by treatment in the form of a homeopathic remedy.

the job Homeopathy is mostly clinic-based, usually in community-based clinics or the outpatient departments of hospitals. There are five dedicated homeopathic hospitals (e.g. The Royal London Homoeopathic Hospital) with either day bed or full-time inpatient wards. Homeopathic consultations are often long, typically an hour for new patient consultations and 15–20 minutes for follow-up visits. Continuity of care is important and individual patients usually see the same doctor throughout their treatment. Homeopathic hospitals usually offer a range of complementary therapies such as acupuncture (p 96) and/or herbal medicine. The specialty does not run an on-call service.

extras All five homeopathic hospitals are centres for teaching and research into homeopathy. Many homeopathic specialists do private practice work, plenty of which is available. Many practitioners use homeopathy alongside conventional medicine (e.g. a GP with a weekly homeopathy clinic).

ⓘ *For further information:*

The Faculty of Homeopathy, Hahnemann House, 29 Park Street West, Luton, LU1 3BE
Tel: 0870 444 3950   Fax: 0870 444 3960   Web: http://www.trusthomeopathy.org

A day in the life ...

09:00   Clinic appointment lasting one hour with a new patient presenting with recurrent abdominal pain without a diagnosis despite numerous investigations

10:00   Follow-up appointments lasting 20-minutes covering a wide range of conditions from arthritis to tiredness

12:30   Time for lunch and catch up with colleagues

13:00   Case conference

14:00   Teaching medical students, doctors or nurses

16:00   Telephone consultations, admin work, research or management meetings

18:00   Home to put your feet up and relax with your family!

myth	New Age mystics using diluted placebos
reality	Pragmatic generalists, filling the effectiveness gaps in conventional medicine with harmless medicines which act differently from placebos
personality	Incredibly enthusiastic, passionate doctors, with great empathic skills and an insatiable love of learning
best aspects	Having the opportunities to really get to know patients and using medicines which cause no harm
worst aspects	Being dismissed by anti-homeopathy colleagues as a quack
route	Homeopathic medicine is not a recognized specialty in the UK; most practitioners train in conventional medicine (GP or hospital specialist) then take the Faculty of homeopathy membership exam
numbers	About 2000 registered practitioners (both doctors and non-doctors); number of unregistered homeopaths is unknown
locations	GP surgeries, community clinics, private practice and five UK NHS homeopathic hospitals

life						work
quiet on-call						busy on-call
boredom						burnout
uncompetitive						competitive
low salary						high salary

Immunology

Immunologists provide diagnostic tests and treatment for patients with a wide range of immunological diseases. Recent progress in immunology has been extremely rapid, both in terms of the understanding of diseases and the treatments available (e.g. monoclonal antibodies); sadly the progress of diseases has also been rapid, with the emergence of HIV. Like haematologists (p 158), immunologists run a diagnostic laboratory service alongside direct clinical practice. Immunologists need to stay abreast of the 'basic science' in order to work in this rapidly moving discipline.

the patients are usually those with multisystem diseases such as immune deficiency and vasculitis or specifically immune-mediated diseases such as allergy. The immune deficiency and vasculitis patients have chronic diseases and are often on ongoing complex treatments, for example immunoglobulin replacement. This means they build a close therapeutic relationship which is sustained over many years. Allergy patients may be seen as one-off episodes or managed by specialist nurses. More complex allergy cases need longer-term, consultant-led management. Some immunologists have a paediatric background, but most only see children in clinics shared with paediatricians.

the work is a mixture of clinical treatment and overseeing laboratory testing. Immunologists are in a privileged position since they are responsible for carrying out the tests on the patients directly under their care. As a result they get to know their patients on a cellular level as well as on a personal level. Immunology centres are almost always based in teaching hospitals and immunologists are usually active teachers.

the job The majority of clinical work is in outpatient clinics two or three times a week; occasionally patients may need admitting, but inpatient care is often shared with another team (e.g. respiratory medicine). There is no on-call work. Immunologists usually work in centres with at least two immunology specialists along with specialist nurses to assist in the clinical work and biomedical scientists and clinical scientists who perform much of the day-to-day laboratory work. Good communication skills are crucial working in this large multidisciplinary team with a broad range of patients.

extras Immunology lends itself to research which can be either basic science or clinical; trainees are encouraged to do an MD or PhD. There are many immunology conferences, often in interesting destinations around the world. Flexible working is possible and fits in easily with training. For those with the time, extra cash can be made through private practice (mainly allergy-focused) or working with pharmaceutical companies.

ℹ️ *For further information:*

British Society for Allergy and Clinical Immunology, 17 Doughty Street, London, WC1N 2PL
Tel: 020 7404 0278   Fax: 020 7404 0280   Web: http://www.bsaci.org

08:00	Read about the use of gene therapy in children with hereditary immunodeficiency
09:00	Immune deficiency clinic; most of the patients are well-known follow-ups, but it's always good to have some new referrals to work up
12:00	Pop into medical admissions unit to see a lady admitted with severe anaphylaxis on the way back to the lab
13:00	Lab has just diagnosed acute leukaemia in a young man; phone the local haematologist with the bad news
16:00	Teleconference with pharmaceutical company about new treatment for inflammatory bowel disease
17:00	Take some MSc exam papers home to mark

myth	Boffins who play with antibodies and never leave the lab
reality	Immunologists provide patient-centred care for patients with complex, life-long illnesses—despite playing with antibodies
personality	Energetic, inquisitive, academic, attention to detail
best aspects	Having to keep abreast of science; complex diseases
worst aspects	Financial constraints mean that it's not always possible to use the newest emergent technologies
route	CT1 Core medical training (p 34) then ST3 Immunology; MRCP and FRCPath (Immunology) exams; alternative route via paediatrics
numbers	130 of which 25% are women
locations	Teaching hospitals

life		work
quiet on-call		busy on-call
boredom		burnout
uncompetitive		competitive
low salary		high salary

Infectious diseases and tropical medicine

Infectious diseases and tropical medicine (IDTM) is second to none for variety and job satisfaction. The IDTM consultant needs thorough experience of acute medical illness, a knowledge of general internal medicine and training in microbiology and virology, immunology, parasitology and therapeutics. Unsurprisingly the training is long and since there is no unique procedure (e.g. endoscopy), private practice earnings will be comparatively low. Expect to be older, wiser and poorer than colleagues, but richer in experience.

the patients The typical patient is young and previously fit, often from overseas (e.g. refugees), so there is a very broad range of ethnic backgrounds and English language ability. Patients are referred from medical admission units (the most exciting patients from acute general medicine, i.e. previously well but with life-threatening infections) or from GPs with less urgent pathology. The relationships forged with most patients and their families will be intense, brief and very satisfying. There is longer continuity of care with patients with chronic infections such as tuberculosis (6–12 months' treatment) and HIV/AIDS (lifelong treatment).

the work ranges from the hyperacute to the diagnostic puzzle. IDTM physicians may be called to the emergency department to manage acutely feverish and septicaemic patients with life-threatening infections such as meningitis. With correct management many of these patients can make a full recovery. Less acute problems include enlarged lymph nodes, swollen joints, rashes, diarrhoea and fevers. These require a systematic and holistic approach, especially since anxiety, depression and fatigue often obscure the true problem or may be the problem itself. Other key presentations include the immunocompromised (e.g. HIV, leukaemia or taking steroids) and colleagues with needle-stick injuries.

the job Work is split between outpatient clinics and wards. Some specialists also mix laboratory research (e.g. molecular biology, parasitology, immunology) with clinical work. Close relationships are maintained with other specialists, especially microbiologists and radiologists; there is a healthy challenge to diagnose patients who have puzzled organ-based specialist colleagues but also the need to seek their expert opinion. On-call is hands-on and busy much of the time.

extras It is a misconception that IDTM physicians can spend their career working six months in the UK and six months abroad; no NHS hospital would tolerate this. Wanderlust is generally satisfied by research projects in the field or working as an overseas doctor (p 220) during a break from training. Subspecialty training (e.g. immunocompromise) is possible in larger centres. Flexible training is difficult to arrange, especially due to the long training required and busy nature of the job. There is some private practice.

ⓘ For further information:

Royal College of Physicians, 11 St Andrew's Place, Regent's Park, London, NW1 4LE
Tel: 020 7935 1174   Fax: 020 7487 5218   Website: http://www.rcplondon.ac.uk

A day in the life ...

08:00 Review the overnight admissions; assess the worryingly ill patients

09:00 Outpatients: urinary infections, complicated pneumonia, tuberculosis, Lyme disease, schistosomiasis, more tuberculosis, sarcoidosis, infected diabetic toe, chronic fatigue syndrome

13:00 No time for lunch, ward round with junior doctors and students, then ITU and ward referrals; get advice from microbiologist; ask radiologist to do biopsy

17:00 Check emails, write manuscript of clinical study in Sudan, see staff nurse who has stuck her finger with a needle in emergency department

19:00 Go home satisfied and grateful not to have caught drug-resistant TB yet

myth	Glamorous international experts who spend months abroad fighting Ebola outbreaks then return to the NHS when they want
reality	An NHS-based specialty with long training and long hours but excellent job satisfaction
personality	Must love hands-on clinical work and also like laboratory work; generalist, academic, calm in an emergency
best aspects	The diagnostic challenge; curing acutely ill patients; lots of teaching; overseas contacts; overlaps with other specialties
worst aspects	Very long training; busy on-calls; almost no private practice prospects
route	CT1 Core medical training (p 34) then ST3 Infectious diseases or topical medicine; MRCP exam; Diploma in tropical medicine and hygiene and PhD/MD also help
numbers	320 of which 25% are women
locations	Hospital-based in larger district general hospitals and teaching hospitals

life					work
quiet on-call					busy on-call
boredom					burnout
uncompetitive					competitive
low salary					high salary

Intensive care

Intensive care is a young specialty, arising in the 1950s with ventilator development, but expanding rapidly with advances in monitoring, organ support and pharmacological treatments. Dealing with the sickest patients in the hospital makes it one of the most challenging, exciting, and occasionally stressful, careers. Most intensive care doctors initially train in anaesthesia, medicine, emergency medicine or general surgery and may continue to work in these specialties too.

the patients All patients are very sick from a disease process, trauma or following surgery. Admissions comprise unplanned emergencies or elective postoperative surgical cases requiring invasive monitoring and organ support. The elderly account for the majority of admissions. Since many patients are ventilated and sedated, communication is limited, but there is intense contact with families.

the work Patients can be referred from any hospital-based specialty, anywhere in the hospital, at any time, with any number of failing organs. Accordingly the range of clinical scenarios is broad and the workload unpredictable. The main objective is to support and optimize the function of failing organs using mechanical and pharmacological support, aided by monitoring systems to follow the patient's progress. Good knowledge of physiology and pharmacology is essential. Patient care also involves practical procedures including intubations, central lines, arterial lines, chest drains and percutaneous tracheostomies. Despite best efforts intensive care mortality is 10–20%, depending on the case mix. Sometimes difficult decisions are made about limiting or withdrawing organ support in patients who fail to respond to treatment, or in whom further support is deemed futile.

the job is based on the intensive care unit with ward reviews of potential admissions. Intensive care beds are an expensive and limited resource so juggling beds is a common problem with prompt discharge of patients once they are well enough. Transfers to other intensive care units happen occasionally due to lack of space or for specialist care. The job involves frequent contact with other specialties and health professionals including the referring team (who usually share care), consultant specialists, physiotherapists, technicians, dieticians, pharmacists and microbiologists. Close working relationships are also needed with the specialist nursing staff, who are vital to each patient's well-being as they care for only one or two patients each shift and are the best monitor of the patient, along with providing continuous care.

extras In between looking after the intensive care unit, consultants return to work in their base specialty (e.g. anaesthetics, acute medicine), undertake research and often teach. There is no scope for private practice, but flexible training is possible. Subspecialization is possible in regional centres with separate intensive care units for cardiac, neurosurgical and paediatric patients.

🛈 *For further information:*

The Intensive Care Society, Churchill House, 35 Red Lion Square, London, WC1R 4SG
Tel: 020 7280 4350   Fax: 020 7280 4369   Web: http://www.ics.ac.uk

08:00	Handover from the previous night; assess bed availability and plan for elective post-operative admissions
09:00	Review patients on intensive care, optimizing care and planning interventions
11:00	Teaching ward round
13:00	Book CT/USS scans
14:00	Review patient on the ward—intubate and ventilate on the ward, insert central line and transfer to intensive care
15:00	Speak to relatives
16:00	Transfer ventilated patient for CT scan accompanied by a specialist nurse
17:00	Informal ward round—make plans for the night
18:00	Admit elective admission from theatre following major surgery
20:00	Hand over to the night team

myth	Playing God in the 'Expensive Scare Unit'
reality	Using sophisticated tools to optimize treatment of the sickest patients
personality	Decisive, realistic, action-orientated, calm in an emergency, good practical skills, communication skills (for relatives), team player
best aspects	Bringing patients back from the brink of death
worst aspects	Realizing that you cannot save them all; bed management
route	CT1 Acute care common stem, anaesthetics (p 28) then ST3 Anaesthetics; FRCS exam alternative route via other acute specialties
numbers	225 (as their main specialty) of which 12% are women
locations	Hospital-based in most district general hospitals and teaching hospitals

life						work
quiet on-call						busy on-call
boredom						burnout
uncompetitive						competitive
low salary						high salary

Journalism and medical writing

Only a lunatic would go into medicine with the idea of becoming a journalist; despite their handwriting many doctors can write well and a few try to extend this beyond patients' notes. Sir Arthur Conan Doyle, the ophthalmologist who wrote Sherlock Holmes, is a classic example. Most medical writers do a modest amount of journalism alongside their medical duties and earn a few thousand pounds a year from this (certainly much less than equivalent time spent in private practice). A few manage to make writing/journalism a full-time job, with clinical medicine a part-time 'hobby'. For a select few, appearances on TV or regular features in newspapers can make them 'household names' (e.g. Dr Hilary Jones and Dr Phil Hammond), earning over £150 000 a year.

getting started Nearly everyone starts by offering articles to medical newspapers and magazines, particularly the three GPs' weeklies: *Pulse*, *Doctor* and *General Practitioner*. It is important to pick a subject that is of interest and at the right level for the readership. The subject will usually be an area of personal interest and specialization. After cutting one's teeth on such publications there is the possibility of submitting to more generalist publications (e.g. via the feature editors of a mother and baby magazine or various well women publications). Most medical journalists learn their craft through trial and error, including the (often) constructive comments of those who turn down their efforts. Regrettably, a high proportion of early pieces are likely to be rejected, but training in medicine prepares you for hard work and occasional disappointment. There are courses in medical journalism (e.g. City University, London), but very few doctors have the time to take them.

the work For the great majority of doctor journalists the work will be getting the odd article into print when they have time away from clinical activities to write it. A few, with a terrific drive to write and incredible persistence, may manage to turn out over a million words a year (that's about 2000 to 3000 pages). The writing can range from specialist articles for medical journals to humorous pieces for newspapers to TV scripts or books. Much of the work entails sitting in front of a computer screen at home or researching the topic on the Internet or in journals. Those who have the ability to produce accurate articles quickly on a wide variety of subjects can do very well. A doctor working for a national newspaper may be expected to produce an accurate, readable article on almost any medical subject at half an hour's notice.

extra Opportunities for writing and journalism are expanding, as are the range of media (particularly websites). It is difficult to make a full-time living this way, but for those who enjoy writing it can be a very rewarding experience.

ⓘ *For further information:*
Medical Journalists Association: http://www.mja-uk.org

A day in the life ...

09:00 Morning clinic

13:00 Lunch with the computer finding the latest information for an article on managing children with a fever for a parenting magazine

14:00 Afternoon clinic

17:00 Home, turn on the computer and start writing the article; important to make the advice safe, but also understandable to a lay audience

19:00 Meal with family

20:00 Back to writing; eventually finish the article and print it for proof-reading tomorrow morning before sending it to a paediatrician for review

To be a 'star,' you really do have to make a decision to spend at least eight hours a day at the keyboard.

But the average medically-qualified journalist is more likely to spend half an hour per day in writing—after finishing her daily toils in general or hospital practice.

myth	Doctors who lounge around all day waiting for a TV interview or occasionally writing a quick article
reality	Mostly full-time clinical specialists who write in their free time; writing is a slow and complex process that requires practice
personality	Fairly extrovert, great love of words, persistent, committed, able to present information in a clear way, empathetic
best aspects	Seeing your stuff in print; seeing someone else reading it
worst aspects	The difficulties in getting paid; rejections from publishers; competition from non-doctor journalists working full-time
route	Initial training in a medical specialty to provide expertise and experience; developing writing skills alongside clinical ones
numbers	About 200, but only a handful work full-time as a journalist
locations	Mostly at home, in front of a computer

life					**work**
quiet on-call					**busy on-call**
boredom					**burnout**
uncompetitive					**competitive**
low salary					**high salary**

Locuming

Locum work is temporary work to fill a gap on a hospital's rota (due to training, sickness, maternity leave, etc.). Duration ranges from one shift to many months. Most doctors will do some locum shifts, often alongside a full-time clinical job (to earn extra money) or alongside a research job (for clinical experience and extra money). It is also a useful option for gaps between jobs (e.g. returning from abroad, unsuccessful ST applications). A small minority choose to work as a 'career locum' due to the freedom, flexibility and relatively high rates of pay; this is also possible abroad, e.g. in Australia or New Zealand (p 69).

the patients Locums can take place in any specialty and almost any hospital so the patients are highly variable. Unsurprisingly this results in almost no continuity of care, which can be a good or bad thing.

the work also varies between specialties and hospitals. Generally the locum is expected to perform the same role as the permanent doctor at the equivalent grade, i.e. a junior doctor with four years experience in general medicine would be expected to do the same job as a CT1–CT2 doctor working there. Like any doctor, locums are expected to consult seniors if they need advice and colleagues/nursing staff for help with the hospital systems (e.g. how to refer a patient). Locums usually do not get training apart from advice on specific cases encountered through the work.

the job Most locums find work through an agency (registration takes a few weeks) or are offered shifts by their own Trust. One of the hardest aspects is dealing with the different systems in each hospital. Almost every one has its own unique computer system for viewing results and sometimes X-rays; furthermore, systems for referring to specialties also vary as do bleep systems, door codes, computer access codes, etc. This can be extremely frustrating, as everything takes longer, and challenging, as it forces doctors to work with unfamiliar protocols. Locums are usually employed to cover specific shifts and are paid by the hour. Many of the jobs offered tend to be antisocial (e.g. evenings, nights and weekends), but it is possible to get contracts for a few months.

extras Locum pay is usually higher than equivalent full-time posts, but there is no paid annual leave, sick leave, study leave, indemnity or pension. Hourly rates and travel costs are negotiable. A few locum agencies have arrangements for funding training courses for those who work many hours for them. The locum has the advantage of choosing when and where they work but is limited by the work available; there are some travel options (e.g. locums in Jersey or the Isle of Man) which often include the cost of a flight.

ⓘ *For further information:*

Medacs Doctors (Locum Agency), FREEPOST BD2364, The Old Surgery, 49 Otley Street, Skipton, North Yorkshire, BD23 1BR
Tel: 0800 442200   Fax: 0800 442220   Web: http://www.medacs.com
NHS Professionals (NHS Locum Agency): http://www.nhsprofessionals.nhs.uk

A day in the life ...

08:45	Arrive on time despite busy traffic and hour drive; try to find parking space
09:00	Find the personnel department/switchboard for bleep and directions
09:15	Arrive on ward, introduced to colleagues, shown computer system
09:30	Start clerking patients; asking colleagues frequent questions about where to find equipment and how to get results; all the variety of any medical job
11:00	Called to emergency department to review 19-year-old with Marfan's and chest pain; diagnose aortic dissection; call surgeons to arrange immediate surgery
13:00	Mini ward round and review/discuss findings with patients
13:30	Quick lunch; try to calculate pay per mouthful
14:00	Outpatient clinic: 8–12 patients alongside seniors
17:00	End of shift; get timesheet signed and head home

myth	A medical mercenary
reality	Provide an essential service, but often not respected by interviewers
personality	Patience, flexibility to work in changing environments, good at following instructions, enjoys travelling, good navigation skills
best aspects	Great variety; chance to see different working practices; flexibility
worst aspects	Limited teaching; work does not count towards training; learning new working practices; no job security; having to prove abilities repeatedly
route	Increased experience and training make job finding easier; training courses help (e.g. ALS); membership exams are a great asset
locations	Almost any specialty, almost anywhere in the country

life						work
quiet on-call						busy on-call
boredom						burnout
uncompetitive						competitive
low salary						high salary

Maternal and fetal medicine

Any doctor can manage a patient, but only a select few can manage two at once. Maternal and fetal medicine focuses on illnesses that affect pregnant women and/or their unborn babies. It is therefore one of the most diverse jobs in medicine. Doctors working in this subspecialty are trained in practices such as using ultrasound to visualize the second patient, the fetus. They also attend specialist clinics, often with specialist physicians, to manage women with pre-existing health care disorders in their pregnancies.

the patients are women of reproductive age (about 15 to 45 years) and their babies (from before conception to after birth). It is this combination of patients that makes the job so interesting. The mother undergoes marked changes in physiology during pregnancy which can affect pre-existing medical problems, whilst the fetus may be affected by the maternal condition or may have problems of its own. The management of both patients is often inextricably intertwined and careful counselling and descriptive skills are often required to explain problems and treatments to prospective parents.

the work There are three main scenarios: (1) women with pre-existing illnesses (e.g. heart disease, renal disease) embarking on pregnancies which pose risks to them and challenges to their doctors. The role of the maternal and fetal specialist is to advise on the feasibility of a successful pregnancy and then provide specialist obstetric care through the pregnancy alongside a medical specialist in the relevant condition (e.g. cardiology). (2) New onset of maternal illnesses during pregnancy; these can be in any system so a broad knowledge of medicine is essential. (3) Illness or malformation in the fetus including poor growth and rhesus incompatibility disease; some problems require fetal therapy (e.g. blood transfusions) or even surgery. The use of ultrasound to visualize the fetus in utero has revolutionized management and this is a key skill of the job.

the job is split between outpatient clinics, focused on maternal and/or fetal health, and high-risk obstetrics, which is the management of labour in the presence of increased risks to the mother and/or fetus. The specialty is very senior-led and consultants have a hands-on approach leading to busy on-calls. Specialists work as part of a multidisciplinary team including paediatricians, clinical geneticists, surgeons and midwives. Good communication between these teams is vital for optimal patient management.

extras Teaching and research opportunities are plentiful and trainees are encouraged to undertake a research project. Flexible training is well established and respected. Private practice is somewhat limited, especially compared to the rest of obstetrics and gynaecology.

ⓘ *For further information:*

British Maternal and Fetal Medicine Society, 27 Sussex Place, Regent's Park, London, NW1 4RG
Tel: 020 7772 6211   Fax: 020 7772 6410   Web: http://www.bmfms.org.uk

08:00 Antenatal ward review and delivery suite handover from night team

09:00 Outpatient clinic: either specialist antenatal clinic or ultrasound clinic

13:00 Postgraduate meeting: highly specialized discussion of an aspect of pregnancy with multidisciplinary team

15:00 Lead consultant on delivery suite: regular reviews of the management of women who are in labour or delivering; requires constant care, vigilance and team work

16:30 Review of patients on the antenatal wards

17:00 Handover to evening team

myth	A career for those who can't choose between paediatrics and obstetrics and gynaecology
reality	Challenging and emotionally charged specialty helping women through difficult pregnancies
personality	Calm, approachable, team player, academic, excellent communication skills, good visual skills
best aspects	Great variety of conditions in both the mother and unborn baby; successful births in complex cases; flexible training options
worst aspects	High emotional content; failure can be catastrophic; babies do not know the difference between night and day
route	ST1 Obstetrics and gynaecology (p 36) then subspecialty training in Maternal and fetal medicine at ST6; MRCOG exam
numbers	270 of which 33% are women
locations	Hospital-based in teaching hospitals and a few larger district general hospitals

life						work
quiet on-call						busy on-call
boredom						burnout
uncompetitive						competitive
low salary						high salary

Maxillofacial surgery

Maxillofacial surgery offers an exciting and challenging career. It is a surgical specialty concerned with the diagnosis and treatment of disorders affecting the face, jaws, mouth and neck. Disorders of the face and jaws affect appearance, social interactions, speech, ability to eat and quality of life. The face is the only part of the body that is not easy to hide, so both the surgeon and the patient will be judged on the scars. The specialty covers generalists in district general hospitals to surgeons with a subspecialty interest working in tertiary centres.

the patients Maxillofacial surgery covers all ages from neonates to the elderly and this diversity in age is reflected in the conditions treated. Specialists tend to see a higher proportion of younger patients than many other surgical specialties. The patients can come from any ethnic or social background. Many of them are relatively healthy apart from their maxillofacial problem.

the work The maxillofacial surgeon's role is to diagnose and manage conditions in the soft and hard tissues of the face. These vary with age: children are treated for facial deformity and cleft palette/lip disorders; young adults often present with facial trauma following sporting accidents, drinking accidents or assault; the elderly often present with cancer, particularly oral cancer which is the sixth most common cancer in men. Other common problems include salivary gland disease, facial deformity, dentoalveolar problems and oral medicine disorders. The surgery is often long and complicated; the face has limited 'spare tissue' so it is essential to correct the problem with the least damage possible. There is wide scope for reconstructive techniques including free microvascular tissue transfer from forearm, thigh, lower leg, pelvis and abdomen.

the job Like many surgical jobs the work is divided between outpatient clinics, operating theatres and the wards. Maxillofacial surgeons frequently work alongside other specialists including orthodontics, oncologists, ENT surgeons, neurosurgeons, ophthalmic surgeons and plastic surgeons. On-calls tend to be relatively mild since there are very few maxillofacial emergencies that justify operating at night.

extras Sub-specialization is common in larger maxillofacial units; the main options are maxillofacial oncology or facial deformity. Clinicians usually maintain a general role in trauma, oral surgery and oral medicine. Academic interests are encouraged during training and university academic appointments are available. Flexible training is difficult, not least because of length of training. There is reasonable scope for private practice though there is some overlap with plastic surgery.

ℹ️ *For further information:*

British Association of Oral and Maxillofacial Surgeons, Royal College of Surgeons of England, 35–43 Lincoln's Inn Fields, London, WC2A 3PN
Tel: 020 7405 8074   Fax: 020 7430 9997   Web: http://www.baoms.org.uk

08:00	Ward round: 15 beds
08:30	All-day theatre list begins with cervical lymph node biopsy in a patient with high grade non-Hodgkin lymphoma; liaise with haemato-oncologist for bone marrow biopsy
10:00	Second case: Caldwell–Luc maxillary antrostomy, biopsy and antral washout, proceeds without incident
13:30	Inhale quick lunch whilst writing operation notes
14:00	Patient with a squamous cell carcinoma of the tongue; requires two maxillofacial surgeons (i) ablative — dental extractions, neck dissection, partial glossectomy (ii) reconstructive — radial forearm free flap
19:20	ITU ward round
19:30	Home/on-call

myth	Glorified dentists who just deal with teeth
reality	Dual-qualified doctor/dentist; interesting, varied surgical specialty involving the head, neck and sometimes rest of body
personality	Highly motivated, good manual dexterity, calm under pressure, team player, able to maintain long periods of concentration
best aspects	Great variety of cases and techniques
worst aspects	Eternal training
route	Requires dental and medical degrees (usually in that order); ST1 Oral and maxillofacial surgery (p 50); MRCS exam
numbers	370 of which 4% are women
locations	Hospital-based in most hospitals

life						**work**
quiet on-call						**busy on-call**
boredom						**burnout**
uncompetitive						**competitive**
low salary						**high salary**

Medical defence organizations

Medicolegal advisory work is an increasingly busy career to be in! In fact, although medical law is often thought of as a fairly modern specialty, protection organizations have been around since 1885. Despite the many changes over the years and increased scrutiny of the profession by the public, media, government authorities and the medical profession itself, the aim of the medicolegal adviser is the same: to provide professional support and expert advice to any member who seeks help.

the 'patients' Members of defence organizations, like patients, vary in age, personality, experience, activities and place of practice. They range from medical students to foundation doctors in their first month of paid employment to GPs with 30 years' experience through to commercially aware cosmetic surgeons. How individuals react in times of stress, or when challenged, varies enormously and can often be unpredictable. The doctors may be experiencing some of the most difficult times of their lives. Some contacts will be brief (a single phone call or letter), while others will be prolonged, spanning a number of years.

the work When imagining the work of defence organizations most people think of claims for compensation (i.e. clinical negligence work). However, medicolegal advisers' workload is much more varied, and it is often the non-claims cases which affect both the profession as a whole and individual doctors on a more personal level. Complaints, GMC investigations, inquests, media scrutiny, disciplinary procedures, ethical dilemmas, interactions with courts or the police and allegations of a criminal nature are all areas in which medicolegal advisers are asked to advise and assist members.

the job is predominately office-based, but involves direct contact with members by telephone, correspondence and in person. There is a degree of travel around the country to attend meetings and hearings with members. Medicolegal advisers work within a team, although on a day-to-day basis they are largely autonomous. There is little scope for promotion as the structure is fairly flat compared to the NHS hierarchy. Once fully trained the advisers have very heavy workloads which increase in complexity commensurate with experience. Of course, individuals naturally develop their own areas of expertise and specialist interest.

extras In addition, medicolegal advisers regularly lecture and run workshops on the potential pitfalls of practice as well as providing educational material on changes in the law and regulation.

ℹ️ *For further information:*

Medical Protection Society (MPS), Granary Wharf House, Leeds, LS11 5PY
Tel: 0845 605 4000   Fax: 0113 241 0500   Web: http://www.medicalprotection.org

08:30	Provide advice on telephone advisory line: take a call from a doctor who has been arrested, reassure and arrange for a solicitor to meet him at the police station in between the other 20 calls
13:00	End of telephone session; catch up with messages waiting for attention and discuss a difficult case with a colleague; grab a sandwich
14:00	Deal with email and postal correspondence
15:00	New cases are allocated; try to deal with cases whilst being constantly interrupted with queries
16:00	Prepare for meeting with member and solicitor the following day
17:30	Head to conference with barrister about a forthcoming GMC case, hoping to get home in time to watch *CSI*

myth	A soft option for doctors who want a hobby
reality	Professional support and expert advice
personality	Objective, analytical, empathetic, sense of humour
best aspects	Assisting and representing fellow professionals in their hour of need; ensuring fair treatment
worst aspects	Blame culture leading to increasing claims
route	Clinical experience, ideally post-membership exams; postgraduate qualification in medical law helps greatly; in house, on-the-job training
numbers	100
locations	Office-based with frequent travel to hospitals, PCT headquarters, courts, counsel's chambers and GMC

life					work
quiet on-call					busy on-call
boredom					burnout
uncompetitive					competitive
low salary					high salary

Medical education

Medical education is a very broad church covering academia, research and its most public face: teaching. The wide variety and range of jobs covered by this specialty means that there is probably a place for anyone with the desire, passion and enthusiasm to change the world. There are a small number of full-time medical educationalists who have followed an academic career path including research (ideally research into teaching methods). A larger number of doctors teach regularly alongside other clinical activities.

the patients Most medical educationalists continue to 'keep their hand in' by seeing patients on a regular basis. This is essential to maintain a degree of respect from trainees and colleagues and a working knowledge of what is happening at the coal face (essential if one is involved with assessment). Patients are increasingly being used as 'experts' in patient/educator programmes.

the work There are two major subdivisions to education: undergraduate and postgraduate. Few people successfully work in both spheres. Within each there are 'fat controllers', who administer curriculum design and training programmes, and the 'luvvies', who design and deliver the materials that the students/trainees receive. Personality, knowledge and interests often dictate where one ends up. Those working as academics must have a love of qualitative research (particularly questionnaires), which for many medics is a totally alien concept.

the job Depending on whether one becomes a fat controller or a luvvie (see the work above) the day can involve either meetings, meetings and more meetings or lectures, tutorials and assessments. Most medical educationalists perform a mixture of these two roles, though as a guide, the sharper the suit, the less likely someone is to have been near a whiteboard, a blackboard or, indeed, a student in the last 24 hours. Those committed to medical education academia need to work their way up through a large education centre, usually in a medical school.

extras Most people involved with medical education in medical schools have an MSc, MEd or PhD in a related field of interest. Whilst this is not essential for many jobs it is becoming de rigueur for new consultants and GPs applying for posts with a specialist interest in education. Other essential qualifications include an understanding partner who will overlook late nights and weekends spent by the computer preparing teaching and assessment materials.

ⓘ *For further information:*

Association for the Study of Medical Education, 12 Queen Street, Edinburgh, EH2 1JE
Tel: 0131 225 9111   Fax: 0131 225 9444   Web: http://www.asme.org.uk

A day in the life ...

00:00	Finish PowerPoint presentation for next day's teaching session
09:05	Late for first lecture with final years (fortunately half of them are later)
10:30	Meeting with dean and administrators
12:00	Grab sandwich whilst attending research meeting
13:00	Problem-based learning (PBL) facilitation with six first year students
15:00	Second lecture of the day, 'Age and ageing', to second year medics
16:10	Catch up with emails and correspondence
17:00	Attend freshers' cheese and wine party
19:00	Home for bath and start preparing course for next week

myth	Those that can do; those that can't teach; those that can't teach become educationalists
reality	An ever-growing, increasingly influential and important specialty that needs inspirational, dynamic individuals
personality	Like Bassett's, 'it takes allsorts'; clear communication, empathy, talent for stating the obvious, able to see the big picture
best aspects	The continual amazement and joy of working with some of the cleverest and most challenging students and trainees
worst aspects	There is about as much respect for great teaching and teachers as there is for the flat earth society
route	Educational experience developed alongside clinical training in any specialty; postgraduate qualifications (e.g. MSc, MEd or PhD) are a great asset; there are numerous training courses
numbers	250 full-time, many more part-time
locations	Medical schools and all postgraduate teaching environments

life		work
quiet on-call		busy on-call
boredom		burnout
uncompetitive		competitive
low salary		high salary

Medical entrepreneur

Many medics have good ideas: most forget them, a few pass them on to others to develop, but it is those who pursue their ideas that are true medical entrepreneurs. An entrepreneur is someone who starts a new business, usually with a new business concept. It is a career that very few expect to follow when starting a medical degree; it favours those with confidence in their own ideas and the mindset to take a risk. The most important attributes are passion and focus. It also helps to know about, or find someone you trust who knows about, accounting. With a good concept and the right management it is one of the few ways a medic can become rich; it is also one of the few ways a medic can become bankrupt.

the patients are ultimately going to be the beneficiaries of the health care product or service that is developed. By focusing on the needs of a patient population as the customers the business should have the best possible chance. Businesses are often full-time jobs so a break from clinical practice is usually necessary.

the work is often mundane with low-key daily rewards (e.g. hiring a new employee, making a new market contact) but it is important to keep an eye on the end goal—to deliver the product or service at a reasonable profit. As the business grows the work becomes more exciting with other employees to do the mundane jobs. Employing good staff and having good systems in place is key to ensuring that daily operations run smoothly, allowing the entrepreneur to focus on the important decisions and tasks, e.g. meeting investors, meeting customers and determining future strategies.

the job will depend entirely on the type of business being started. In general, much of the time will be spent in an office but some time will be spent outside it, either selling the idea to venture capitalists, selling the product or service or travelling to appointments. It is important to have the right temperament to handle customers, employees, suppliers and investors; this is similar to a clinician dealing with patients, colleagues and managers. An entrepreneur has complete autonomy to make decisions since it is their business, though it is important to keep investors (and for larger businesses, the board) content.

extras It is impossible to know where the journey will go! A successful business may lead to further ventures, world travel, management positions in other businesses or early retirement. An unsuccessful one may lead to a strategic retreat to clinical medicine.

ⓘ *For further information:*

There is no formal college or association, but these books may provide inspiration:
The black swan: the impact of the highly improbable by Nassim Nicholas Taleb
The tipping point: how little things can make a big difference by Malcolm Gladwell
Blink: the power of thinking without thinking by Malcolm Gladwell
Finance for non-financial managers by Gene Siciliano

A day in the life ...

08:00	Breakfast meeting with a potential customer or influencer
09:00	Deal with emails on Blackberry as they come in to prevent being overwhelmed by the end of the day (less of an issue when starting up)
10:00	Book travel and meeting requests (no PA yet)
11:00	Write the marketing blurb for newsletter and new company brochure
12:00	Update spreadsheets: Profits and Losses (P&L), Cash Flow, Balance Sheet
13:00	Team lunch
14:00	Calls to politely harass suppliers who have not yet delivered
16:00	See potential customers (often on the road)
18:00	Drinks with colleagues; networking

myth	It's difficult and really risky
reality	It's difficult and really, really risky
personality	Outgoing 'salesperson' personality balanced by absolute integrity, calm and logical decision-making, business sense, leader
best aspects	Seeing the first product/idea come to fruition; seeing people use it; seeing the money in the bank from the first sales; being in charge
worst aspects	Bankers and bureaucrats, who always seem to say 'No'
route	There is no defined route: go with the flow and follow passions
locations	Worldwide (anywhere with good Internet access)

life						work
quiet on-call						busy on-call
boredom						burnout
uncompetitive						competitive
low salary						high salary

Medical ethics

Believe the hype: medical ethics is *the* up-and-coming specialty in medicine. The rise of new technologies, our ever-increasing ability to delay death, the changing public expectations of doctors and medicine and the inclusion of medical ethics in medical school curricula and membership examinations make medical ethics a vital part of medical practice and education. This field is wonderfully varied and includes grappling with difficult decisions, teaching medical students and health care professionals, appearing on radio and television, speaking at conferences and writing in academic journals.

the patients The medical ethicist can be asked to consider cases involving elderly patients in palliative care one day, severely disabled neonates the next and dishonest medical students the day after. Ethical issues can arise in virtually all fields of medicine, from dermatology to neurosurgery. In an educational role, they teach medical students, as well as doctors, nurses and other health care professionals. Direct contact with patients is uncommon.

the work Medical ethicists, like other specialists, are involved in many types of activity. They often sit on clinical ethics committees which help resolve ethical dilemmas arising in hospitals. As experts in a growing field, they are often invited to give talks at medical conferences. They are solicited by journalists to give opinions on topical medico-ethical cases. They take part in debates on television, radio, newspapers and public institutions. They write articles in academic journals on their research interests, which could be anything from truth-telling in the doctor–patient relationship to the multiple understandings of autonomy. Most medical ethicists teach medical students, set and mark exams and attend meetings on educational matters.

the job Medical schools are the homes of many ethicists, although some can be found in philosophy and law departments. Medical ethicists spend most of their time in the office and lecture theatre, although some occasionally venture on to the wards to give talks to clinicians. Many institutions can only afford one full-time medical ethicist (and some even less!), although several are blessed with more. Part-time opportunities also exist.

extras It would be fair to say that the life of the average medical ethicist is a pleasant one, although this of course depends on the level of support the institution provides for teaching, marking and other tasks. If you acquire a good reputation in the field you will be invited to join prestigious committees, travel across the world to give talks and write articles in renowned publications.

ℹ️ *For further information:*

UK Clinical Ethics Network, Ethox Centre, University of Oxford, Badenoch Building, Old Road Campus, Headington, Oxford, OX3 7LF
Tel: 01865 287893   Fax: 01865 287884   Web: http://www.ethics-network.org.uk

09:00	Arrive at work; revise session on medical errors for teaching at 10 a.m.
10:00	Teach second year medical students
11:30	Accept Sky News' request for comment on story of terminally ill 10-year-old boy
12:30	On air ... for 3 minutes
13:30	Back in office; work on article on confidentiality for medical journal and meet first year student about possible special study module on ethics
15:00	Attend meeting about next year's finals examination
17:00	Clinical ethics committee meeting at hospital

myth	Airy fairy types who always have an opinion without actually giving an answer
reality	Provide rigorous and reasoned analyses of thorny problems to improve patient care
personality	Analytical, articulate, broad-minded, academic, generalist
best aspects	Helping medical students, health care professionals and members of the public appreciate the moral dimensions of medicine
worst aspects	Medical students and doctors who dismiss ethics as blindingly obvious or irrelevant to medical practice
route	Medical degree followed by masters or PhD in medical ethics
numbers	60
locations	Medical schools, although sometimes philosophy or law departments

life						work
quiet on-call						busy on-call
boredom						burnout
uncompetitive						competitive
low salary						high salary

Medical law

Medical law requires a unique mindset: someone who spends six years training in one profession, only to discover that their true vocation requires a similar length of training in another. As well the double qualification (which is likely to please parents if not wallets) the medical lawyer has a truly unique range of expertise. In many ways medical law is one of the oldest medical specialties; people sued each other in Biblical times for messing up and haven't stopped since. It is also one of the last specialties for true generalists since doctors from any specialty (or their patients) may need legal advice at some point.

the patients cover a wider range than those in other specialties, including those not yet born, those who were never born, those who are not yet dead and those who are dead.

the work varies depending on the type of law. There are three main roles: (1) Full time lawyers work either as solicitors or as barristers to assert a client's legal rights (e.g. suing a Trust after the administration of intrathecal vincristine). This involves meeting clients, preparing cases by obtaining medical records, sifting through the medical records, identifying and instructing experts, negotiating on behalf of clients and occasionally going to court. (2) Medicolegal advisors work in Trusts or for defence organizations (p 180); they use their knowledge of the law to respond to inquiries from doctors about clinical situations with legal implications (e.g. consent). They also formulate policy documents and are the first port of call following a medical disaster or when a complaint is received (e.g. a doctor has just given intrathecal vincristine; what should be done from a legal viewpoint?) (3) Risk managers work full time to look into care 'systems' and why they may have failed (e.g. how was a doctor able to give intrathecal vincristine). Each departments usually has a part-time 'risk lead' who is trained to evaluate patient safety and investigate problems and complaints when they occur. This would form a small part of their job plan—the rest of the time they would work as a clinical specialist.

the job is mostly office-based, but all medical lawyers, regardless of their role, may find themselves travelling to interview doctors, other health care staff and patients. Much time is spent writing or checking other people's writing.

extras Medical lawyers may receive frequent invitations to speak from all manner of medical specialties. They become involved in Trust hierarchy including being present at all stages of high-level strategic planning. Regular teaching is required for everyone from consultants to students. Legal qualifications can be studied for part-time (takes twice as long); part-time work is possible.

ℹ️ *For further information:*

Faculty of Forensic and Legal Medicine, 3rd Floor, 116 Great Portland Street, London, W1W 6PJ
Tel: 020 7580 8490   Web:http:// www.fflm.ac.uk

A day in the life of a medicolegal advisor

08:00	Arrive at work to clear emails whilst it is quiet
09:00	First meeting: prepare a doctor for giving a statement to a solicitor
10:00	Travel to coroner's court with team of nurses and doctors
11:00	Sit through coroner's case
12:00	Leave coroner's court and travel back to work
13:00	F1 teaching programme: teaching doctors about careful note-keeping
14:00	Clinical governance meeting
15:00	Telephone advice to a consultant surgeon about a difficult consent issue
16:00	Review risk management policy on antenatal ward
17:00	About to leave when consultant physician sits down to talk about concerns regarding one of his trainees

myth	Failed medics whose only skill is reading doctors' handwriting
reality	Working medic, specializing in failed medics
personality	Confident, well-prepared, articulate, sympathetic, academic
best aspects	Can make a real difference to patients and colleagues in distress
worst aspects	Seeing the same avoidable situation happen repeatedly to different patients or doctors
route	F1 essential but training up to Royal College membership at least is usually required. Law conversion (1 year full time) then lawyer qualification (2 years full time) then find a suitable job; risk manager training is quicker (2-year part-time masters)
Locations	Mostly office-based; part-time work is available

life						work
quiet on-call						busy on-call
boredom						burnout
uncompetitive						competitive
low salary						high salary

Medical management consulting

Are there any doctors who don't think they could spend taxpayers' money better within the NHS? This medical specialty tackles such interminable problems on a daily basis. Doctors who go into management consulting leave behind the patient interaction, but enter into health care's business world. The scope is broad and includes subjects such as supply and demand of NHS equipment, the finances of a Foundation Trust or information governance of electronic patient records, often bridging the gap between the commercial and the public sectors.

the patients/clients The success of any management or change programme requires the proper engagement of the people it will affect. With a clinical background and hospital experience, doctors are ideally placed to liaise with patients, nursing staff, the Royal Colleges and even the ministers at the Department of Health. Management consultants are also trained in business skills to negotiate with pharmaceutical, medical device and IT companies.

the work Management consulting work often means filling in the gaps that clients cannot manage themselves. Whether this involves a strategic analysis of market competitors, sourcing a particular blood product or training the work staff to use a new IT system, there is a need to adjust to a number of differing roles. However, as individual expertise develops, consultants tend to focus on particular aspects of project delivery and learn to maximize their potential for subject matter expert roles, for example, medicolegal reviews.

the job Teams are allocated according to the specific requirements of each project, so a management consultant may find themselves working with a wide variety of other consultants, from both within their own firm and beyond. For public sector projects these teams can be very large indeed, sometimes creating the feeling of too many cooks! Much of the work rapidly becomes familiar, with project plans, workshops, stakeholder meetings and deadlines guiding day-to-day activities. Consultants are often out and about visiting the client at their workplace before spending a few days at the office, or working from home, to consolidate their findings. Where the client base is not within a commutable distance, it is normal to spend time 'enjoying' living out of hotel rooms.

extras There are always plenty of options for professional development in management consulting. Passing on some medical insight from experience of the NHS, or helping to train the new recruits each year, is always welcomed. Flexible working is frequently accommodated and some doctors can even keep their hand in with clinical work by continuing some NHS sessions.

For further information:

Institute of Business Consulting: http://www.ibconsulting.org.uk
Management Consultant Association: http://www.mca.org.uk

A day in the life ...

08:00	Travel to client site
09:00	Run workshop to review specific treatment options with relevant clinical personnel; identify areas for improvement and associated difficulties
12:30	Working lunch, chatting to workshop attendees
14:00	Back to the office: plan suitable solutions and materials for the client in an internal team meeting
15:00	Liaise with client to problem-solve issues that have arisen
17:00	Manage the ever-growing email stream
18:00	Head home with (nearly) no chance of being disturbed

myth	Overpaid ex-docs who love their suits and are demons at PowerPoint
reality	Medically trained managers, with a real understanding of the stresses and strains of patient care, are what the NHS really needs
personality	Generally assertive, 'can do' attitude, independent thought, good business sense, good communication skills, organized
best aspects	Great variety and being part of the fast-moving business world; uncovering and improving the sticking plaster solutions that hold the NHS together; no on-calls!
worst aspects	Learning the basic consulting skills before advancing through the grades: it means doing the business equivalent of F1 and F2 years
route	Medical experience is essential: foundation programme at least, ideally post-membership; most management consulting firms have structured career progression programmes; a good MBA helps
locations	Office-based, lots of travel; some working from home is often possible

life		work
quiet on-call		busy on-call
boredom		burnout
uncompetitive		competitive
low salary		high salary

Medical manager

The title of medical manager encompasses several roles and varies between organizations. Over the past few years, the perception of medical managers has changed considerably. The role is now seen less as a betrayal of clinical responsibility than as one that is essential to an organization's focus on quality of care. Success, however, will only come with a proven track record as a clinician who has experienced and shared the working lives of colleagues within the Trust.

the patients Although most medical managers continue to have an active clinical practice, the clinical workload is often reduced in favour of managerial activities in larger organizations. None the less, the reason that these clinicians that are really effective as medical managers is their demonstrable and actively communicated commitment to improving the overall quality of patient care. The life of any manager is beset with problems (or challenges, depending on mindset), but the solutions to problems can only be delivered effectively by placing the patient at the centre of one's thinking.

the work varies according to the role. There is increasing involvement in corporate affairs as one progresses from being a clinical lead for a specialty, through being a clinical director to being a medical director. It is essential that training is undertaken to provide the knowledge and skills associated with these roles during this transition. At all levels, medical managers need to understand how to manage colleagues and teams in order to deliver the Trust's objectives. This requires detailed and multidisciplinary understanding of how each specific section of the organization works and how best to harness all staff to work towards a common goal.

the job involves many meetings. If these are managed effectively, it is in these meetings that vital communication necessary to deliver service development takes place. Understanding the dynamics of meetings is vital to the job and the manager needs to develop their communication and leadership skills, particularly for chairing meetings. With increasing seniority managers become more involved in corporate management and need to learn more about business planning and financial and budgetary management. It is important to explore a range of training opportunities to acquire this knowledge.

extras Training and development programmes for managers are widely available and provide a great opportunity to learn from others. Local networks of medical managers, many of them fairly informal, are of considerable assistance in discussing issues and improving personal performance. There is no greater tonic than knowing others have just the same problems to cope with.

ⓘ *For further information:*

British Association of Medical Managers (BAMM), Petersgate House, St Petersgate, Stockport, Cheshire, SK1 1HE
Tel: 0161 474 1141   Fax: 0161 474 7167   Web: http://www.bamm.co.uk

A day in the life ...

08:30	Chair Clinical Management board
10:30	Answer clinical query from colleague
11:00	Attend Hospital Infection Control Committee
13:00	Executive Directors' weekly meeting
16:00	A mixture of clinical and managerial catching up

myth	Ex-clinicians who have gone over to the dark side
reality	Doctors who make a difference to patient care at an organizational level
personality	Determined, eternally optimistic, able to express ideas coherently, business-minded, sociable
best aspects	Making changes to improve quality of care
worst aspects	Being performance-managed by people who have never done the job; endless meetings, not always chaired well
route	Consultant/GP-level training; local appointment, best aided by a formal development course, e.g. the Fit to Lead programme from the British Association of Medical Managers
numbers	1400 of which 30% are women
locations	All hospitals and Trusts (acute, mental health and primary care) require medical managers although the roles may vary

life					work
quiet on-call					busy on-call
boredom					burnout
uncompetitive					competitive
low salary					high salary

Medical microbiology

Medical microbiology encompasses bacteriology (the largest microbiology specialty), virology (which has its own training programme, see p 288), mycology and parasitology. Most microbiologists are really bacteriologists, with some training in the other specialties. Microbiology has sometimes been regarded as a Cinderella specialty which deals in organisms with long Latin names. However, recent changes in the epidemiology of infectious diseases, government targets and media interest have resulted in some bugs becoming household names (e.g. MRSA). This ever-increasing clinical and public profile means microbiologists are frequently being asked for their input and are also getting more invitations to hospital balls!

the patients Unlike most other clinical specialties, microbiologists are mainly advisory to clinical colleagues working in all health care settings. Microbiological clinical review of any patient in any specialty may be prompted by: a call for advice from the clinician; a positive laboratory result; a laboratory test request; or as part of a routine ward round (e.g. intensive care). The range of specialties makes the job very interesting and varied, although a specific interest in infections in a particular specialty can be developed. Some microbiologists do run clinics, e.g. hepatitis clinics.

the work The main role of a microbiologist is as an interface between the clinical areas of the hospital and the microbiology laboratory. They are also responsible for the functioning of the microbiology department and the interpretation of microbiological tests. The work frequently involves hands-on bench work for the more complicated tests and diagnoses. The clinical role of the microbiologist, including infection control, is increasing. Time is also spent teaching all grades of staff as well as undergraduates.

the job Greater laboratory centralisation means that microbiologists increasingly cover multiple sites. Microbiologists work within multidisciplinary teams including the laboratory staff (e.g. clinical scientists), other specialists and the infection control team. The split between the laboratory, wards, clinics, infection control, management and teaching varies greatly between jobs as does the on-call experience (which is largely for telephone advice) and the requirement for weekend and bank holiday laboratory attendance.

extras Many microbiology trainees choose to study for additional qualifications during their training period (e.g. MSc, Diploma in tropical medicine and health). There are numerous opportunities for teaching, research and subspecialization. Flexible training is becoming more common. Opportunities for private work do exist but are limited.

ⓘ *For further information:*

The Royal College of Pathologists, 2 Carlton House Terrace, London SW1Y 5AF
Tel: 020 7451 6700   Fax: 020 7451 6701   Website: http://www.rcpath.org

A day in the life ...

09:00	Interpretation of culture results, phoning results, answering clinical queries
10:30	Laboratory bench round and collection of results for ward round
11:00	Ward round, e.g. ITU, oncology, infectious diseases
12:15	Departmental clinical meeting with trainees, laboratory representative and infection control nurses to discuss cases from all clinical areas visited
13:00	Lunch
14:00	Authorization of laboratory results and investigation of unusual results
15:30	Infection control committee, laboratory management meeting or teaching
17:00	Read and respond to email correspondence, e.g. a new government target
17:30	Leave for home to prepare for evening class in 'Dealing with the Press'

myth	Boring backroom boys (and girls) obsessed with hand-washing and antibiotic resistance
reality	Working alongside front line troops in the ongoing battle against bugs
personality	Academic, analytical, generalist, happy away from acute medicine
best aspects	Fast-developing subject with a wide range of career options
worst aspects	Limited use of IT systems in some laboratories slows the reporting of lab results and can lead to incessant chasing from junior doctors
route	ST1 Medical microbiology/virology–microbiology (p 40); FRCPath exam
numbers	810 of which 40% are women
locations	Hospital-based (within a laboratory) in larger hospitals, but often covering more than one hospital site

life					work
quiet on-call					busy on-call
boredom					burnout
uncompetitive					competitive
low salary					high salary

Medical oncologists

Medical oncologists specialize in treating cancer patients with an array of systemic therapies (e.g. chemotherapy, hormone therapies and biological targeted compounds) compared with clinical oncologists (p 118), who use similar therapies along with radiotherapy, and haematologists (p 158) who treat leukaemia and lymphoma. Many cancers are treated without radiotherapy so medical oncologists still offer a complete approach to patient care. Those who are attracted to a career in medical oncology are often driven by its academic background and the desire to introduce new treatments through clinical trials.

the patients Most cancers are more common in people over the age of 60 so the patient population is often elderly; accordingly an ability to assess fitness for a proven intervention is essential. Cancer can affect any social class and all cultural backgrounds (though some ethnicities are prone to certain types of cancer). The needs of a deferent life-long smoking ex-miner pose a completely different challenge to those of a highly strung, alternative medicine advocate with breast cancer. Having to explain difficult prognoses, complex treatment schedules, let alone the concept of randomization, can be quite a challenge.

the work Medical oncologists treat solid tumours (as opposed to leukaemia and lymphoma). The most common cases are lung, colon and breast and these require systemic treatments at all stages of the disease. Many oncologists subspecialize to treat specific types of cancer (e.g. breast) whilst at superregional centres there are subspecialists in rare cancers (e.g. osteosarcoma). At one extreme the treatment aims to cure (adjuvant treatment) but more commonly treatments are given to palliate or relieve symptoms and prolong survival. The work is always rewarding when a difference is made to someone's life.

the job Until recently this rare breed of physician could only be found in larger teaching hospitals; cancer services are now expanding rapidly into most district general hospitals. The majority of clinical work is outpatient based; inpatient stays are reserved for severe symptoms (treatment side-effects or from the underlying disease) or infusional regimens unsuitable for outpatients. On-calls tend to be relaxed with most calls dealt with by phone. Oncology is a very supportive environment with close multidisciplinary teams (which discuss every referral, usually after the diagnosis has been made) and cooperation with other specialties.

extras Research is actively encouraged and the large cancer charities are an excellent source of funding for PhD or MDs. Teaching opportunities for both undergraduates and postgraduates are plentiful. For a medical specialty private practice can be very lucrative.

ⓘ *For further information:*

Association of cancer Physicians (ACP), Dept of Medicine, Royal Marsden NHS Trust, Downs Road, Sutton, Surrey, SM2 5PT
Tel: 020 8661 3276   Fax: 020 8643 0373   Web: http://www.cancerphysicians.org.uk

A day in the life ...

07:30	Admin and paperwork catch-up
08:00	Lung cancer multidisciplinary meeting; discuss new referrals and developments in current cases
09:30	Lung cancer clinic; one new patient, while the rest are follow-ups well known to the team
14:00	Answer emails and post whilst eating a sandwich
15:00	Chemotherapy prescribing with chemotherapy specialist nurse
15:30	Ward round of oncology unit
17:00	Sign clinic letters then home
17:30	Drive home

myth	Boffins out of touch with reality who spend all the drug budget
reality	Driven, hard-working physicians always keen to practice evidence-based medicine for patients with serious diseases
personality	Academic, enthusiastic, committed, diplomatic, accommodating
best aspects	'Complete' specialty: close liaisons with research staff whist maintaining genuine holistic care of patients
worst aspects	Few medical oncologists, so many are split between two hospitals miles apart; life can be lonely and demanding in smaller units practicing as a single-handed specialist
route	CT1 Core medical training (p 34) then ST3 Medical oncology; MRCP exam
numbers	350 of which 30% are women
locations	Hospital-based in most district general hospitals and teaching hospitals

life			●		work
quiet on-call		●			busy on-call
boredom		●			burnout
uncompetitive			●		competitive
low salary				●	high salary

Medical politics

Medicine is more than a job, it is a professional career. The training is demanding and the commitment lifelong, so it is important that doctors play a part in shaping the future of the profession itself. Taking part in medical politics offers a chance to take control of the direction for medicine. It is possible to be involved in medical politics at all stages of a career, from being a medical student through to retirement. Along the way one forges close friendships and gains a huge support network of other students/doctors; it can also be enormous fun. Many medical politicians cut their teeth at medical school as prominent members of the university medical society or local doctors' committee. Be warned: asking a question about finance entails a significant risk of ending up as treasurer!

the patients/colleagues Clinical medicine exposes a doctor to a wide variety of colleagues, each with their opinion on how the medical world should work. Medical politics provides an introduction to a much wider group of colleagues who will be only too ready to warn and advise! It is not without reason that gaining consensus on an issue in medicine is known as herding cats.

the work Whatever branch of medicine is of interest, there is a trainee or specialty association keen to attract active engagement from representatives of the profession. Most of the Royal Colleges encourage junior doctors, as well as fully trained doctors, to participate in their activities. The British Medical Association (BMA) has specific committees for all branches of medicine, including medical students. The Junior Doctors Committee (JDC), like those for GPs, staff and associate specialists and consultants, negotiates pay and conditions of service for all.

the job It is possible to pitch involvement in medical politics at a level that works for the individual. All levels of medicine need representative advice from appropriate doctors. This may be local, through the local/hospital medical society; specialty-specific, through the association or college; or national, through the union (the BMA) or on national advisory bodies. Being involved in committees or political meetings at any level encourages excellent communication, the need to make points persuasively and organisational skills (running conferences or even protests). Speed reading and sifting skills are also important as there are always agendas and minutes to read with important details hidden in the minutiae. The best can think on their feet, negotiate, persuade and amuse in less than three minutes.

extras Many national level bodies offer personal development in relevant skills (e.g. media training). Some organizations include opportunities for international travel.

ⓘ *For further information:*

British Medical Association, BMA House, Tavistock Square, London, WC1H 9JP.
Tel: 020 7387 4499   Fax: 020 7383 6400   Web: http://www.bma.org.uk
Local medical committees, specialist societies, Royal Colleges

05:30	Up early to catch train to London
06:30	Read meeting papers on the train and clear emails from previous night
08:00	Breakfast meeting with Royal College President
09:00	Meeting with committee secretary
10:00	Chair the committee
13:00	Working lunch with leading members of a clinical association
14:00	Attend a meeting on a new national strategy; try to ignore the buzzwords
17:00	Meet the Minister to update her on the committee's position
18:00	Phone calls to colleagues on the way to working dinner

myth	Dull docs trying to escape medicine for meetings and the love of hearing their own voice
reality	Committed colleagues trying to improve all aspects of what doctors do, from ways of working to pay and conditions
personality	Confidence, conviction, ability to listen, ability to weigh up evidence and opinion, organized, excellent time management
best aspects	The opportunity to make a real difference and improve medicine and the lives of doctors
worst aspects	Those who won't get involved but will always give their opinions; dull and seemingly endless committees; requires a significant time commitment to do it well
route	Occurs alongside medical training/work; initial involvement in local committees gradually working up to national ones
numbers	Several thousand at some level; <100 as their main role
locations	Meeting-based with frequent travel and meals out

life		work
quiet on-call		busy on-call
boredom		burnout
uncompetitive		competitive
low salary		high salary

Merlin

Merlin is an international medical aid agency which offers one of the most rewarding opportunities available to a doctor. The projects are diverse, from emergency response teams in the aftermath of an earthquake to mobile clinics in refugee camps or helping to re-establish a hospital in a country after years of conflict. Wherever they end up, the doctor will be sharing valuable skills and helping to save lives, whilst experiencing new challenges and enhancing their skills. At times of major emergencies (e.g. earthquakes), it's a case of all hands on deck and all doctors are needed (even those without previous experience of aid work). Longer-term projects require previous experience of living or working in a developing country along with post-graduate qualifications in public health, tropical medicine or health systems management.

the patients Merlin works in Africa, Asia and the Middle East, so there is no 'typical' patient base. However, the majority of Merlin's programmes serve neglected and isolated communities, where the existing health facilities and the levels of morbidity and mortality are often shocking. In some countries language differences and low literacy levels mean that interpreters are essential.

the work *Emergency responses* the work depends on the specific disaster and the previous state of health of affected communities. For example, after an earthquake the initial work will be trauma (fractures, infected wounds) whilst helping to prevent disease outbreaks with mass vaccination campaigns. *Longer placements* (e.g. rebuilding a health system) the work includes supervising local staff at a clinic, hospital ward rounds and performing operations. Malaria, respiratory infections and diarrhoeal diseases are extremely common. Training and supervision of local health staff is key; this can be challenging due to poor education or motivation, so doctors need to be adaptable and innovative.

the job *Emergency responses* Short-term intense contracts (e.g. 1–2 months). Doctors need to hit the ground running and pitch in wherever needed, from setting up a tented clinic to working in makeshift camps for displaced people. *Longer placements* Posts last 6–12 months with possible extensions. The role is split between hospital work and administration (e.g. meetings with partner organisations, the Ministry of Health, or donors), queries, reports, checking drug supplies and training events. Wards may be over-stretched, with patients on the floor. There may be no laboratory or imaging so clinical judgement is essential.

extras include experiencing life in some of the most neglected and isolated parts of the world; learning about different cultures; working with a wide variety of people from all over the world; and, most of all, making a real difference for people who might otherwise have no hope of getting professional medical care.

For further information:

Merlin, 207 Old Street, London EC1V 9NR
Tel: 020 7014 1600   Web: http://www.merlin.org.uk

myth	Triaging a queue of starving mothers and children to decide who may live or die
reality	Making a real difference to the lives of people who are desperately poor and have limited options
personality	Committed, able to cope in difficult situations, interested in new experiences, flexible, innovative, good clinical judgement
best aspects	Making a big difference despite few resources; getting to know far-removed cultures and places; being part of a close team
worst aspects	Missing family and friends and, occasionally, creature comforts
route	At least ST3/post-membership in a specific specialty; diploma in tropical medicine and/or masters in public health (or similar) is desirable alongside previous developing world experience
locations	Site of a disaster or a hospital in a developing country

life		work
quiet on-call		busy on-call
boredom		burnout
uncompetitive		competitive
low salary		high salary

Metabolic medicine

Metabolic medicine is a new adult subspecialty of chemical pathology (p 112), however the specialty is already well established in paediatrics. It deals with patients with deranged chemical processes; these may be genetic (errors of metabolism), acquired (diabetes) or iatrogenic (parenteral nutrition). Metabolic medicine specialists diagnose and manage this complicated group of patients.

the patients Metabolic medicine covers adults from ages 18 years onwards, from the young with familial hypercholesterolaemia to elderly patients on parenteral nutrition seen in intensive care settings. The patients are usual referred by other hospital specialists (e.g. endocrinologists and cardiologists). Alongside the patients in clinic there are requests for advice about patients under other specialists or in the community.

the work The diversity is enormous but broadly covers five main areas: lipid disorders and cardiovascular disease, diabetes, metabolic bone disease and renal stones, nutrition and obesity and adult inherited metabolic disease. Large specialist hospitals may require subspecialization in one of these areas while a smaller hospital may need a more general overview. Many metabolic medicine consultants also work as chemical pathologists with the responsibility of running a diagnostic laboratory.

the job There is a roughly equal split between outpatient clinics and laboratory-based work; some consultants may also attend ward rounds (e.g. nutrition round of patients in intensive care on parenteral nutrition). The specialty is very much senior-led though within the laboratory there are specialist biochemical scientists and clinical scientists to process the majority of samples. On-calls are usually not too onerous and the majority of problems can be dealt with over the phone. Much of the job entails liaison with other specialists or directly with patients so communication skills are vital.

extras There are usually lots of opportunities for teaching medical students, junior doctors, biomedical scientists and other ancillary staff. Academic interests are encouraged and a research project is an essential part of training as a chemical pathologist. Flexible training is well established within the specialty and the lifestyle is compatible with family life. Private practice is very limited.

ℹ️ *For further information:*

The Royal College of Pathologists, 2 Carlton House Terrace, London, SW1Y 5AF
Tel: 020 7451 6700   Fax: 020 7451 6701   Web: http://www.rcpath.org

A day in the life ...

08:00	Review of abnormal specimen results on the laboratory IT system
09:00	Outpatient lipid clinic: 5 new patients and 15 familiar faces
13:00	Review of equipment tenders with laboratory managers over lunch
14:00	Authorization reviews (checking that the descriptions of complicated laboratory results are correct before sending them out)
15:00	Clinic notes, dictating letters and researching the literature on the more unusual cases
16:00	Teaching medical students
17:30	Review laboratories' work schedule for evening, depart for home

myth	Test tubes, pipettes, large glasses and bow ties
reality	Busy specialty with emphasis on patient contact but time to pursue interesting cases and own research interests
personality	Good communication skills, team work, sense of humour, academic, systematic
best aspects	Good variety, ability to reassure patients
worst aspects	Pathology is highly automated and can be monotonous; constant battle with managers fixated about cutting budgets
route	ST1 Chemical pathology (p 112); FRCPath and MRCP exam; the route via core medical training is not yet defined
numbers	40 of which 20% are women
locations	Mostly teaching hospitals and specialist hospitals.

life					work
quiet on-call					busy on-call
boredom					burnout
uncompetitive					competitive
low salary					high salary

Neonatology

Neonatology is a subspecialty within paediatrics dedicated to the care of newborn babies, sick babies and premature babies. A neonatologist or 'baby doctor', is trained specifically to deal with the most complex and high-risk situations. It is a hands-on, consultant-led specialty based on teamwork rather than hierarchy. Communication with and support of parents is paramount.

the patients The neonatologist is responsible for babies in the neonatal intensive care unit (NICU) as well as on the postnatal ward. Approximately 10% of the deliveries have some problems requiring admission to neonatal intensive care. The very preterm infants with immature organ systems require constant monitoring and expert care for a few months before they are ready for discharge. Term newborns may have different problems, often complex and less predictable (e.g. perinatal asphyxia, birth defects, infections or genetic disorders). Infants may be followed up in the neonatal outpatient clinics for the first couple of years (until walking and talking).

the work Neonatology is technically challenging, not least of all because of the size of the babies. Diseases in the newborn period reflect the unique neonatal physiology, thus presenting challenges in diagnosis, management and treatment. Day-to-day work entails a combination of practical skills (e.g. airway management, assisted ventilation, umbilical catheterization) and clinical management (e.g. prescribing parenteral nutrition, managing neonatal emergencies). Whilst newborns are resilient, ethical-legal dilemmas involving end of life decisions and palliative care are not uncommon. Neonatologists also work closely with obstetricians in pre-birth counselling and delivery planning of high-risk pregnancies.

the job The neonatologist's time is split between neonatal intensive care, postnatal wards, deliveries, follow-up clinics for high risk neonates after discharge, patient-related administrative work, parental discussions and attending clinical or educational meetings. The job is based on collective effort in a multidisciplinary team structure involving dieticians, physiotherapists, nurse specialists and paediatric surgeons. The specialty is highly consultant-supervised and is frequently busy 24 hours a day. Some units require consultants to be resident when on-call and this is likely to increase.

extras There are plentiful opportunities for teaching medical students and junior doctors. Flexible training/job sharing is well respected. Private practice is almost non-existent. There are opportunities for overseas travel both for work and research training programmes. Academic interests are encouraged but not essential (unless a trainee hopes to work in a tertiary unit).

🛈 *For further information:*

Royal College of Paediatrics and Child Health, 50 Hallum Street, London, W1N 6DE
Tel: 020 7307 5600   Fax: 020 7307 5601   Web: http://www.rcpch.ac.uk

myth	Babies don't talk back
reality	People do it for the love of it and the buzz of NICU; stakes are high, responsibilities huge, with emotions running high
personality	Empathy, sensitivity, patience, ability to handle stress, team player; caters for wide mix from the obsessive–compulsives, to high-tech geeks, to the calm and unflappable
best aspects	Dynamic, challenging and multifaceted job in a supportive multidisciplinary environment; close rapport with parents
worst aspects	Babies don't know the difference between night and day; intense workload; heavy and unpredictable out-of-hours on-call commitments
route	ST1 Paediatrics (p 38) then subspecialization; MRCPCH exam
numbers	320 'pure' neonatologists, 1200 mixed with general paediatrics
locations	Hospital-based found in most hospitals

life						work
quiet on-call						busy on-call
boredom						burnout
uncompetitive						competitive
low salary						high salary

Neurology

So you want to be the doctor that brain surgeons turn to for advice? While many students rate neurology as one of the most interesting subjects, many junior doctors exhibit a degree of 'neurophobia'. The specialty suits devilishly determined thinkers who can weigh up information and target tests to explain a patient's symptoms. Neurologists are skilful clinicians with healthy teaching and research interests. It has been said that a textbook of neurological treatments would be slimmer than Kate Moss, but this is rapidly changing. For example, the range of treatments for epilepsy and Parkinson's disease are expanding and there are new arrivals such as immunotherapy for multiple sclerosis and clot-busting drugs for stroke.

the patients Neurological conditions account for 20% of general medical admissions. The patients are generally younger than in many other medical specialties. Anxiety symptoms commonly complicate neurological presentations and communication difficulties are a frequent challenge. Speaking to witnesses of blackouts is essential; the telephone becomes more important than the tendon hammer (although neurologists do quite like the tendon hammer). Job satisfaction comes from assessing new cases and the long-term care of patients with chronic, and sometime disabling, illnesses.

the work The spectrum of diagnoses is broad, ranging from those of the brain and spinal cord to those of nerve and muscle. Presentations range from headache, epilepsy and stroke (common and manageable) to motor neurone disease and Huntington's disease (rare and incurable). The conditions are often fascinating and require detective work to diagnose.

the job Neurology overlaps with many other disciplines, so being a well-rounded generalist is important. Being in the diagnostics business, the neurologist forges close links with pathology, radiology and particularly neurophysiology and neurosurgery. Most neurologists work in teams and can develop a special interest; this can range from esoteric bench work (e.g. mitochondrial laboratory research) to practical bedside approaches (e.g. wheelchair rehabilitation). Even for super-specialists, most neurology work occurs in the clinic room and there are relatively few inpatient beds. On-call is less intense than elsewhere in medicine since it is confined to neurology, despite initial training in general medicine.

extras Neurologists are usually keen teachers and lecturers, often to be found quizzing students on nerve roots or eye movements. Historically, research was needed for trainee posts, but increasingly research projects are started during specialty training. Those who wish can find good opportunities for private practice, particularly in metropolitan areas. Flexible training is also possible.

ℹ️ *For further information:*

Association of British Neurologists (ABN), Ormond House, 27 Boswell Street, London, WC1N 3JZ
Tel: 020 7405 4060   Fax: 020 7405 4070   Web: http://www.abn.org.uk

A day in the life ...

08:00	Get in early to meet with specialist nurse who is preparing an audit presentation
09:00	'First fit' clinic; telling people that they must stop driving is always difficult
10:00	Trainee pops into clinic for advice about a ward referral; MRI scans reviewed together
12:00	Eat sandwiches while reviewing a journal article prior to publication
13:00	Multidisciplinary team meeting
14:00	Weekly ward round: a patient with a head injury is very agitated; speak with worried parents on the ward
16:30	Give Botox to help with a spastic arm at the end of the round
19:30	On-call at home but disturbed only once: trainee calls to ask for advice about patient with myasthenia

myth	Brainiacs who care only about diagnosis
reality	Brainiacs who care about patients
personality	Pub-quiz loving, family-orientated, academic, generalist, good memory, methodical, analytical
best aspects	Intellectual stimulation; rewarding patient contact
worst aspects	Low cure rate juxtaposed against high patient expectations
route	CT1 Core medical training (p 34) then ST3 Neurology; MRCP exam
numbers	900 of which 20% are women
locations	Hospital-based, mostly in teaching hospitals but expanding into district general hospitals

life						**work**
quiet on-call						**busy on-call**
boredom						**burnout**
uncompetitive						**competitive**
low salary						**high salary**

Neurosurgery

The title of this book suggests that there is something special about neurosurgery and it doesn't take a rocket scientist to work out why. The central nervous system is complex, unforgiving, functionally mysterious and rarely understood at medical school, yet it is the seat of the soul. Doctors who want to spend their days working within it must therefore be very clever (questionable), brave (probably), foolhardy (possibly) and arrogant (undoubtedly).

the patients are those of all ages from premature infants to the geriatric population with structural nervous system problems. Most large centres split the paediatrics off from adult work with dedicated paediatric neurosurgeons.

the work Congenital anomalies such as spina bifida, hydrocephalus, tumours, cerebral haemorrhage, trauma and spinal degenerative disease make up the bread and butter work. Esoteric subspecialties of movement disorders, psychosurgery, pain and epilepsy are there for those who are interested. Whilst the adult workload is increasing with the ageing population, there are some threats to the specialty on the horizon. Already aneurysm surgery has been virtually replaced by interventional neuroradiology. Tumour, pain and movement disorder work is vulnerable to a 'medical breakthrough'. Spinal neurosurgery may become the province of spinal surgeons with orthopaedic and neurosurgical training. The golden age of neurosurgery may have already passed or may be just one new technique around the corner...

the job Neurosurgeons hunt in packs in large regional centres, usually attached to teaching hospitals. Most serve around a dozen district general hospitals, with catchment populations of 2–3 million, although there are a handful of smaller units serving half as many. The duty neurosurgeon will therefore spend a lot of their day fielding telephone calls and juggling more patients than beds. This is nothing new; it is said that an ST1 trainee in neurosurgery needs only two words of English ('No beds'), whilst an ST4 trainee needs just four ('Terribly sorry, no beds'). This doesn't change as you move up the ladder. Neurosurgery is consultant-led, with decisions and surgery, even in the middle of the night, requiring the consultant to be awake and in the hospital.

extras It is an academic subject with many opportunities for research and teaching. There is plenty of private practice, both clinical and medicolegal, so a financially poor neurosurgeon is a rarity. Flexible training is virtually non-existent so can be difficult to organize.

ⓘ *For further information:*

Society of British Neurological Surgeons, 35–43 Lincoln's Inn Fields, London, WC2A 3PE
Tel: 020 7869 6892   Fax: 020 7869 6890   Web: http://www.sbns.org.uk

A day in the life ...

07:45   Meeting in radiology to review all emergency CT/MRI scans sent by image link from district general hospitals; emergency admission prioritized

08:15   Ward round: begins in ITU then moves on to neurosurgery ward

09:00   Theatre or clinic; most theatre lists are all day long with 1–4 cases; day case neurosurgery is a case that takes all day!

12:30   Dream of a lunch break—a technically possible historic rarity

18:00   Review theatre cases and evening ward round; may have emergency operating to do

19:00   Look at paperwork in office; send email to wife asking her to say goodnight to kids for you

myth	Arrogant, self-important chaps with fighter pilot mentality
reality	Increasing number of girls with arrogant, self-important fighter pilot attitude to match the chaps
personality	How many neurosurgeons does it take to change a light bulb? One: they hold it still whilst the world revolves around them!
best aspects	You ARE a brain surgeon; very challenging and satisfying workload; Ferrari dealers love you
worst aspects	Currently more qualified trainees than there are consultant jobs; high divorce rate; heavy on-calls, even as consultant
route	ST1 Neurosurgery (p 50); FRCS exam
numbers	420 of which 5% are women
locations	Hospital-based; mostly regional centres in teaching hospitals

life		work
quiet on-call		busy on-call
boredom		burnout
uncompetitive		competitive
low salary		high salary

Nuclear medicine

Few people realize that it's not just assassins who have the chance of giving radioactive isotopes to people (though Polonium is still hard to come by)! The specialty of nuclear medicine uses radioactive substances to look at physiological processes in disease, aid diagnosis and offer treatment for chronic or life-threatening diseases. The field is developing rapidly including new radio-isotopic therapies for lymphoma and neuroendocrine tumours.

the patients Nuclear medicine covers all ages from 0–100. In the same day a nuclear medic may be trying to diagnose biliary atresia in a neonate and finding out why a 100-year-old has heart failure. Patients come in all sizes, shapes and colours with a great variety of diseases. Some may only be seen once, though many with chronic diseases (e.g. renal disease or cancer) may come many times within a year. Good communication skills are needed to explain to patients, who are often quite anxious, why they need to be temporarily radioactive.

the work Much of the work is computer-based as image optimization and manipulation are needed for accurate diagnosis. There is a significant amount of patient contact each day, for example stressing a patient for a cardiac study or explaining why they need treatment with radioiodine for their hyperthyroidism. There is some lab work and, if involved in radionuclide therapy, outpatient and ward work.

the job tends to be 9–5 with no on-call. Patient preparation, such as cardiac stressing, usually occurs in the morning with imaging in the afternoon, followed by reporting. As with all diagnostic specialties there is a major commitment to multidisciplinary meetings. The department is run by a team which includes physicists, radiopharmacists, nuclear medicine technologists, nurses and reception staff.

extras There are no subspecialties in nuclear medicine, but some people develop areas of special interest such as nuclear cardiology, thyroid clinics, joint cancer clinics or osteoporosis clinics; a range of inpatient work can also be developed. Flexible training and senior part-time posts are common. There is very limited private practice but there are numerous opportunities for research, which is encouraged.

🛈 *For further information:*

British Nuclear Medicine Society, Regent House, 291 Kirkdale, London, SE26 4QD
Tel: 020 8676 7864   Fax: 020 8676 8417   Web: http://www.bnmsonline.co.uk

08:30   Multidisciplinary team meeting

09:30   Cardiac stressing

12:30   Management or education meeting accompanied by lunch

13:30   Private study or research

14:30   See three patients with hyperthyroidism and arrange I-131 for treatment

15:30   Admit and treat an inpatient with I-131 mIBG for phaeochromocytoma (not every day, sometimes it's a paraganglioma or carcinoid tumour!)

16:30   Reporting

17:30   Go home, on time, almost every night!

myth	Live in the gloomy recesses of the radiology department, dress oddly and glow in the dark; possibly related to orcs and goblins
reality	Blend of advanced science and clinical skills for the good of the patients; jury out on the orc/goblin ancestry
personality	Academic, generalist, team player, easy-going
best aspects	Rapid growth in positron emission topography (PET) CT and new therapies mean this is an exciting time for nuclear medicine
worst aspects	Some old equipment; ever-changing government targets in diagnostics; limited private practice
route	CT1 Core medical training (p 34) then ST3 Nuclear medicine; MRCP exam; alternative route via clinical radiology
numbers	275 of which 25% are women
locations	Hospital-based in larger district general hospitals and teaching hospitals

life						**work**
quiet on-call						**busy on-call**
boredom						**burnout**
uncompetitive						**competitive**
low salary						**high salary**

Obstetrics

Although a specialty in its own right, obstetrics is combined with gynaecology (p 156) in most consultant appointments. However, as smaller maternity units close, the larger units may employ more dedicated obstetricians without gynaecological commitments. The work entails emotional highs and lows; great happiness may swiftly be followed by the sadness of a pregnancy loss.

the patients vary from worryingly young to worryingly old! Demographic changes mean higher numbers of older mothers who often have concurrent medical problems, placing them at greater risk. Similarly the advances in assisted conception mean many more multiple pregnancies with their associated dangers. Whilst most mothers and their pregnancies are healthy, some have serious medical problems including diabetes, hypertension and cardiac disease, to name a few. These patients require intensive management, often involving multiple specialists to ensure good outcomes and minimise risk.

the work Antenatal clinics are busy and problems vary from minor to life-threatening. Helping to deliver a baby has few rivals in the job satisfaction league; when all goes well it is hugely rewarding, but sometimes tragedy strikes. A good obstetrician must be adept at communicating with mothers of all backgrounds and beliefs at times of both happiness and great stress. A cool head is essential to organize the labour ward and keep the team of midwives, doctors and others all working together. Some obstetricians will specialize further in maternal and fetal medicine (p 176).

the job There are few quiet obstetric jobs. Nights are as busy as days and stamina is required. Consultants are increasingly present on the labour ward. Obstetricians enjoy a combination of medicine and surgery (the national Caesarean section rate is over 20%). There is plenty of interaction with the other specialists and continued exposure to general medical and surgical problems in obstetric patients. There is plenty of opportunity to develop a niche specialty in obstetrics such as cardiac disease, diabetes or HIV.

extras Obstetrics is a practical specialty and there is nothing to compare with the hands-on experience. Teaching of medical students, junior doctors, midwives and other specialists is a continual, essential part of the job. Academic obstetrics is a challenge in this era of molecular research, but audit, evidence-based obstetrics and protocol development are essential to department improvement. Private obstetrics is unusual outside the M25 and private practice insurance premiums are high and getting higher. Flexible training is well established.

ℹ For further information:

Royal College of Obstetricians and Gynaecologists, 27 Sussex Place, Regents Park, London, NW1 4RG
Tel: 020 7772 6200   Fax: 020 7723 0575   Web: http://www.rcog.org.uk

A day in the life ...

08:00   Joint morbidity meeting with neonatologists

09:00   Antenatal ward round

09:30   Antenatal clinic: admit a hypertensive primigravid woman

12:30   Called to see patient with placenta praevia and further bleeding

13:00   Trainee teaching session

14:00   Labour ward: elective Caesarean; *in utero* transfer of preterm labourer (i.e. transfer to a hospital with a suitable level of neonatal intensive care); 'lift out' with forceps

17:00   Hand over to late shift and head home

20:00   Write protocol on the management of gestational diabetes

myth	Back-to-back Caesarean sections for those who are 'too posh to push'
reality	Obstetrics is one of the foremost specialties in pushing forward evidence-based medicine; there is a huge variety of pathology and it is an immensely practical subject
personality	Cool head under pressure, able to prioritize, teamwork, good communication skills, good practical abilities, patient
best aspects	There is nothing more satisfying than delivering a baby
worst aspects	Babies cannot tell night from day; medicolegal concerns; unreasonable patient expectations
route	ST1 Obstetrics and gynaecology (p 36); MRCOG exam
numbers	3100 (combined with gynaecology) of which 33% are women
locations	Hospital-based in vast majority of hospitals

life				●		work
quiet on-call				●		busy on-call
boredom				●		burnout
uncompetitive		●				competitive
low salary				●		high salary

Occupational medicine

Occupational medicine is all about the two-way interaction between health and work. The diversity of people and their employment contexts offers an enormous variety of clinical problems to solve. Occupational physicians deal not only with individual patients (employees) but also a wide range of managers (employers), employee representatives and colleagues in other specialties and disciplines. Some work within the NHS, but most work either for in-house services or for independent occupational health providers that serve a number of different employers. Some are contracted directly by employers.

the patients are usually employees of an organization for whom the occupational physician provides a service. Most patients are referred by their managers or self-referred. Referrals from GPs and other specialists are rare, but the UK government's Health, Work and Well-being strategy aims to promote health through employment in all people of working age, potentially broadening the scope of occupational medicine. Patients' expectations about the doctor–patient relationship may be different from that in other specialties. They may not have chosen to be referred so the challenge is to build rapport and trust.

the work A functional as well as a diagnostic medical model is appropriate in assessing the interaction between health and work. What can the employee do, or not do, considering their current state of health? What will enable them to do more or do it better? Occupational physicians need good negotiating and influencing skills in order to achieve positive outcomes for employees and employers. A clear understanding of consent and confidentiality issues and relevant employment law are vital.

the job Occupational physicians usually work as part of multidisciplinary occupational health teams, including specialist occupational health nurses, psychologists, administrators and sometimes physiotherapists, ergonomists, occupational hygienists and safety practitioners. Occupational physicians may be called on to give advice about environmental issues including the effect of an organization's activities on the natural environment. On-call requirements vary, but part-time work is possible and work–life balance is usually good.

extras Occupational physicians working in teaching hospitals or academic centres may teach undergraduates and train postgraduate doctors specializing in occupational medicine and participate in research. There are also opportunities to be involved in national level work and media exposure. Flexible training is usually possible and there are opportunities for private practice. Overseas placements are available with larger multinational corporations.

🛈 *For further information:*

The Faculty of Occupational Medicine, 6 St Andrew's Place, Regent's Park, London, NW1 4LB
Tel: 020 7317 5890   Fax: 020 7317 5899   Web: http://www.facoccmed.ac.uk
Society of Occupational Medicine: http://www.som.org.uk

A day in the life ...

08:00	Drop kids off at school and travel to work
09:00	Clinic: six patients referred by their managers because of sickness, absence or concerns about their health at work
12:00	Meeting with senior nurse to discuss operational issues
13:00	Lunchtime meeting with CEO and Director of human resources, interrupted by call to sort out employee with acute psychosis
14:00	Environmental working group or health and safety committee
15:00	Case conference to discuss absence management issues with managers and human resources advisors
16:00	Meeting with occupational health trainees
16:30	Media interview: journalist writing an article about repetitive strain injury
17:00	Take home papers for tomorrow's meeting to read on the train

myth	Agents of the capitalist system forcing the sick to work
reality	Specialists finding the right balance whilst advocating for their patients
personality	Listening skills, team player, problem-solving skills, flexibility, able to manage uncertainty, ability to understand different perspectives, non-judgemental
best aspects	Finding workable solutions; every story is different
worst aspects	The common misconception that occupational health services just send people 'off sick'
route	CT1 Core medical training (p 34) or ST1 GP Vocational training (p 32) then ST3 Occupational medicine; MRCP, nMRCGP or diploma in occupational medicine
numbers	800 of which 20% are women
locations	Office-based in NHS or large corporations

life		work
quiet on-call		busy on-call
boredom		burnout
uncompetitive		competitive
low salary		high salary

Ophthalmology

Medical schools have always provided relatively limited opportunities for undergraduates to experience ophthalmology in their busy curriculum, although clinical demand, expressed as referral rates from primary care, is high and growing rapidly. Eyesight is extremely important and it is the ophthalmologist's job to protect and preserve it.

the patients An ophthalmologist manages all kinds of patients, from premature neonates (screening for, and treating, retinopathy of prematurity) to centenarians (who get cataracts and appreciate the restoration of vision and colour). Generally an ophthalmologist's patients are well, apart from their eye problems. The ability to improve or restore a patient's sight is a rare privilege. Some patients have long-term conditions (e.g. glaucoma and diabetic retinopathy), allowing lasting clinical relationships to form.

the work Ophthalmologists are both physicians and surgeons to the eye and the structures around it including the lids, orbit, lacrimal system, optic nerve and visual pathway. The range of diagnoses is enormous, however there are unique diagnostic tools to help including biomicroscopes, indirect ophthalmoscopes, lasers, ultrasound and fluorescent photography. Cataract surgery accounts for 50–60% of surgical procedures and is usually done under local anaesthetic. Operating on the eye sometimes seems more like jewellery work, with sparkles, twinkles, bright lights, fractions of a millimetre between triumph and disaster and the magnified virtual world of the operating microscope. High-tech modern surgical instruments enable the surgeon to produce routinely excellent results and to take the credit.

the job Outpatient clinics represent 50–70% of working time and are often relentlessly busy and routinely overbooked. The rest of the time is spent in theatre, reviewing patients post-op or the usual consultant paperwork. Ophthalmologists routinely liaise with other specialties including ENT, plastic surgeons, neurologists, neurosurgeons, paediatricians and endocrinologists.

extras Most units include teaching and research as an integral part of the weekly programme. Ophthalmologists generally develop a special interest such as retinal disease, paediatric ophthalmology and ocular motility, glaucoma, corneal disease, oculoplastic surgery or neuro-ophthalmology. Work is usually split between general ophthalmology, including cataract surgery, and the specialist field. Flexible training is more acceptable than in other surgical specialties and there is a higher proportion of women than in most. Private practice is common and highly lucrative, largely due to cataract surgery.

ⓘ *For further information:*

The Royal College of Ophthalmologists, 17 Cornwall Terrace, London, NW1 4QW
Tel: 020 7935 0702   Fax: 020 7935 9838   Web: http://www.rcophth.ac.uk

08:00	Post-op ward round: six patients from yesterday following three cataracts, one eyelid repair and two trabeculectomies
09:00	Eye casualty: chap with arc eye, child with dog bite to lower lid
10:45	Called out to administer IV fluorescein (fluorescein angiography)
11:15	Back to eye casualty
12:30	Back on to the ward to clerk patients for the afternoon list
13:00	Journal club in the seminar room with lunch
14:00	Theatre: 5 cataracts and one squint; includes working in the eyes of patients whilst they are awake and talking
17:30	Catch up with notes; waiting for dictation from yesterday's clinic
18:00	Half an hour working on an audit
18:30	Buy the new trainee a drink at the 'rehydration clinic'

myth	Obsessives who just take out cataracts
reality	A wonderful micro-world of specialist skills and procedures, many unique to the specialty
personality	Excellent fine coordination, excellent binocular vision, good communications skills (patients usually conscious)
best aspects	Unique combination of intellectual, clinical and surgical challenge; the opportunity to make patients very happy
worst aspects	There is never enough time to do the job as well as desired
route	ST1 Ophthalmology (p 50); FRCOpth exam
numbers	1800 of which 20% are women
locations	Hospital-based, found in the majority of hospitals

life		work
quiet on-call		busy on-call
boredom		burnout
uncompetitive		competitive
low salary		high salary

Orthopaedic surgery

The *BMJ* once published a report comparing the hand sizes of surgeons and primates.[1] It concluded that orthopaedic surgeons were evolutionarily less developed than other surgeons and in fact much closer to our hairy ancestors. The typical 'orthopod' is seen as male, monosyllabic and money-orientated. Thankfully this view is being revised. Technical developments, increasing numbers of female surgeons and robust research output are redefining the mould of the orthopaedic surgeon. A career in orthopaedics offers the technical demands of a rapidly progressing surgical specialty together with high levels of job satisfaction and options for academic activity.

the patients The ages of the patients vary depending on the subspecialty. The majority of patients seen by surgeons who specialize in joint replacement will be 60+, while those specializing in sports injuries and limb reconstruction will focus on a younger adult population. The subspecialty of paediatric orthopaedics treats patients from infancy to adolescence. Apart from children's orthopaedics, the majority of orthopaedics is based on 'episodes of care' where a patient requires, say, a hip replacement, and then is not seen for a couple of years until another joint causes problems. Prolonged continuity of care is decreasing but rest assured, the problem patient will always find their way back to clinic. One of the great things about elective orthopaedics is that the patients are generally well.

the work Most orthopaedic surgeons split their time between elective work, e.g. pre-planned surgery for arthritis, and trauma work, e.g. broken bones. Some posts are purely elective, leaving the trauma work to a linked team of surgeons (see Trauma surgery, p 280). Time is divided between clinics, operating lists, on-call commitments and admin.

the job Orthopaedics requires good manual dexterity, a problem-solving mindset and a sense of responsibility. The responsibility inevitably felt for patients means a roller-coaster of emotions about individual surgical outcomes. The opportunity to restore a patient's quality of life is unparalleled and patients are often very appreciative of the outcome. Conversely, when something goes wrong, the responsibility lies squarely on the surgeon's shoulders. A level head and an ability to self-appraise are essential to see one through to retirement.

extras Research interests are increasingly common, as is helping bioengineering to develop new surgical implants or soft tissue engineering models. Private practice is common and pays well.

ℹ️ *For further information:*

British Orthopaedic Association, 35–43 Lincoln's Inn Fields, London, WC2A 3PE
Tel: 020 7405 6507   Fax: 020 7831 2676   Web: http://www.boa.ac.uk
British Orthopaedic Trainees Association: http://www.bota.org.uk

---

[1] Fox JS *et al.* Are orthopaedic surgeons really gorillas? *BMJ* (1990) 301(6766): 1425–6.

08:00   X-ray meeting or ward round

09:00   Clinic; this may be a fracture clinic for acute injuries or an elective clinic seeing patients with problems relevant to one subspecialty (e.g. shoulder problems)

12:30   Review patients who are due for surgery

13:30   Theatre; operating list of elective cases including a hip replacement

17:30   Finish theatre; review the post-op patients

18:00   Home or office to address administration pile (typically large)

myth	As strong as an ox and half as bright
reality	Neither of the above! Technical aptitude is more important than strength and academic prowess is needed to beat the competition, since increasing numbers have MDs or PhDs
personality	Confident, practical, focused, driven, do not typically suffer fools lightly, competitive
best aspects	Surgery is enormously fun; you make people better; great toys
worst aspects	Tiring; increasingly competitive; both elective and trauma surgery can take much longer than anticipated which can affect home/family plans at short notice
route	ST1 Surgery in general, trauma and orthopaedic surgery (p 48) then ST3 Trauma and orthopaedic surgery; MRCS exam
numbers	3200 (combined with trauma surgery) of which 3.5% are women
locations	Hospital-based, found in most hospitals

life						work
quiet on-call						busy on-call
boredom						burnout
uncompetitive						competitive
low salary						high salary

Overseas aid

Unlike almost any other career, medicine is useful all over the world. Overseas work can be a full-time career or an interesting side arm to a more conventional career. Either way it is important to plan how it will fit into a career, both in terms of taking time off (p 68) and choosing an appropriate specialty. For full-time work consider public health (p 248), tropical medicine (p 168), general practice (p 144), acute medicine (p 98) or emergency medicine (p 130). These specialties are all also useful for shorter-term work, but so are many other specialties, such as paediatrics (p 224), obstetrics (p 212), gynaecology (p 156) and anaesthetics (p 100). There are many options but it is important to consider finances, family commitments and the type of work involved.

the patients in resource-poor countries present many challenges. Language barriers, late presentation and sheer numbers all commonly compound the lack of medical supplies. Problems depend on the situation but poor nutrition, infection and exposure are common, especially following natural disasters.

the work depends on the scenario and employing agency. This is an opportunity to make a *real* difference to many lives. It may be saving the life of an earthquake victim, preventing a cholera outbreak in a refugee camp or planning aid on a huge scale to save thousands (without actually meeting them). The day-to-day activities vary with specialty (e.g. ward rounds, clinics, theatres) but there is usually an emphasis on teaching to empower communities to continue the work once the visiting doctor leaves.

the job There are three main options: (1) Voluntary work organized directly with a specific overseas hospital providing specialist services (e.g. clinics and training for local staff) for a fixed period of time. (2) Clinical or public health work through a non-governmental organization (NGO) e.g. Merlin (p 200), Médecins sans Frontières, Red Cross or VSO (p 290). They may provide a limited wage though this will probably not cover a mortgage back home. They usually require a certain level of experience (e.g. ST3 and post-membership) and a minimum time commitment (e.g. 2–12 months). (3) Work for a governmental or larger organisation (e.g. World Health Organisation) with opportunities for political and managerial roles. Significant clinical experience is required, this work is mostly office-based although it is usually well paid.

extras This is not a career for those looking for private practice or super-specialization. The main advantages are travelling, experiencing different cultures, making a difference to a community and expanding clinical skills. There are also some limited options for research.

🛈 *For further information:*

World Health Organisation: http://www.who.org
The Red Cross: http://www.redcross.org.uk
Voluntary Services Overseas: http://www.vso.org.uk
Merlin: http://www.merlin.org.uk
Medécins sans Frontières: http://www.msf.org
Red-R: http://www.redr.org.uk
Medics Travel: http://www.medicstravel.org

A day in the life in a refugee camp ...

06:00	Wake up to the sounds of the camp stirring
07:00	Breakfast and planning session with other staff
08:00	Review of sickest patients in the inpatient tent
10:00	Start clinic: a triage is run by local nurse but the patient line stretches far into the distance; see patients with translator
13:00	Pause for lunch and case discussion with colleagues
13:30	Back to clinic; by sunset over 100 patients have passed through
18:00	Called to see a women in obstructed labour; forceps delivery
20:00	Evening meal with colleagues then straight to bed for much-needed sleep

myth	An easy life escaping from work to go travelling
reality	Can be, but can also be the hardest work imaginable, often with little, and sometimes no, reward
personality	Independent thinker, sense of social responsibility, calm, flexible, good clinical skills, patient
best aspects	Seeing the world; being involved in the heart of a community and really making a difference
worst aspects	Being helpless in a resource-poor environment or where a man-made situation causes continuing harm
route	Public health (p 44), general practice (p 32), medicine (p 34, with the diploma of tropical medicine and hygiene)
locations	Anywhere in the world from hospitals, community projects and field tents to the offices of NGOs or the World Health Organisation

life						**work**
quiet on-call						**busy on-call**
boredom						**burnout**
uncompetitive						**competitive**
low salary						**high salary**

Paediatric surgery

Paediatric surgery is still the most varied surgical career. The patients range from premature neonates to adolescents, and although children can become very ill very quickly they have a strong tendency to bounce back and the vast majority are curable. The surgery covers almost everything except the heart, bones and brain, so it includes abdominal, thoracic, trauma surgery, some neurosurgery, some plastic surgery, transplantation, endoscopy, laparoscopic surgery and a tiny amount of cancer surgery. Most surgeons work in tertiary centres, but the system is changing and district general hospitals (DGH) may employ paediatric surgeons to cover their routine work and reduce the need to transfer children.

the patients Paediatric surgeons give advice on antenatally diagnosed problems and operate on children from 500g (birth at 25 weeks gestation) to 75 000g (16-year-old adolescents). Most patients are under 5 years old, so communication with the whole family is automatic and essential. Although some neonatal problems require continuous follow-up for 16 years, most children are cured or their management is shared with paediatricians. Disability is an increasing source of complex surgery, as increasing efforts are made to improve the quality of life of these children (e.g. prevent vomiting, create a continent bladder, ensure faecal continence).

the work There are three main subgroups: (1) Neonatal surgery, performed on babies with congenital anomalies (e.g. an absent anus or misconnected oesophagus) (2) Older children with acquired or congenital problems (e.g. appendicitis or problems related to cerebral palsy) (3) The largest group are simple conditions only requiring day case surgery either in a tertiary unit or a DGH (e.g. circumcision or inguinal hernia). Surgery takes place against on a background of daily ward rounds, twice-weekly clinics (often in the local DGH) and regular teaching meetings.

the job Like many surgery jobs, time is split between theatre, clinics and the wards. The service has always been very consultant-led, so an on-call rota of 1:4 to 1:7 will include more night and weekend work than most specialties. Most paediatric surgeons work closely with the relevant paediatricians, including neonatologists, and have specialist paediatric nurses as part of the team.

extras Under- and postgraduate teaching is a constant feature, but academic posts are rare. Private practice is minimal. Paediatric urology is now almost completely separate and treats complex kidney, bladder and genital abnormalities (e.g. neurogenic bladder or hypospadias). Flexible training is possible and easier than in many surgical specialties.

ℹ️ *For further information:*

The British Association of Paediatric Surgeons, 35–43 Lincoln's Inn Fields, London, WC2A 3PE
Tel: 020 7869 6915   Fax: 020 7869 6919   Web: http://www.baps.org.uk

08:00	Ward round and see patients for theatre
08:30	Theatre list: three day cases—inguinal hernia, sigmoidoscopy, excision of thyroglossal cyst and one inpatient—insert gastrostomy for child with feeding problems and cystic fibrosis; review patients post-op
13:00	Leave for DGH; eat lunch in car
14:00	Outpatients in DGH; 12–15 patients of which 6–8 are new (presenting with acquired and congenital problems) and 7–9 old (post-op follow-up for minor surgery (one-off) or major surgery (long-term))
18:30	Home; after supper, correct draft of paper for publication

myth	Manic surgeons with Pooh ties and waistcoats doing circumcisions
reality	The most varied surgical specialty, as almost all surgical subspecialties are possible and the patients range from small babies to adolescents; thinking paediatricians who can operate
personality	Ability to communicate with infants, children, adolescents, parents and grandparents, good practical skills, calm in an emergency
best aspects	Huge variety of work, every week of your entire career you can see something new; minimal cancer work and very few deaths
worst aspects	Still considerable night and weekend work as a consultant; everyone thinks that you are wealthy because you are a surgeon, but private practice is minimal
route	ST1 Surgery in general, paediatric surgery (p 48) then ST3 Paediatric surgery; FRCS exam
numbers	240 of which 15% are women
locations	Hospital-based in large tertiary hospitals and a few DGHs

life						work
quiet on-call						busy on-call
boredom						burnout
uncompetitive						competitive
low salary						high salary

Paediatrics

Paediatrics offers one of the most diverse jobs in medicine. In a single week a paediatric registrar might intubate a premature baby, diagnose coeliac disease in a toddler, resuscitate a teenager with meningitis and counsel parents on coping with their child's newly diagnosed diabetes. And all of this takes place with *Finding Nemo* in the background! The specialty includes generalists in district general hospitals, community paediatricians and tertiary centres with specialist services.

the patients Paediatrics covers children from birth to the age of 16–19 years; about 75% of the case load is under 5 years of age. In smaller centres paediatrics includes newborn babies (neonates), though in larger hospitals this is a separate specialty (p 204). One of the main challenges of paediatrics is dealing with such a wide range of patients, from toddlers' tantrums to ultra-cool teenagers. Along with the children, the paediatrician also needs to communicate effectively with parents for the history and management plan. Families are often followed up for many years.

the work The diverse range of patients is reflected in the range of illnesses. Paediatricians are generalists in the truest sense and only the biggest hospitals have outright specialists. Infectious diseases make up the majority of the workload, particularly children with fever and the yearly bronchiolitis epidemic. The majority of patients make a rapid and full recovery. Non-accidental injury is uncommon, but must stay in the back of the mind all the time and can create difficult dilemmas.

the job There is an equal split of ward- and clinic-based medicine. The specialty is very senior-led so that consultants have a hands-on approach, however this does mean that telephone calls in the middle of the night are relatively common. Regular liaison with paediatric dieticians, physiotherapists, occupational therapists, play specialists and nurse specialists is essential.

extras There are plentiful opportunities to teach medical students and junior doctors. Academic interests are encouraged but not essential (unless hoping to specialize). Private practice is somewhat limited and depends on the adequacy of local services. Flexible training is well established and respected.

ⓘ *For further information:*

Royal College of Paediatrics and Child Health, 50 Hallum Street, London, W1N 6DE
Tel: 020 7307 5600   Fax: 020 7307 5601   Website: http://www.rcpch.ac.uk

08:30	Handover from night team
09:00	Ward round: 21 beds, 8 children discharged
11:30	Called to review septic child in admission unit
12:00	Radiology meeting
13:00	Paediatric grand round
14:00	Outpatient clinic: eight families seen; called in middle of clinic to discuss further management of septic child
16:30	Mini ward round and review of three new admissions
17:30	Hand over to evening team and head home to more kids!
19:00	Spend evening reviewing latest Disney DVDs

myth	Big kids swinging tiny stethoscopes and wearing Disney ties
reality	True generalists managing all manner of conditions in patients from 24 weeks' gestation to 16–19 years
personality	Sense of humour mandatory, calm, approachable, excellent communication skills with all age groups, patient
best aspects	Great variety; high cure rate in most areas; flexible training options are well established
worst aspects	Can have high emotional content—failure can be catastrophic; limited scope for private practice; babies don't know the difference between night and day!
route	ST1 Paediatrics (p 238); MRCPCH exam
numbers	3900 of which 45% are women
locations	Hospital-based specialty found in most hospitals

life		work
quiet on-call		busy on-call
boredom		burnout
uncompetitive		competitive
low salary		high salary

Pain management

Pain management is a specialty that has evolved over the last 30 years and embraces both the care of patients in the peri-operative period and those who have long-standing problems associated with trauma, nerve injury and chronic disease. In 2007 the Faculty of Pain Medicine was established within the Royal College of Anaesthesia to ensure a dedicated training pathway. Most consultants supervise teams of specialist pain nurses who provide the continuity for inpatient care. The ideal environment is that of a multidisciplinary team with consultants having primary responsibility for coordinating the care of those with chronic pain. The focus of activity is changing, with specialist services being provided in tertiary centres whilst many services are being devolved to Primary Care Trusts who are providing exciting opportunities for service development.

the patients are of all ages but the majority are over 40 years with a female predominance. Aside from pain issues, most patients are generally healthy, though they may have limited mobility. As its name suggests, chronic pain can last a long time so there is significant continuity of care.

the work Chronic low back pain is the single largest diagnostic group, while others include nerve injury (neuropathic pain), trauma, degenerative joint disease and cancer. The emphasis is on pain management rather than cure. Great importance is placed on dealing with the emotional and psychological responses to pain and distress. Techniques are developed and therapies provided to encourage greater independence among patients. Improving activities of daily living and developing coping strategies are key elements of care. Psychological support, combining cognitive behavioural therapy and pain management programmes, is essential.

the job There is a mixture of ward-based activity, outpatient clinics and theatre sessions for procedures. It is a consultant-run service supported by specialist pain nurses and nurse consultants. On-calls are usually relaxed but where specialized services such as spinal cord stimulation or implanted drug delivery systems are developed the days can be long. Pain management programmes require integration with specialist support from physiotherapists, psychologists, physicians, neurosurgeons and rheumatologists.

extras Pain is a 'hot' subject for the pharmaceutical industry and there are many opportunities for clinically based research and academic involvement. Teaching at undergraduate and postgraduate levels is common and educational travel is encouraged through the 10 000-member-strong International Association for the Study of Pain (IASP). Private practice is in the 'regular earnings' category.

ℹ *For further information:*

Faculty of Pain Medicine, Royal College of Anaesthetists, Churchill House, Red Lion Square, London WC1R 4SG
Tel: 020 7092 1726 Web: http://www.rcoa.ac.uk/

A day in the life ...

07:45	Review new referral letters and requests for medicolegal reports
08:30	Meet with nurse specialists and review new inpatient referrals
09:00	Outpatient clinic, mixture of new and old patients, interspersed by phone calls from GPs and patients
12:00	Review patients seen on the wards with nurse specialists
13:00	Meet palliative care team, review joint patients
14:00	Procedure session in dedicated theatre suite
16:00	Meet office manager to discuss service capacity issues
16:45	Discuss day issues with PA and review latest dictated notes and letters
17:45	See two new outpatients in private wing or one case for a medical report
19:15	Head for home and large G and T!

myth	Ex-anaesthetists sticking TENS machines on whingers
reality	A physician-based discipline requiring a wide range of medical knowledge
personality	Calm, approachable, easy-going, good interpersonal and communicating skills, good listener, patient
best aspects	Wide diversity of medical and social problems; ability to get to know the patients and develop a personalized style of service
worst aspects	Very tiring and can be an emotional drain; few cures and some angry and frustrated patients
route	CT1 Anaesthetics (p 30) then ST3 Anaesthetics with subspecialization; FRCA exam; route may change to core medical training with dedicated ST programme in the future
locations	Hospital-based, found in larger district general hospitals and teaching hospitals

life					work
quiet on-call					busy on-call
boredom			☺		burnout
uncompetitive					competitive
low salary					high salary

Palliative medicine

Palliative medicine deals with patients and families in crisis. It is the medical component of multidisciplinary palliative care. All patients have serious, advanced illness and their needs tax clinical, medical and psychological skills in order to relieve their distress. The specialty evolved from hospice medicine and has grown very rapidly, especially since publication of the NHS Cancer Plan.

the patients Most patients referred will be beyond cure, although some may have intractable symptoms requiring your skills. Although many are elderly, there are a surprisingly large number of seriously ill younger adults. Paediatric colleagues may occasionally seek your opinion and support. Families are your secondary patients, as they are very much part of the caring team. Very few patients have absolutely no social attachments. The duration of direct contact with patients may be short but it is intense and significant.

the work Palliative medicine grew out of cancer care and the majority of patients will have advanced cancer, especially in community and hospice practice. However, increasing pressure to diversify means that general hospital palliative physicians are now seeing as many as 40% non-cancer patients. Outcome measures clearly reflect appropriate expectations such as adequate symptom control, patient and family satisfaction and achievement of preferred place of care (e.g. the patient's home). The work will comprise detailed clinical assessment, therapeutic intervention, sophisticated teamwork and education. The areas of medicine which are crucial include solid general medicine, pharmacology, oncology, psychology and communication skills.

the job Palliative medicine is practiced in the community, in general hospitals and in specialist units (hospices). Posts will have differing mixtures of these components. Team work within palliative care is essential and sophisticated. Clinical nurse specialists, particularly those who can prescribe, are key colleagues within the team. Close liaison with general practitioners and fellow consultants is essential to success and makes the job interesting, challenging and supportive. Palliative physicians will often be in the position of assisting colleagues when they have reached the limit of their expertise.

extras Opportunities exist for teaching and for enlarging the rather small research base. Palliative insights are welcomed outside medical circles, for instance in sociology, psychology, philosophy and ethics. Foreign travel to describe UK practices is often requested as palliative care is a new specialty originating in the UK. Private practice is virtually non-existent but flexible training is well established.

ℹ️ *For further information:*

The Association for Palliative Medicine of Great Britain and Ireland, Bellis House, 11 Westwood Road, Southampton, SO17 1DL
Tel: 023 8067 2888   Web: http://www.palliative-medicine.org

08:30   Journal club with staff at hospice

09:30   Admission meeting to confirm requests for hospice beds that day

10:00   Multidisciplinary team meeting for inpatients

11:30   Ward round with trainee, senior nurse seeing patients and families

13:00   Meet visiting foreign doctor over lunch

13:45   Travel to general hospital

14:15   Seminar with F1 doctors about ethics at the end of life

15:30   Hospital ward visits with clinical nurse specialist (CNS)

16:30   Home visit with community CNS and district nurse

19:00   Home for supper and to review communication skill teaching strategy

22:15   Call from hospice night nurse with drug dose query

myth	Hand-holding pious do-gooders
reality	Demanding medically and psychologically; one of the most intensely clinical specialties, with a strong team philosophy
personality	Caring, compassionate, able to handle raw emotions, empathy mixed with degree of toughness, well balanced, team player
best aspects	Genuine gratitude from patients and relatives; opportunity to help in people's life crises; emphasis on team work; work takes place in hospitals and in patients' homes
worst aspects	Psychological battle fatigue; nursing philosophy that views palliative medicine as only opioid prescription; fear that delay until tomorrow may be too late
route	CT1 Core medical training (p 34) or GP vocational training (p 32) then ST3 Palliative medicine; MRCP or nMRCGP exam
numbers	500 of which 60% are women
locations	Mixture of hospitals, specialist units and the community

life			●			**work**
quiet on-call			●			**busy on-call**
boredom				●		**burnout**
uncompetitive				●		**competitive**
low salary		●				**high salary**

Pharmaceutical medicine

Pharmaceutical medicine is a specialty based in the pharmaceutical industry or regulatory bodies that researches, develops and regulates medicines, as opposed to Clinical pharmacology and therapeutics (p 120), which is a hospital-based specialty using pharmaceutical knowledge to inform individual patient management. Pharmaceutical physicians (the doctors working in pharmaceutical medicine) help to ensure that everything to do with a medicine is as safe and as effective as possible from the first time it is given to humans to the last prescription dispensed before it is discontinued. Generally pharmaceutical physicians are not involved with direct clinical care, but an encyclopaedic knowledge of medicine and a generous dose of previous clinical experience are essential.

the patients Pharmaceutical physicians do not have patients themselves, but all patients treated with drugs are in some way their responsibility.

the work There are four main roles: (1) Promoting drugs that have gained a product licence or marketing authorization from a regulatory authority; this involves training sales representatives, reviewing proposed advertisements and picking the brains of leading academics to ensure the company maximizes the medical usefulness of its products; (2) Designing, running and reporting clinical trials of a new drug; this entails travelling to visit the academic researchers who are putting their patients into company-sponsored clinical trials; (3) Working in a clinical pharmacology unit doing ward-type work with healthy volunteers who are given drugs under tightly controlled conditions to work out their pharmacokinetic and pharmacodynamic properties; (4) Working for a regulatory authority (e.g. MHRA, the Medicines and Healthcare products Regulatory Agency) to determine the uses of a new drug, how it should be prescribed and to review side-effect reports to decide whether a previously unrecognized side-effect of a treatment has been reported or if a change to the prescribing information is required.

the job is largely office-based though often with frequent travel. Pharmaceutical physicians work alongside a team of pharmacologists, pharmacists, statisticians and marketing/advertising staff. There is no specific on-call, but since it is a business environment there may be demands on time outside office hours.

extras Most pharmaceutical companies are global research-based organizations so there are opportunities to travel and work abroad. Jobs are generally well paid with generous benefits packages unknown in clinical practice. Part-time and freelance work are real possibilities. There is even the possibility of moving onwards and upwards and becoming a business manager.

ℹ *For further information:*

Faculty of Pharmaceutical Medicine, 1 St Andrews Place, Regents Park, London, NW1 4LB
Tel: 020 7224 0343   Fax: 020 7224 5381   Web: http://www.fpm.org.uk
British Association of Pharmaceutical Physicians: http://www.brapp.org.uk

A week in the life ...

Mon	Day in office: emails, teleconference, advert review, research meeting
Tue	Fly to Glasgow to discuss a new clinical trial with a specialist, meetings with research nurse, hospital pharmacist etc.
Wed	Morning in office: emails, literature search; afternoon at meeting in Heathrow hotel to plan next year's programme of education meetings
Thur	Day in office: run training session for sales representatives, phone call to follow up a serious adverse reaction, review report on subgroup analysis of a major clinical trial, update PowerPoint for tomorrow's meeting
Fri	Train to Bristol to give a presentation at a formulary committee meeting of a PCT considering adding company's new drug to their formulary

myth	A glorified drug rep who has sold their soul to industry
reality	Cutting-edge designer and regulator of medicines
personality	There are niches for all personality types from the 'bold as brass' to the 'safe pair of hands'
best aspects	Resources available to support creative scientific thought
worst aspects	Box-ticking and paperwork
route	Can apply to industry jobs anytime after the foundation programme but common route is CT1 Core medical training (p 34) then ST3 Clinical pharmacology and therapeutics; MRCP exam
numbers	700 of which 40% are women
locations	Office-based almost anywhere in the world, usually in big cities

life		**work**
quiet on-call		**busy on-call**
boredom		**burnout**
uncompetitive		**competitive**
low salary		**high salary**

Plastic and reconstructive surgery

Plastic surgery combines the ability to perform complex (and often curative) procedures with an aesthetic eye. The surgery itself requires dexterity, and intimate knowledge of anatomy, disease processes and healing mechanisms. Often reconstructive procedures are one-offs using core skills to approach and solve a unique surgical problem, for instance with a bespoke microsurgical transfer of a piece of tissue from one part of the body to another.

the patients encompass the entire age range, from newborn infants with cleft lip and palate and toddlers with accidental burns, right through to adults with traumatic injuries to the hands or face or various cancers of the skin and soft tissues that require reconstruction. Cosmetic surgery is largely reserved for the fee-paying patient, though the NHS still covers cosmetic defects following trauma and where there is a proven functional or psychological indication. The majority of patients are young and fit and make a good recovery; a few disorders can be life-threatening (e.g. melanoma or severe burns). There is a good mix of short treatment episodes and those that require long-term follow-up (e.g. complex reconstructions and cancers).

the work is extremely variable; emergency work is mainly trauma or burns including hand injuries, severed tendons and nerves and maxillofacial injuries. The elective work is mostly reconstructive, and can range from relatively quick surgery to improve hand function to long and complex procedures with multiple surgeons from a range of specialties. Operations for skin cancers can often be performed under local anaesthetic, which is safer and allows the surgeon to chat to the patient. Most emergencies can be dealt with by middle grades or wait until the next day, however there is always the potential of severe injuries or burns requiring immediate consultant care in the middle of the night (e.g. amputated digits requiring long microsurgical transfers to be reattached).

the job is a mix of operating theatres and clinics; there are also multidisciplinary team meetings or combined clinics for complicated reconstructions requiring several specialists. Contact with a wide range of specialists is common including breast surgeons, maxillofacial surgeons, orthopaedic surgeons and paediatric surgeons, physiotherapists and occupational therapists.

extras There is much research into tissue regeneration, scarring, skin cancer, bioengineering and transplantation, accompanied by numerous conferences. Sub-specialty interests are encouraged (e.g. paediatric plastic surgery or hand surgery, p 160). Cosmetic surgery is expanding globally and there is the potential to be very busy in the Golden Nugget of private practice out-of-hours.

ℹ️ *For further information:*

British Association of Plastic and Reconstructive and Aesthetic Surgeons (BAPRAS), 35–43 Lincolns Inn Fields, London, WC2A 3PE
Tel: 020 7831 5161   Fax: 020 7831 4041   Web: http://www.bapras.co.uk

A day in the life ...

08:00	Check desk and emails before anyone else gets in to disturb me
08:30	Ward round of overnight emergency admissions
09:00	Outpatient clinic: see a mixture of general plastic surgical cases and then a joint case with the breast surgeons of a woman considering an immediate breast reconstruction at the time of mastectomy
12:30	Grab a sandwich from the WRVS canteen and review an article
13:00	Go to day surgery unit and see patients for afternoon list
13:30	Set up music on iPod for the afternoon list before the anaesthetist arrives
13:45	Five day surgery cases
18:00	Private clinic: three new patients (including urgent new diagnosis of melanoma which is excised immediately) and six follow-ups
21:30	Arrive home to find family watching recorded episode of *Nip Tuck*

myth	Bunch of smoothies in pin stripes doing nose jobs
reality	Complex surgery including trauma, burns, cancer, cleft lip and palate, hand surgery and breast reconstruction
personality	Perfectionist, excellent fine coordination, excellent vision, fastidious, practically minded, artistic eye
best aspects	Varied case load; results easy to appreciate; satisfied patients; healthy private practice for those who want it
worst aspects	People thinking plastic surgeons are a bunch of smoothies doing nose jobs, especially at PCT level
route	ST1 Surgery in general, plastic surgery (p 48) then ST3 Plastic surgery; FRCS exam
numbers	700 of which 12.5% are women
locations	Hospital-based, found in most hospitals

life		work
quiet on-call		busy on-call
boredom		burnout
uncompetitive		competitive
low salary		high salary

Pre-hospital medicine

As its name suggests, pre-hospital medicine is about managing a patient prior to transportation to hospital. The aim is to get a suitably equipped and skilled doctor to the patient as soon as possible allowing life-saving and pain-relieving interventions. The majority of practitioners are GPs offering a voluntary on-call service for their local area, major incidents or large sporting/recreational events. Some emergency departments offer pre-hospital services and there are currently four helicopter-based units in the UK (UK HEMS). It is a stimulating and challenging career requiring many diverse skills from remote area survival and a knowledge of vehicle construction to anaesthetics and emergency medicine. It combines decision-making under stress with the ability to work alone, but equally the need to work as a team member with many ancillary services.

the patients The age range is broad, from childbirth (literally) right through to death (sometimes imminent). It may range from caring for one patient to triaging and 'doing the best for the most' in a major incident with several hundred patients at once. Despite expectations of one-off clinical contact, if done in the context of being a GP, the practitioner may remain in contact with the patient and their family for years, with the incident forming the basis of a close clinical relationship.

the work is widely variable. It may include thrombolysing a patient with an MI in their living room, directing traffic to protect non-medical colleagues at a non-injury road accident or being happily bored in the sun at a sporting event. The doctor must be able to care for themselves in potentially hostile environments to ensure that they are relaxed enough to use their clinical skills; this entails being physically fit and mentally robust.

the job is in some ways perfect: no outpatients, no booked surgeries, no ward rounds, in fact sometimes an excuse to leave a consultation! The job offers almost total autonomy and the callout systems have evolved for the needs of different parts of the country. Cities offer a higher workload but with more immediate back-up, whilst rural areas have long transport times to definitive care and limited resources which frequently involve thinking out of the box and emergency services being backed up by vets, farmers or agricultural contractors.

extras The majority of the work is voluntary except for a handful of emergency department or helicopter-based specialists. Teaching is often stimulating and fun. There is great overlap with expedition medicine (p 134), offering exciting travel opportunities. Meetings with peers can be stimulating; there is a need for more quality research but this can be practically and ethically difficult.

ℹ️ *For further information:*

Faculty of Pre-hospital Care, Royal College of Surgeons of Edinburgh, Nicolson Street, Edinburgh, EH8 9DW
Tel: 0131 527 1732   Fax: 0131 557 6406   Web: http://www.rcsed.ac.uk/
British Association for Immediate Care (BASICS): http://www.basics.org.uk

A day in the life ...

09:30	General GP clinic: 10 minute consultations
10:52	Pager sounds in the middle of discussing treatment for Mr Jones' high blood pressure; five-car pile-up on motorway two minutes ago
10:53	Apologize to Mr Jones; receptionist will try to cancel remaining patients
11:06	Arrive at scene via hard shoulder with green light and siren; quick triage: one not breathing (dead), one in respiratory distress, six walking wounded; start primary assessment on patient with respiratory distress
11:20	Needle decompression of tension pneumothorax; ambulance arrives; work with paramedics to stabilize the patient and treat the others
12:30	Accompany patient with pneumothorax to emergency department
13:30	Arrive back at GP surgery for lunch and afternoon clinic...

myth	Rambo of medicine; wears underwear outside flame-resistant trousers
reality	Being cold and wet in a dirty ditch at night feeling lonely whilst making life-saving clinical decisions
personality	Calm, confident team player who knows their strengths and weaknesses, willingness to listen and learn, problem-solving skills
best aspects	Feeling you may have made a difference, if only by being present and supporting your colleagues in the other emergency services
worst aspects	When emergency department staff, with no concept of the job, ignore the handover but offer gentle suggestions of how to do it 'properly'
route	No fixed route; training in anaesthetics, emergency medicine, acute medicine and general practice all help; diploma in immediate medical care from the RCS Edinburgh pre-hospital care faculty (see opposite)
locations	Anywhere, any time in any weather; often GP-based in remote areas

life						work
quiet on-call						busy on-call
boredom						burnout
uncompetitive						competitive
low salary						high salary

Prison medicine

Prison medicine is a GP specialty offering vital primary care services to prisoners; as a job this is fascinating, demanding, exciting, challenging and, at times, frustrating. A prison doctor will see more pathology in a week than a regular GP will see in a month and the scope for improvement and developmental work is enormous. Imprisonment can be a window of opportunity to sort out complex health care issues from substance misuse to chronic disease; a healthier prisoner returned to society is also less likely to offend again.

the patients There are approximately 80000 prisoners in the about 150 prisons throughout the UK, however each year over 200000 men, women and juveniles pass through the system. The population tends to be young with a higher proportion of men. Prisoners have unique health needs; there is a high incidence of mental illness (prevalence of 90%), personality disorders, substance and alcohol misuse, blood-borne viruses (particularly hepatitis C), smoking-related diseases, self-harming behaviour, sexually transmitted infections, dreadful teeth and generally poor health with little previous care. Prisons are to disease what Kew Gardens is to plant conservation.

the work Prisons and prison populations vary. Local prisons are for 'acute' prisoners from local courts or police cells. The prison doctor's work here is focused on substance misuse/withdrawal, assessing mental state, self harm and preventing suicide and medical issues relating to self-neglect. In long-stay prisons the problems are more like those encountered in general practice, with chronic disease management being the mainstay of the work and with an increasing emphasis on care of the elderly. A strong drug subculture leads to constant pressure to prescribe opiate and sedative medication. In female prisons there is a very high incidence of intravenous drug usage, STIs, hepatitis C and cervical pathology. Throughout prisons poorly controlled chronic conditions (e.g. diabetes, epilepsy, asthma, COPD) pose a particular challenge; there is often no identifiable GP, chaotic attendance at hospital appointments and disorganized clinical notes.

the job The majority of the work is clinic-based in prisons; there are often small secure inpatient wards for mild acute illness; those with serious acute illness are transferred to standard hospitals with a police escort. The job is supported by many specialists including mental health teams, substance abuse services, public health and infection control units.

extras All GPs working in prisons will have some sessions in mainstream primary care. The pay is similar to general practice, but the diversity of experience is much greater.

ⓘ *For further information:*

Royal College of General Practitioners, 14 Princes Gate, Hyde Park, London, SW7 1PU
Tel: 020 7581 3232   Fax: 020 7225 3047   Web: http://www.rcgp.org.uk

A day in the life ...

08:00   Emails and papers

08:15   Morning meeting with management, doctors, nurse manager, pharmacy, substance misuse and mental health; review of past 24 hours

09:00   Clinic appointments for prisoners

11:30   Visit segregated prisoners (bad and mad prisoners, often a fine dividing line)

12:00   Admin and lunch

13:00   MDT with psychiatrists, CPNS and other mental health specialists

14:00   'Code black' emergency (unconscious); OK this time, but CPR skills are essential

14:30   Substance misuse clinic

16:00   MDT with health promotion, blood-borne viruses team

18:00   New arrivals; acute medicine, drugs, alcohol, trauma, etc. (paid extra for session)

20:30   Home

myth	Medicine for the brave; dodging murderers to deliver paracetamol
reality	Medicine for the clinically brave treating the broadest mix of pathology seen anywhere in the NHS; challenging, exciting and rewarding on both an individual and public health level
personality	Sense of humour, enthusiasm, non-judgemental, interested in ethical and legal issues, generalist, strong personality
best aspects	The variety: every day is completely different
worst aspects	Sometimes all the patients want is pills
route	GP Vocational training (p 32) then subspecialisation; nMRCGP exam; training in mental health and substance misuse both help
locations	Prisons, there are about 150 around the country

life					**work**
quiet on-call					**busy on-call**
boredom					**burnout**
uncompetitive					**competitive**
low salary					**high salary**

Psychiatry: child and adolescent

Child and adolescent psychiatry is a fascinating branch of medicine covering the assessment and treatment of a wide range of mental health problems in children and adolescents up to 18 years old. It requires skills in assessment, mental state examination, therapeutic approaches and psychopharmacology. There is the added complexity of developmental and family perspectives but the benefit of lengthy assessment and follow-up appointments; an essential luxury compared to other specialties.

the patients are all under 18, though their families are normally integral to assessments and follow-up work. Increasingly only those with significant mental health problems are seen by Child and Adolescent Mental Health Services (CAMHS) whilst less severe cases are managed through a range of community resources. Most patients will require at least four sessions but many, particularly those with enduring mental illness, will require follow-up over years.

the work Presenting problems vary according to the age of the patient. Younger children often present with neurodevelopmental problems, e.g. autism or hyperkinetic disorder (ADHD), whereas adolescent problems are often similar to those seen in adult psychiatry, e.g. anorexia, depression or psychosis. The clinical work may be with the child/adolescent on their own, with their family or occasionally with a group of children or adolescents. Away from the clinics time is spent in team meetings, supervising other team members and in multi-agency meetings (including school staff). Consultant child and adolescent psychiatrists are also often involved in teaching and service developments.

the job The majority of child and adolescent psychiatrists' work is in outpatient clinics, though a small number work in inpatient units. Recently, specialized posts have developed, e.g. adolescents or neurodevelopmental disorders. On-calls for consultants are increasing, but are far from universal; they are generally not busy and most cases require telephone advice only. CAMHS take a multidisciplinary approach to which psychiatrists contribute through mental state examination, psychopharmacology knowledge and expertise in psychotherapeutic approaches (e.g. cognitive behavioural therapy). Liaison with other specialties (e.g. paediatrics, adult psychiatry and emergency medicine) is common.

extras Recent years have seen an expansion in the field including increased opportunity for subspecialization. There are good opportunities for teaching and research and excellent meetings and conferences to support continuing professional development. Flexible training is well established and the specialty is family friendly. Child and adolescent psychiatry is not the career of choice for those with aspirations of private practice (though there are a few opportunities).

ⓘ *For further information:*

Royal College of Psychiatrists, 17 Belgrave Square, London, SW1X 8PG
Tel: 020 7235 2351   Fax: 020 7245 1231   Web: http://www.rcpch.ac.uk

A day in the life ...

08:30 Phone calls to schools to discuss progress of children seen in clinic

09:00 New patient assessment in clinic; 3-year-old with delayed speech being assessed for autism, parents anxious but very helpful

10:30 Follow-up clinic

14:00 Team meeting with discussion of new cases seen over the last week

15:00 Meeting with other professionals involved in development of specialist learning disabilities team

16:30 Advice to a team member assessing adolescent who has self-harmed

16:45 Deal with phone calls/emails/post; dictate assessment report

18:00 Watch *The Simpsons*, play computer games and listen to thrash metal in an attempt to keep up with adolescents' cultural reference points

19:00 Admit defeat: watch *Newsnight* supping Horlicks and wearing slippers

myth	'Soft' specialty exploring cutting-edge developments in helping children keep their mattresses dry at night
reality	Severe and enduring mental health problems are common in children and adolescents and correct management can have dramatic effects; bed-wetters are usually seen by paediatricians
personality	Sense of humour, excellent communication skills, interested in people, calm, pragmatic, good at team work
best aspects	Fascinating and varied, patient improvement often facilitated through the family, development of therapeutic skills
worst aspects	Families who are reluctant to attend/engage; child abuse cases
route	CT1 Psychiatry core-training (p 42) then ST4 Child and adolescent psychiatry; MRCPsych exam
numbers	1150 of which 55% are women
locations	Mostly clinics in the community (e.g. large health centres); some hospital-based clinics and a few inpatient units

life						work
quiet on-call						busy on-call
boredom						burnout
uncompetitive						competitive
low salary						high salary

Psychiatry: general adult

Psychiatry is fascinating; there are no two ways about it! Friends, family and many others, even including one's surgical colleagues, often share this fascination. Psychiatrists are in a very privileged position. Patients confide in them and tell them their most personal and private concerns. This confidence does not occur automatically but is achieved partly through advanced training in communication and interviewing skills and partly because in psychiatry there is more time (and a greater inclination) to ask and to listen.

the patients Adult psychiatry covers patients from 17 to 65 years of age, with a very broad range of conditions and backgrounds. Patients may be hallucinating, suffering alarming delusions, unable to stop compulsive checking, experiencing panic attacks, uninhibited and grandiose or in the pit of depressive despair. They may have been referred because of chronic physical symptoms for which there is no apparent organic cause. The list of possibilities goes on and on, and no two cases are the same. The overriding theme in adult psychiatry is variety.

the work Psychiatry is not an easy option. The work can be challenging and requires sustained concentration and thought regarding the problems which present. Because no blood test or scan will yet differentiate between different diagnoses (e.g. paranoid schizophrenia and mania) psychiatrists need to rely in large part on their knowledge, experience and clinical acumen. They work very closely with other members of a multidisciplinary team, including nurses, occupational therapists and social workers, to take a biopsychosocial approach to dealing with the patient's problems. The challenge of elucidating the relevant features of the presentation, generating a meaningful formulation and putting together an effective multidisciplinary treatment plan is central to what makes psychiatry so enjoyable.

the job There are several subspecialties to choose from, including community psychiatry, addictions, forensic psychiatry (p 140), liaison (general hospital) psychiatry and psychotherapy (p 246). Each has its own particular mix of disorders and therapeutic approaches, ranging from the biological (an ever improving array of medications as well as modified electroconvulsive therapy) to the psychological (including cognitive behavioural therapy and psychodynamic psychotherapy). Referrals come from several sources, including GPs, hospital doctors, social workers, police and various other agencies.

extras There are many opportunities for teaching (medical students, junior doctors and other health care professionals) and for research (not just in academic centres). Private practice is also possible, whether in an NHS consultant's own time or by working for a private mental health service provider.

ⓘ *For further information:*

Royal College of Psychiatrists, 17 Belgrave Square, London, SW1X 8PG
Tel: 020 7235 2351   Fax: 020 7245 1231   Web: http://www.rcpsych.ac.uk

A day in the life ...

08:30   A cup of coffee with the team and review of new referrals, allocating each to the most appropriate team member for assessment

09:30   Seeing a patient with schizophrenia with a community psychiatric nurse; assessment of risk (e.g. suicidal ideas) and management options

10:30   Teaching junior colleagues

11:30   Phone call with GP about managing a patient with complex depression

12:00   Sandwich lunch while discussing an idea for improving the service

12:30   Case conference presented by an ST2 and followed by an interesting and helpful exchange of ideas amongst all grades of psychiatrists

13:30   Sort out mail and go through emails

14:00   Clinic; one new patient assessment and several interesting follow-ups

17:00   Home, not on-call too often and not too onerous when on

myth	'Mad' doctors assessing 'mad' patients
Reality	Diverse, challenging work making important decisions about patients' management and risk
personality	Excellent communicator, team player, empathetic
best aspects	Variety of psychiatric conditions, investigations and treatment options; options for research and subspecialization; teamwork
worst aspects	A heavy workload in some jobs with the possibility of burnout, although this is lessened by effective team working
route	CT1 Psychiatry core-training (p 42) then ST4 General adult psychiatry; MRCPsych exam
numbers	4800 of which 30% are women
locations	Depends on the subspecialty area; may include community clinics, hospital inpatients or secure units

life					work
quiet on-call					busy on-call
boredom					burnout
uncompetitive					competitive
low salary					high salary

Psychiatry: old age

Why on earth would anyone want to work with mad old people? Mental health problems are particularly common among the elderly and the specialty of old age psychiatry has developed over the last 30 years in recognition of the unique needs of older people, whether they live in the community or in a hospital. Two-thirds of NHS beds are occupied by elderly patients and at least half of these have a mental health problem. The most striking facet of the specialty is the wide range of patients, care settings and illnesses that the job covers.

the patients Most old age psychiatry services see people after they reach the age of 65 years, though people who develop dementia before that age are often under the care of old age psychiatrists too. The patients come from all backgrounds, since mental health (and dementia in particular) pays no respect to gender, race or social class. There are important links to be forged with family members (spouse, siblings, children and occasionally parents), carers and wider social networks. Contact can be as a one-off, but more often takes place over several years, meaning that therapeutic relationships can evolve and mature over time.

the work is wonderfully varied, but common themes are person-centred care, independence and choice. Depression and dementia are common in late life, and no two patients present in the same way, leading to diagnostic and management challenges. One of the core roles is using specialist knowledge and skills to construct and help deliver complex packages of care that keep people at home; this entails a lot of work interfacing with other organizations such as social services. Other conditions include delirium, alcohol misuse, schizophrenia and pretty much every other mental disorder in the book.

the job is usually based in the community within a multidisciplinary team of psychiatrists, CPNs, social workers, psychologists and occupation therapists. 'In the community' means just that, with a lot of assessments carried out at home. There are usually a couple of outpatient clinics each week. A small inpatient population (usually divided into beds for functional or organic disorders) requires input including a ward round once or twice a week. On-call can be shared with colleagues from other psychiatric specialties, though some centres have a separate rota for old age psychiatry. Either way the on-call is rarely busy.

extras Old age psychiatry is generally an under-researched area, so opportunities are readily available, particularly in service evaluation and delirium. There is a Nobel Prize waiting for the person who sorts out dementia! Medical students like old age psychiatry placements for the wide range of opportunities and enthusiasm shown by all staff. Flexible training is well established.

ⓘ *For further information:*

Royal College of Psychiatrists, 17 Belgrave Square, London, SW1X 8PG
Tel: 020 7235 2351   Fax: 020 7245 1231   Web: http://www.rcpsych.ac.uk

08:30	Turn up at the community unit, pop the kettle on and check mail
09:00	Memory clinic, working with a nurse and Alzheimer's Society worker to assess and monitor patients and carers; includes mid-morning break for coffee and biscuits
12:30	Case conference at the psychiatric hospital
14:00	Community team meeting to allocate new referrals and review caseloads
15:00	Supervision of a trainee
16:00	Visit paranoid woman at home who believes her neighbours are pumping gas into her flat; discuss with her GP and agree to ask a CPN colleague to visit
17:30	Arrive home, confident that there will be no disturbance from work; reflect on an excellent career choice!

myth	Herding demented old folk into nursing homes
reality	Helping older people maintain their independence and mental health
personality	Good team player, strong leadership qualities, sense of humour, caring, good communication skills, patient
best aspects	Fascinating variety of problems and the ability to make a real difference for a marginalized group of people
worst aspects	Endless assessments of capacity, often requested in error; the need to continually remind others why your service is important
route	CT1 Psychiatry core-training (p 42) then ST4 Old age psychiatry; MRCPsych exam
numbers	1050 of which 40% are women
locations	Community-based throughout the country

life						work
quiet on-call						busy on-call
boredom						burnout
uncompetitive						competitive
low salary						high salary

Psychiatry of learning disability

Learning disability (LD) psychiatry is a rewarding and varied specialty offering mental health services to a patient group with complex needs. The term 'learning disability' is used in the UK rather than 'mental retardation' in the USA or 'intellectual disabilities' in most of Europe. Care of those with LD has moved away from institutional settings (e.g. the asylums of Victorian times) towards a community-based setting with a wide range of services tailored to individuals. LD psychiatry is appealing to people who enjoy the continuity of working with the same people for long periods and who function well in multidisciplinary teams.

the patients People with learning disability are defined as having an IQ of less than 70 since childhood with a deficit in social functioning. This may be due to autism, a recognized syndrome, or may have no known cause. Overall about 3% of the general population meet this definition; many also have communication difficulties or physical disabilities. Most LD psychiatrists see patients with mental health problems from 18 years upwards (younger patients with LD maybe seen by child and adolescent psychiatrists, p 238 but are sometimes seen by LD psychiatrists who specialize in seeing children). Their carers and family are essential as a source of information as well as for management and support.

the work Many psychiatric disorders are over four times more common in those with learning disabilities. Diagnosis can be extremely challenging due to difficulties in communication and understanding, so the specialty requires excellent clinical skills and an ability to integrate many different sources of information. Neuroses (e.g. generalized anxiety disorder, obsessive–compulsive disorder) and challenging behaviours are especially common, but the full range of general psychiatric disorders are seen including depression, bipolar disorder and schizophrenia. Epilepsy is extremely common in this population (about 30%) so knowledge of epilepsy management and pharmacology is essential.

the job is largely community-based and LD psychiatrists work in a wide range of settings including day centres, patients' own homes, community clinics, hospitals and occasionally police stations. Due to the complex nature of the client group, community teams consist of a broad range of professionals including psychologists, nurses, occupational therapists, physiotherapists, dieticians, speech therapists, social workers and care managers. Compared to most specialties the on-call workload is quite light.

extras There are plenty of opportunities for both teaching and research; academic interests are encouraged but not essential. Private practice is relatively limited but income can be supplemented by doing medicolegal work. Flexible training is well established.

ⓘ *For further information:*

Royal College of Psychiatrists, 17 Belgrave Square, London, SW1X 8PG
Tel: 020 7235 2351   Fax: 020 7245 1231   Web: http://www.rcpch.ac.uk

A day in the life ...

09:00   Team meeting to discuss the latest referrals and difficult cases including a person with learning disabilities and diabetes who is refusing treatment

10:30   Community clinic: one new patient who has recently become very disturbed when left alone; several follow-ups with a variety of mental health problems

13:30   Mental Health Act assessment of patient presenting with psychotic illness and learning disabilities who is displaying aggressive behaviour and refusing medication

15:00   Inpatient clinical team meeting to review the management of each of the patients

17:30   Leave for home

myth	Dolling out Prozac in asylums
reality	A community-based specialty with the potential to make a big difference to disadvantaged individuals
personality	Tolerant of uncertainty, easy-going, patient, non-judgemental, empathetic, positive, team player, excellent communication skills
best aspects	The field of LD is filled with caring and enthusiastic people; patients are very rewarding to work with
worst aspects	Funding disputes, especially for complex cases
route	CT1 Psychiatry core-training (p 42) then ST4 Psychiatry of learning disability; MRCPsych exam
numbers	450 of which 45% are women
locations	Mixture of community- and hospital-based settings

life					**work**
quiet on-call					**busy on-call**
boredom					**burnout**
uncompetitive					**competitive**
low salary					**high salary**

Psychotherapy

For those really interested in what makes people tick, psychotherapy is the ideal career. Psychoanalytic psychotherapy is essentially the study of relationships. It uses the relationship between therapist and patient as the vehicle for therapeutic change. Above all else it is a human encounter, 'being with' rather than 'doing to'. Working closely with people and observing them develop, often after the most appalling circumstances, is an extraordinarily moving experience. Patients are increasingly demanding psychological therapies. The challenge for the profession is how to provide improved access with limited resources.

the patients People come with the whole range of human difficulties: mental illness (particularly personality disorders and complex, long-standing problems), psychosomatic illness, profound neglect, abuse and trauma. Behind these presentations are fundamental problems in relating to 'the self' and others which can be traced back to their earliest experiences in the family. These ways of relating are reviewed in the therapeutic relationship, which is then used as a safe place for exploration and understanding, linking past experiences with present symptomatology. This enables the patient to develop new and more satisfying relationships. Finding and making these links is like being part of an unfolding drama which therapist and patient write together using the psychoanalytic model as a frame of reference. Thus, no two therapies are ever alike. This is what makes being a psychotherapist endlessly fascinating.

the work Therapy can be of any duration from a single session to several years; it is common to have weekly sessions for 3 to 24 months. It can be practiced individually, in couples, in families or in groups. A typical psychological therapies department is multidisciplinary (doctors, nurses, psychologists and occupational and other therapists) and provides a range of therapeutic models. Medical psychotherapists traditionally train in psychoanalytic psychotherapy although some now train in cognitive and cognitive analytic therapy.

the job The consultant will see the most complex patients for assessment and therapy. A significant proportion of time will be spent providing supervision, teaching, training and consultation to other mental health staff and GPs. Additionally, the consultant will usually have a role as the head of department, in clinical leadership and in department development.

extras There are good opportunities for private practice, though these are not always lucrative. An essential aspect of training is personal therapy to deal with unresolved conflicts and painful memories, which hinder emotional and psychological development. It is essential we know as much about ourselves, our strengths and our weaknesses, in order not to impose our own solutions on our patients. It is, above all, an awe-inspiring and humbling experience.

ⓘ For further information:

Royal College of Psychiatrists, 17 Belgrave Square, London, SW1X 8 PG
Tel: 020 7235 2351   Fax: 020 7245 1231   Web: http://www.rcpsych.ac.uk

A day in the life ...

09.00	Supervise trainees
10.30	See a patient dealing with issues regarding childhood emotional abuse
11.30	Referrals meeting (with coffee)
12.30	Departmental or academic meeting (with lunch)
14.00	New assessment of a patient presenting with obsessive–compulsive symptoms
16.00	Dealing with latest crisis or government 'initiative' (with tea)
17.00	Group therapy

myth	Middle-aged men talking to young, attractive articulate women about their sexual fantasies
reality	There are no stereotypes; a long training requiring dedication and self-motivation; always interesting, demanding, frustrating and satisfying by turns
personality	Well-balanced, curious about the human mind, introspective, thoughtful, patient, tolerant, capacity to enjoy life
best aspects	It is uplifting to encounter hopefulness and courage in adversity; continues to be fascinating throughout one's career; what could be more interesting than talking to people about life?
worst aspects	Can be emotionally and psychologically draining; it is never as easy as it sounds; government interference with inappropriate targets and simplistic solutions
route	CT1 in Psychiatry core-training (p 42) then ST4 in Psychotherapy; MRCPsych exam
numbers	330 medical psychotherapists of which 50% are women
locations	Outpatient departments in the community or in hospitals; there are a few specialist residential units

life		work
quiet on-call		busy on-call
boredom		burnout
uncompetitive		competitive
low salary		high salary

Public health

Most doctors focus on one patient at time. Public health considers groups of people. It may be a population defined by geography, age or disease. Instead of treating illness, public health is about preventing illness. It aims to find ways of helping people to improve their health, especially the most vulnerable and those who are least likely to receive care or services. The job is mainly about the long term; how can people be encouraged to take more exercise? How can the rise in TB be stopped? What are we going to do if there is flu pandemic?

the patients While about 6 billion people could benefit from public health interventions, the actual specialists have no direct patient contact. Public health is about working with people and systems to achieve change. This may be working with GPs, hospital specialists, teachers, schools, the police, politicians or the public. Public health is practiced everywhere. One day it may be going into a school to discuss an outbreak of meningitis, next doing a radio interview on teenage pregnancy then visiting the local authority to talk to local councillors.

the work is about making populations healthier. This may be by introducing a health promotion programme such as stopping smoking or stopping the increase in childhood obesity. Health protection is a major part of the work, such as following up an outbreak of food poisoning or Polonium poisoning or even saving the nation from some new disease such as Avian flu or SARS. Assessing data and looking at the evidence are fundamental because public health is about putting research and evidence into practice.

the job Instead of a ward, public health clinicians are office-based, though they are often at meetings or working in the community. Words and data replace the stethoscope. Communication and influence are the tools of the trade to make change happen. The work is very varied and can take place in all sorts of places. Some doctors specialize and work with one group of people or a small range of diseases. Others are generalists and relish the managerial and political aspects of the job as the Director of Public Health for a PCT. Others teach or are researchers.

extras There are many opportunities for teaching, writing, media work, researching or developing national policy. Flexible training is well established and respected. There is very limited scope for private practice.

For further information:

Faculty of Public Health, 4 St Andrews Place, London, NW1 4LB
Tel: 020 7935 0243   Fax: 020 7224 6973   Web: http://www.fphm.org.uk

A day in the life ...

08:30	Reply to emails, go through some papers with the secretary
10.00	Spend time with other members of staff discussing various issues
11.00	Attend meeting with the education authority about teenage pregnancy
12:00	Launch a new chlamydia service at the local Boots
13:00	Visit a group of GPs to talk about smoking cessation services
14:00	Meet with PCT colleagues to discuss management issues
15:00	Make a number of phone calls, reply to emails, talk to staff
16:00	Chair a meeting to review the PCT breast screening figures
16:30	Leave the meeting early to participate in a telephone conference with the HPA about a food poisoning outbreak in the local hospital
17.45	Go home, read the papers for tomorrow's meeting at the local hospital

myth	Doctors who prefer committees to patients
Reality	A wide-ranging specialty from communicable disease, through health service quality to health improvement; working with the NHS and a wide range of other organizations
personality	Sees the bigger picture, optimistic, relishes a challenge, 'can do' attitude, sociable, mathematical skills
best aspects	Great variety; very flexible; special interests encouraged; most people have more than one job in the specialty during their career; on-call is minimal except in communicable diseases
worst aspects	Takes a long time to see results; subject to regular reorganization and change; little private practice
Route	ST1 Public health medicine (p 44); MFPH exam
Numbers	1550 of which 45% are women
locations	PCTs, health authorities, universities, Department of Health, Health Protection Agency, potentially anywhere...

life		work
quiet on-call		busy on-call
boredom		burnout
uncompetitive		competitive
low salary		high salary

Radiology: diagnostic

As its name suggests, diagnostic radiology is about finding out what is wrong with patients. The increasing range and complexity of imaging techniques (X-ray, ultrasound, CT, MRI, nuclear isotopes) means that physicians and surgeons cannot maintain a breadth of knowledge about all the possible ways to image the body, so they are more and more dependent on the expertise of the imaging specialist to select the appropriate methods and interpret the results. Because of the range of patients involved, the radiologist needs an encyclopaedic knowledge of clinical medicine, surgery, pathology and therapeutics. A firm grasp of imaging technology is important, but anyone who thinks that machines are more fun than people should seek alternative work.

the patients Radiologists investigate everybody else's patients and deal with all types of organic disease. The degree of contact with patients varies immensely; in some sessions the radiologist may never see the patients (reporting stacks of images obtained by radiographers or imaging technicians), whilst in other sessions (ultrasound, contrast X-ray procedures) radiologists may spend longer with the patient than the clinician who requested the test. A significant factor is that contact with patients is episodic and transitory—the patients are passing through.

the work In a smaller district general hospital, the radiologist will deal with a wide range of patients, cover all types of disease and use many imaging methods. In larger centres subspecialization usually means the radiologist will specialize with clinical teams (e.g. paediatrics, gastroenterology) rather than having an interest in a particular investigative technique (e.g. CT or MRI).

the job Doctors in radiology divide their time between performing procedures on patients, interpreting the results of other procedures performed by radiographers and interacting with doctors and GPs about the choice of investigations and the significance of the results obtained. Radiology departments are multidisciplinary and require teamwork. The proportion of radiology work carried out outside normal office hours is increasing steadily, so most consultant posts involve a significant on-call commitment.

extras The radiologist will typically have a major role in clinical multidisciplinary meetings. There are many opportunities for undergraduate and postgraduate teaching. Research is either technically based (improving diagnostic procedures) or aligned with clinical investigation. Private practice works well for some and can be lucrative. Flexible training is well established and part-time work can often be accommodated at consultant level.

ℹ️ *For further information:*

Royal College of Radiologists, 38 Portland Place, London, W1N 4JQ
Tel: 020 7636 4432   Fax: 020 7323 3100   Web: http://www.rcr.ac.uk

A day in the life …

08:30	Check correspondence and emails, reply to the urgent ones
09:00	CT session; review and report previous evening's outpatient CTs, while supervising and reporting morning CT patients; session interrupted by multiple visits from medical and surgical colleagues to discuss cases
13:00	Grab a quick sandwich then start afternoon ultrasound session early to deal with acute abdominal patient from emergency department and urgent post-op cases from surgical wards
14:00	Patients for ultrasound, 15 minutes per examination
17:00	Dictate ultrasound reports and phone through urgent or unexpected results to clinical teams before heading home, if not on-call

myth	Bad-tempered, vitamin D-depleted introverts who just say 'no' and prefer to be left alone in dark rooms
reality	Clinical detectives finding out what's wrong with patients using a range of almost magical tools
personality	Good communication skills, excellent visual skills, accommodates most types from the obsessive (reading mammograms for two hours and never making a mistake) to the technical whizz (designing their own MRI sequences)
best aspects	A rich variety of patients and types of illness; collaboration with a wide range of clinical specialties; contact with patients is usually at the most interesting stage of their illness
worst aspects	Prioritizing requests with limited time and resources and every doctor in the hospital wants their patients investigated first
route	ST1 Clinical radiology (p 46); FRCR exam
numbers	3900 of which 30% are women
locations	Hospital-based in most hospitals

life		work
quiet on-call		busy on-call
boredom		burnout
uncompetitive		competitive
low salary		high salary

Radiology: interventional

Interventional radiology is a career in image-guided surgery. It is hospital-based, interacting with all clinical teams and performing a wide variety of emergency and elective cases. Tasks range from embolization following an acute haemorrhage secondary to trauma to electively repairing someone's abdominal aortic aneurysm via small incisions in the groin and insertion of an endograft. It is diverse, stimulating, satisfying and definitely cutting edge. The equipment and technology is state-of-the-art and new procedures and equipment are constantly being developed and under evaluation.

the patients The patients are drawn from all age groups and referred from all specialties. Inserting a Hickman line for central venous access into an infant with leukaemia may be followed by inserting a stent into the bile duct to palliate malignant pancreatic disease in an elderly patient. A good relationship with the patients is essential to treating them well. While the work requires direct contact with the patient, this contact is episodic so they are only under the care of an interventional radiologist for a couple of hours at most.

the work The diverse range of patients is reflected in a wide referral base and the extremely wide range of procedures. There is no body cavity that cannot be reached with a CT-guided needle and a good strong arm! The common theme throughout the work is choosing the most appropriate imaging technique to accurately guide the needles and catheters to intervene in locations that other specialists just can't reach. Many of the procedures use local anaesthetic so patient communication is essential.

the job Approximately 30–50% of the job is spent operating in the special procedures room. The rest of the time is split between studying images (ultrasound, CT or MRI) to plan procedures or assess outcomes and meeting with patients (in- or outpatients) to assess pre-procedure or counsel post-procedure. The specialty is very senior-led so consultants have a hands-on approach assisted by trainees. The increasing importance of the interventional radiologist in managing acute and emergency patients means there is an increasing demand for on-call (often 1:5 or 1:6 as part of a network). Regular liaison via multidisciplinary meetings with all referring clinicians is an important part of the job.

extras There are plentiful opportunities for teaching medical students, junior doctors and trainees. Academic interests are encouraged. Many of the procedures being performed may be new or in development and therefore participation in registries and trials is important. Private practice is available though there is some competition with other specialties (e.g. cardiology). Flexible training is well-established and respected.

ℹ️ *For further information:*

British Society of Interventional Radiology, Lavinia Gittins, 4 Verne Drive, Ampthill, Bedford, MK 45 2PS
Tel: 01525 403026   Fax: 01525 751384   Web: http://www.bsir.org

A day in the life ...

08:30 Pre-operating meeting of team (trainee, radiographers and nurses), planning of cases and organisation of list; there may be emergencies to accommodate

09:00 Operating list (usually 4–5 cases, although variable, as one complex case can occupy an entire list); most cases have been pre-clerked and consented in outpatients

13:00 Mulitidisciplinary meeting (e.g. vascular surgery, renal medicine or gastrointestinal)

14:00 Teaching trainees

15:30 Outpatient clinic: new case referrals and follow-up appointments

17:00 Clinical review of morning cases and dictation of reports

18:00 Home to play space invaders to improve hand-eye coordination

myth	Geeky types who 'dyno-rod' patients in dark rooms in the basement
reality	Dynamic career with wide range of interactions with all hospital specialties; opportunity to make a difference by performing new procedures in a minimally invasive way
personality	Thorough, patient, calm in emergencies and able to handle stressful situations, generalist, excellent practical skills
best aspects	Great variety; high success rate with low complication rates and high level of job satisfaction
worst aspects	Complications: though uncommon they can be catastrophic (e.g. death or disabling stroke in 2–3% of cases of patients having carotid artery stents inserted for atherosclerosis)
route	ST1 Clinical radiology (p 46); FRCR exam
numbers	450
locations	Hospital-based in most hospitals, but full-time subspecialists only in teaching hospitals and larger district general hospitals

life					work
quiet on-call					busy on-call
boredom					burnout
uncompetitive					competitive
low salary					high salary

Rehabilitation medicine

Rehabilitation medicine is about the prevention, diagnosis, treatment and rehabilitation management of people with disabling conditions and comorbidity across all ages. The specialty offers a well-rounded mixture of inpatient care, outpatient care and practical procedures.

the patients are adults of all ages, although some also see children (e.g. spinal cord injury, amputee rehabilitation). The rehabilitation medicine consultant works across all phases of illness and disability from acute management of ventilator-assisted individuals, to rehabilitation, to reintegration into the community with domestic, leisure and employment activities. Rehabilitation is often a slow process leading to long continuity of care of the patient and their family.

the work Although approximately 10% of the UK population experience a disability, rehabilitation medicine consultants generally see patients with complex disabilities including brain injury (traumatic and non-traumatic, e.g. subarachnoid haemorrhage and stroke), multiple sclerosis, spinal cord injury, musculoskeletal disorders and amputation. As well as managing the specific condition, rehabilitation medicine promotes function, activities and participation (including quality of life). This will include medical interventions (e.g. prescribing for bowel, bladder and sexual function impairment or phantom limb pain); interventions (e.g. botulinum toxin injection for spasticity) and preventing and managing secondary complications (e.g. pulmonary embolism, osteoporosis). The work also includes discussing prognoses and devising realistic rehabilitation programmes.

the job Most consultants have a combination of inpatient work in a dedicated specialist unit, inpatient liaison for patients in other hospital settings, outpatient clinics and outreach or liaison with the community. Rehabilitation medicine is often multispecialty and always multidisciplinary; much of the time will be spent in a team environment. The multidisciplinary team (MDT) consists of many professionals including physiotherapists, occupational therapists, nurses, psychologists, social workers, orthotists, engineers and others. Team working with a wide range of colleagues is a constant and essential part of the job. Service development is usually a larger part of the job than in many other specialties. On-call arrangements vary, but are usually relaxed, requiring occasional phone advice.

extras There are good opportunities for teaching and research. Potential research fields are broad and include basic science, interventional work and technological or psychosocial research. Medicolegal work is available to top up funds, though there is limited scope for private practice.

ℹ️ *For further information:*

British Society of Rehabilitation Medicine, c/o Royal College of Physicians, 11 St Andrews Place, London, NW1 4LE
Tel: 01992 638865   Fax: 01992 638674   Web: http://www.bsrm.co.uk

A day in the life ...

08:00	Emails and admin
08:30	Ward round of rehabilitation unit and referrals on other wards
10:00	Teaching review with junior doctors
11:00	Multidisciplinary team meeting to discuss a patient's management
12:00	Office work and lunch
13:30	Outpatient clinic, mostly follow-up appointments
16:00	Ward work/procedures/family discussions
18:00	Home

myth	Glorified physiotherapists helping stroke victims learn how to use wheelchairs
reality	A field of medicine where massive improvements in quality of life are seen, allowing patients to live far more independently
personality	Able to see the long-term picture, team player, patient, good communication skills, realistic
best aspects	Very satisfying to improve patients' functional abilities and quality of life; relatively small specialty so colleagues know each other well and good opportunities for collaboration
worst aspects	Can be frustrating; improvements are slow for some; lack of resources when so much more could be done
route	CT1 Core medical training (p 34), GP vocational training (p 32) or CT1 Surgery in general (p 48) then ST3 Rehabilitation medicine; MRCP, nMRCGP or FRCS exam
numbers	325 of which 25% are women
locations	Mostly based in specialist hospitals but practice in district general hospitals and the community are increasing

life					work
quiet on-call					busy on-call
boredom					burnout
uncompetitive					competitive
low salary					high salary

Renal medicine

Renal medicine is a challenging but rewarding medical specialty. It is still relatively new with lots of innovations constantly being introduced, whether it is in the field of dialysis, transplantation or chronic kidney disease management. It is probably the only specialty where a failed organ's function can be replaced by a machine or replaced through transplantation with great success. Renal physicians are not merely 'washing machine techs'.

the patients Adult nephrology involves a wide age range of patients with different ethnic backgrounds and a broad disease spectrum, ranging from hypertension or diabetes to complex glomerulonephritis. The patients are younger than many expect: the median age of a patient on haemodialysis is 65; on peritoneal dialysis, 59; and at transplant, 50. Renal physicians get to know their patients and families very well as the majority of patients remain under long-term follow-up.

the work There is never a dull day in renal medicine. Work ranges from managing acute renal failure in ITU to giving advice on hypertension in a clinic. Chronic renal failure accounts for a large proportion of the workload; in the UK there are about 24 500 adults on dialysis treatment and about 18 500 patients with functioning renal transplants. The main problems in a dialysis unit are usually related to IV access (e.g. thrombosed fistula or sepsis). Transplant centres manage acute transplant problems including surgical complications or rejection. Challenging cases include complex vasculitides with renal involvement where a prompt diagnosis and treatment can save both the patient's life and their kidneys.

the job has a good mix of both inpatient and outpatient clinical medicine. The specialty is mainly consultant-led with multidisciplinary team support. Strong leadership qualities and good communication skills are essential for working in a team comprising dialysis staff, physiotherapists, occupational therapists, social workers, transplant coordinators and managers. Renal patients often have multiple medical conditions requiring liaison with other specialists. On-calls can be busy and there is no escape from telephone calls in the middle of the night.

extras There are plenty of opportunities for teaching and research in renal medicine. Clinical or basic science research is encouraged but not a must nowadays. The UK Renal Registry (http://www.renalreg.com) offers unique epidemiological renal research opportunities. Private practice is minimal outside London. Flexible training is possible.

ℹ *For further information:*

The Renal Association, Durford Mill, Petersfield, Hampshire, GU31 5AZ
Tel: 0870 458 4155   Fax: 0870 442 9940   Web: http://www.renal.org

08:30	Check emails and letters; try to reduce paperwork pile
09:00	Ward round: 22 patients (with 7 outliers and 2 on ITU)
12:00	Medical student teaching
13:00	Lunch and drive to satellite unit
13:30	MDT meeting in the dialysis unit
14:00	Outpatient clinic
17:30	Board rounds (i.e. talk through inpatients), check results and hand over
18:00	Back to office for a further admin blitz
19:30	Home to enjoy a delicious steak and kidney pie

myth	Overly clever doctors obsessed with numbers (creatinine)
reality	Fairly clever doctors obsessed with patients
personality	A mild obsessive neurosis is essential, calm, approachable, sense of humour, academic
best aspects	Variety; keeps you on your toes; true long-term patient care
worst aspects	Friday afternoon referrals when people knew about the abnormal renal function since Monday morning!
route	CT1 Core medical training (p 34) then ST3 Renal medicine; MRCP exam
numbers	650 of which 20% are women
locations	Hospital-based in teaching hospitals and big district general hospitals; often provide services to a community-based dialysis unit

life		work
quiet on-call		busy on-call
boredom		burnout
uncompetitive		competitive
low salary		high salary

Reproductive medicine

Reproductive medicine (RM) is a subspecialty of obstetrics (p 212) and gynae-cology (p 156). It deals with all problems of reproduction, including surgical management (e.g. endometriosis and tubal disease), medical management (e.g. failure to ovulate), assisted reproduction (IVF and the various offshoots) and a great deal of counselling. The specialty only really began in 1978 with the birth of the first child conceived by IVF; now over 1% of babies born in the UK are conceived in this manner.

the patients RM patients are typically young and come in pairs. Many will never have seen a doctor for reproductive concerns before and they are dealt with as couples, rarely as individuals. Most couples don't expect to have difficulties conceiving and feel cheated, exposed and very hurt as inevitably their friends are having babies. RM entails discussing intimate details of the couple's personal life and coping with the emotions that accompany their failure to conceive. This leads to a close working relationship and it often takes a long time to achieve a single conception, let alone a family. It is especially rewarding to be able to help with the conception and see the pregnancy right through to delivery.

the work The core work is IVF, but this involves taking a history, examining the couple, arranging investigations and then discussing the various therapeutic options. No single treatment fits all because no treatment guarantees success and couples may have ethical concerns (e.g. creation of spare embryos). Overall, per treatment success rate is about 25%, but this depends on many factors, not least of all the female's age. Surgery may be offered as both a primary treatment and as an adjunct to IVF. Laparoscopic excision of advanced endometriosis presents significantly more challenges than the most complex computer game.

the job In the UK, much assisted reproduction is carried out in the private sector, although all regions have an NHS service. Most consultants will work in both. Success in RM necessitates working as part of a multidisciplinary team with embryologists, scientists, specialist nurses and counsellors. IVF units (whether NHS or private) are tightly regulated by the Human Fertilisation and Embryology Authority. Clinical on-call varies but usually involves being on-call as part of the general rota for gynaecology; some also cover the obstetric service.

extras Training is usually carried out at the end of a general training in obstet-rics and gynaecology and includes two clinical years and one research year. There is wide scope for clinical and laboratory-based research and teaching is core to the work. Because of the inadequate funding for IVF in the UK most doctors have both NHS and private practices (which can be lucrative).

🛈 *For further information:*

The Society for Reproduction and Fertility, SRF Business Office, Procon Conferences Ltd, Tattersall House, East Parade, Harrogate, North Yorkshire, HG1 5LT
Tel: 01423 564488   Fax: 01423 701433   Web: http://www.ssf.org.uk

A day in the life ...

07:30	Early morning clinic for ovulation induction and cycle monitoring
09:00	IVF session, outpatient clinic or operating list: there is a great deal of variation from day to day, usually with the creation of a life or two at some point
12:00	Management or teaching session
13:00	Lunch (a historical oddity in many specialties)
14:00	Second clinical session: could be NHS or private
17:00	Home; no lives saved, but maybe a few created...
Night	On-call: usually quiet, unlike obstetrics colleagues

myth	Acting as God and playing with life
reality	Only assisting—more like an angel than a god...
personality	Calm, easy-going, good communicator, accepting of beliefs and views of others, empathetic
best aspects	The look of disbelief on a patient's face when she is told she is finally pregnant
worst aspects	Failure of NHS to provide adequate funding to treat all couples
route	ST1 Obstetrics and gynaecology (p 36) then subspecialty training in reproductive medicine at ST6; MRCOG exam
numbers	180 of which 33% are women
locations	Tertiary level hospitals and private clinics

life		work
quiet on-call		busy on-call
boredom		burnout
uncompetitive		competitive
low salary		high salary

Respiratory medicine

For those who believe that variety is the spice of life, respiratory medicine may be the best career. Lungs can go wrong in so many different ways and in so many different people. Respiratory physicians deal with diseases that are infective, malignant, acute or chronic, ranging from the acutely life-threatening to the seemingly trivial (though not to the patient). They see a wide range of patients and work with many other specialties, often as part of the multidisciplinary team.

the patients vary in age, ethnic background and demographics; they range from adolescents with asthma to the elderly with chronic obstructive pulomnary disease (COPD). Like many medical specialties there are a disproportionate number of elderly patients. Anyone from a lord to a labourer can develop respiratory disease but certain diseases have predilections for particular social groups (e.g. industrial diseases). The variety of patients adds to the interest of the specialty as well as providing challenges. The skills involved in communicating with the adolescent with asthma are very different from those required in telling someone they have lung cancer. Many patients can be dealt with in one or two outpatient visits or during a single hospital stay; others will require long term follow-up.

the work There is a large chronic disease component to chest medicine and these patients will sometimes have a personality partly shaped by their disease. COPD, asthma and lung cancer constitute the majority of the workload, but even within these there is much variety. Respiratory medicine requires many practical skills, including bronchoscopy, pleural aspirations, chest drains through to interventional bronchoscopy and medical thoracoscopies.

the job Respiratory medicine is based on the wards and in outpatients. Since chest disease is common, respiratory wards tend to be filled with respiratory rather than general medical patients. Most chest physicians will undertake 2–3 ward rounds a week and provide consults for patients on non-medical wards as well as attending radiology and multidisciplinary meetings. In a larger hospital subspecialization is usual (e.g. parenchymal lung disease or sleep apnoea). One important trend is the movement of services into the community. It is likely that in the future all respiratory physicians will spend some of their time managing patients in primary care facilities. Many respiratory consultants also spend part of their time managing high-dependency units.

extras While it is not a specialty for getting rich, there is private medicine available. Opportunities for research are abundant and there are a number of excellent research centres in the UK. There is plenty of scope for teaching, both within hospitals and in the community.

ℹ *For further information:*

The British Thoracic Society, 17 Doughty Street, London, WC1N 2PL
Tel: 020 7831 8778   Fax: 020 7831 8766   Web: http://www.brit-thoracic.org.uk

A day in the life ...

08:00	Catch up with paperwork, emails and journal reading
09:00	MDT and lung cancer clinic, break bad news to two patients that they have lung cancer; the treatment is often palliative
13:00	Chest X-ray meeting discussing the most interesting cases/images
14:00	Respiratory ward round with juniors; mixture of teaching and management decisions
17:00	Admin
18:00	Home

myth	'Chrony-bronys' who have smoked themselves into hospital and will never leave because of the few treatments available
reality	A wide variety of chest diseases, only some of which are due to smoking; there are now many treatments available and their use requires skill and experience
personality	Easy-going, laid back, good communicator, calm in an emergency, good practical skills
best aspects	The variety; the mixture of acute and chronic conditions
worst aspects	Inpatients require a high level of social support after discharge which takes time and creates many 'bed blockers'
route	CT1 Core medical training (p 34) then ST3 Respiratory medicine; MRCP exam
numbers	1200 of which 20% are women
locations	Hospital-based in the majority of hospitals

life		work
quiet on-call		busy on-call
boredom		burnout
uncompetitive		competitive
low salary		high salary

Rheumatology

Unless you are unusually clumsy, rheumatology involves no orifices or blood – something of a rarity in a clinical specialty. Rheumatology is a multi-disciplinary specialty that deals with disorders of the connective tissues. This is commonly joints but can be any part of the body's structural components (e.g. skin, bones, etc.). These diseases are often multisystemic making diagnosis a complicated but fascinating task. Although pain is a very common symptom in outpatients, patients present in a wide variety of ways.

the patients All ages and populations suffer from the rheumatic diseases, from the very young with juvenile arthritis to the very elderly; no age is immune. On the whole, patients with chronic problems tend to form a very personal relationship with their rheumatologist and usually have a very good outlook on life. A substantial number of patients are seen regularly and form close clinical relationships with the department. Carers are very frequently involved and interaction with them forms a major part of the management plan.

the work The most common diseases are inflammatory and non-inflammatory arthritides (e.g. osteoarthritis and rheumatoid arthritis) but a substantial number of patients have connective tissue diseases with multiple organs systems affected (e.g. systemic lupus erythematosus [SLE], scleroderma). Any disease that affects the joints, muscles, tendons, ligaments, bones or other connective tissues may present. Diagnosing, managing and treating these disorders can be a complicated business requiring good clinical and investigative skills. The work also includes monitoring immune suppressive therapies and numerous procedures such as joint and soft tissue injections, nerve blocks and skin and muscle biopsies. Ward rounds, ward consults, meetings, teaching and research fill the rest of the day.

the job About half the time is spent in outpatient clinics with the remainder split between the wards and administration. The multidisciplinary team is key and includes nurses, physiotherapists, podiatrists and occupational therapists. Contact with other specialties is common, in particular orthopaedics, neurology, renal medicine, chest medicine and gastroenterology. The on-calls are rarely onerous and usually involve telephone advice unless combined with general medicine.

extras Subspecialization is possible in larger centres including paediatric rheumatology, metabolic bone diseases and musculoskeletal and sports medicine. Research opportunities are widespread in both basic science (rheumatologists have a good reputation for transferring treatments from the lab bench to the patient) and clinical research. Many areas have large private practices, but it is not as lucrative as for some other medical specialties.

For further information:

British Society for Rheumatology, Bride House, 18–20 Bride Lane, London, EC4Y 8EE
Tel: 020 7842 0900   Fax: 020 7842 0901   Web: http://www.rheumatology.org.uk

08:30	Dealing with email queries about rheumatic diseases and treatment from GPs
09:30	Multidisciplinary ward round
11:00	Multidisciplinary meeting with trainees and allied health professionals
12:00	Admin over lunch
13:00	Hospital grand round
14:00	Outpatient clinic with patients every 15 minutes and supervising a junior doctor and a nurse
18:00	Go home for a nice glass of wine (good for the joints!)

myth	Steroid pushers inventing ever-more complex antibody tests only they can understand
reality	A lot of diseases come under the rheumatology umbrella and most of these can be controlled with appropriate treatment
personality	Team players, easy-going, good communication skills
best aspects	The variety of symptoms dealt with; long-term clinical relationships with patients
worst aspects	People assuming you do nothing (rheuma-holiday) or just treat rheumatoid arthritis
route	CT1 Core medical training (p 34) then ST3 Rheumatology; MRCP exam
numbers	850 of which 30% are women
locations	Mainly hospital-based in most hospitals; some community clinics

life						work
quiet on-call						busy on-call
boredom						burnout
uncompetitive						competitive
low salary						high salary

Royal Air Force medicine

The Royal Air Force (RAF) offers one of the most challenging careers in medicine. Where else can a doctor be trained to respond to any clinical challenge anywhere on (or above) the Earth? RAF doctors lead their own medical team and make a genuine difference not only to UK servicemen and their families, but to people all across the world that genuinely need help. The majority of RAF doctors work in a general practice role, however a smaller group train as hospital specialists in specialties of benefit to the armed forces.

the patients Within RAF bases the patients are generally younger than in NHS general practice, but their range of pathologies is just as wide. A high proportion of young families emphasizes the importance of appreciating illness in the social context. Overseas the patients may be victims of terrorism, war, famine, floods or poverty. Beat that as an opportunity for challenge and professional satisfaction!

the work The RAF is a close community and the general practice role extends beyond the consulting room. Senior Medical Officers may become involved in any circumstance that affects the physical or psychological well-being of service personnel or their families. Patients are both interested in their own health and motivated to make a swift recovery. Doctors are actively supported by a full primary health care team, but other in-house RAF specialists can also provide fitness and dietary advice or wider social support when required. The medical work is similar in nature to general practice in the NHS or other military settings.

the job The job is all about maintaining a healthy Royal Air Force 'fit for task'. This is achieved both through normal consultations and through opportunistic health promotion in the patients' workplace. Getting out and about is actively encouraged and doctors play a full part in the life of the station, both professionally and socially. After all, how better to understand what medical challenges pilots face than by flying with them, or to appreciate how Air Traffic Controllers divide up the sky than by watching them at the top of 'The Tower'?

extras After gaining the necessary experience, RAF general practitioners may become GP trainers or decide to subspecialize in occupational medicine, aviation medicine, sports medicine, public health or medical management. There are widespread opportunities for training in medicine and other skills. Teaching is also an important role since the Senior Medical Officer is responsible for the medical team.

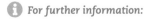 **For further information:**

RAF Medical and Dental Liaison Officer
Tel: 01400 266811   Web: http://www.raf.mod.uk

A day in the life of a Senior Medical Officer in the RAF ...

08:00	Meeting with senior members of primary health care team to plan the day
09:00	General practice clinic of military patients and their families; every case is different, but home visits are rare
11:00	Undertake aircrew medicals: 'Is he fit to fly a £20m, fast jet?' It's your call ....
12:00	Head to the gym, home for lunch or pop into the Officers' Mess for some chat
13:00	Visit the engineering section to conduct an occupational medicine inspection in conjunction with the local Health and Safety Advisor
14:00	Collect kit from the medical centre and head to the sports fields to provide medical cover for a station rugby match
17:00	Head home after checking emails (and cheeky beer to celebrate the rugby win)

myth	Hooray Henrys with handlebar moustaches who think *Top Gun* is the best film ever made and who will only stay in 5* hotels
reality	Generalists with wide experience of occupational, aviation, sports and travel medicine; it is possible that *Top Gun* is the best film ever made
personality	Motivated, flexible, sense of humour, sociable, calm under pressure
best aspects	Great variety; professional satisfaction alongside genuine respect and gratitude from patients; excellent training and careers advice
worst aspects	Domestic flexibility (you can be posted anywhere for months at a time); the need for a body clock that can adapt to different time zones
route	Military cadetship during, or immediately after, medical school (p 18)
numbers	60 in primary care and 50 in secondary care; 17.5% are women
locations	**Primary care** RAF stations throughout the UK as well as Cyprus and the Falkland Islands; **Secondary care** seven Ministry of Defence Hospital Units in UK; **Both** current deployments, e.g. Afghanistan

life		work
quiet on-call		busy on-call
boredom		burnout
uncompetitive		competitive
low salary		high salary

Royal Navy medicine

For those who want a varied, challenging job that stretches their clinical abilities, the Royal Navy may be ideal. On top of the clinical work the job also develops leadership skills and offers the opportunity to practice in exciting environments. Most doctors within the Royal Navy work as general practitioners with the added bonus of specialist training in diving or aviation medicine; a few work as hospital specialists in Military Defence Hospital Units (MDHU) found in certain NHS hospitals.

the patients are mainly service personnel aged between 17 and 50 years based in 'shore establishments' in the UK and abroad, or at sea in surface ships or submarines. There are a few family practices where spouses/partners and children of service personnel are also treated. Hospital doctors look after NHS patients except when on deployment, when patients include UK service personnel, service personnel from coalition forces and entitled civilians.

the work Most doctors in the navy work as Medical Officers, essentially GPs to Navy personnel on bases or on ships; a few work as hospital specialists in a range of specialties. Both roles include the opportunity to work in many different and exciting environments. Royal Navy ships are often first on the scene after hurricanes and earthquakes and frequently offer humanitarian aid. Some doctors work in air stations and look after aircrew serving in the Royal Navy. There are regular operations with other nations providing an opportunity to travel widely.

the job varies according to the type of doctor. Hospital specialists will have a very similar role to their non-military counterparts (ward rounds, clinics, etc.), whilst Medical Officers lead a more 'military' lifestyle with mostly clinic-based practices. The patients are generally fit, so much of the job entails keeping them in good health (health education) with timely treatment of routine and emergency conditions in order to maintain an effective force. In air stations there is a bias towards aviation medicine and in diving establishments towards diving medicine. There is a drive to rehabilitate and support those with remediable problems to full fitness as quickly as possible.

extras Doctors are actively encouraged to follow their passions (within the needs of the service) and broaden their horizons, with unrivalled access to sports facilities (even onboard ships!). Opportunities for travel and adventure abound. On top of training as a doctor, there is support and encouragement to develop new skills and gain extra qualifications.

🛈 *For further information:*

The Royal Navy: Tel: 08456 07 55 55   Web: http://www.royalnavy.mod.uk

10:00	Standeasy (coffee break)
10:30	Appointments ranging from minor injuries to care of chronic conditions
11:30	Administration
12:00	Lunch
13:30	More appointments
14:15	Standeasy/administration
14:45	Further appointments
15:45	Administration
16:30	Command brief (overview of ship's programme and commitments)
17:00	Circuit training
19:00	Dinner

myth	Doctors dressed in white shorts treating seasick sailors
reality	Diverse combination of general practice and remote medicine
personality	Personable even in a confined space, sense of humour, patient, calm, approachable, leadership skills, motivational skills
best aspects	Fantastic lifestyle including travel with enormous variety of work and environments; excellent training opportunities; sense of camaraderie; excellent social life; great sports facilities
worst aspects	Lots of time away from home; long hours seven days a week when at sea; limited second opinions
route	Military cadetship during, or immediately after, medical school (p 18)
numbers	50 in primary care and 70 in secondary care; 10% are women
locations	**Primary care** Shore establishments in the UK and overseas; ships, submarines (men only) or air stations; **Secondary care** seven Ministry of Defence Hospital Units in UK

life						work
quiet on-call						busy on-call
boredom						burnout
uncompetitive						competitive
low salary						high salary

Sexual and reproductive health

This specialty was previously called family planning, though the name and role have moved on. Contraceptive services are still key (e.g. providing advice, fitting intrauterine devices [IUDs] and implants), but many clinics now cover community gynaecology, the management of sexually transmitted infections (essentially community-based genitourinary medicine) and psychosexual work. The career involves a broad range of activities from counselling skills to minor surgery.

the patients Anyone over the age of puberty; and occasionally under. While the core patient group is young women, services also cover men (STI screening and management) and older women (contraception, smears, menopause issues). Inner city clinics particularly may witness a vibrant range of ethnicities, languages and cultures including the homeless, commercial sex workers and newly arrived immigrants. Many of the patients are healthy, but some management of chronic conditions is required, especially HIV. While most of the patients are seen sporadically there are a few who require regular services over many years. Overall young people are a noisy challenge; the ability to treasure the oddities of human behaviour is needed to survive.

the work is mostly preventative, including holistic contraception and well woman services, sexual health promotion, cervical cancer screening, sexual health screening, outreach work for vulnerable groups and young person clinics. Some centres provide diagnostic and treatment services (e.g. ultrasound examinations, colposcopy or hysteroscopy examination). Counselling services for psychosexual problems, vasectomy, female sterilization and termination of pregnancy are also undertaken by some services. For those with ethical doubts about termination of pregnancy it is still feasible to work in sexual and reproductive health, but unease about postcoital contraception is harder to accommodate.

the job The vast majority of the work is in community outpatient clinics; often in different locations on different days. Clinics also include a number of procedures (e.g. inserting IUDs). There is no on-call, but late evenings and Saturdays are expected. Teaching, administration and management often form a large part of the job. There is regular interaction with a number of specialties including genitourinary medicine, public health, GPs, school nurses and gynaecologists.

extras Flexible training is popular and the lifestyle fits well with family life. There are ample opportunities for teaching (GPs, nurses, medical students and hospital trainees). Many larger departments have research interests, but it is by no means a career requirement. Private practice is extremely limited but there are opportunities for medicolegal work if one is interested.

ℹ️ *For further information:*

Faculty of Family planning and Reproductive Healthcare of the RCOG, 27 Sussex Place, Regent's Park, London, NW1 4RG
Tel: 020 7724 5534   Web: http://www.ffprhc.org.uk

09:00	Check emails, post, messages in office
09:30	Drive to clinic listening to Radio 4
10:00	Mixed walk-in clinic: pills, IUDs, chlamydia, warts
12:30	Drive back to office
13:00	Lunch at clinical audit meeting on teenage pregnancy management
14:00	IUD/implant clinic
17:30	Home unless covering evening clinic (17:30 to 20:00)
18:30	Catch up on paperwork and emails
19:00	Enjoy evening with a well-planned family!

myth	Part-timers in sensible shoes limited to providing contraception
reality	Diverse, mentally and physically demanding work with an interesting but often challenging population
personality	Relaxed, team-orientated, level-headed, non-judgemental, flexible, communication skills
best aspects	Broad range of activities; supportive team spirit in clinic teams; good degree of control over working pattern
worst aspects	Limited resources; seen as an easy option
route	ST1 Obstetrics and gynaecology (p 36) then subspecialization into Sexual and reproductive health at ST5; MRCOG exam
locations	Community-based, often with travel to outlying clinics

life						work
quiet on-call						busy on-call
boredom						burnout
uncompetitive						competitive
low salary						high salary

Ship's doctor

Being a ship's doctor is not all about looking good in a white uniform, although that does help a lot! The job is varied and demanding. Ship's doctors are highly trained clinicians working in state-of-the-art facilities, making challenging management decisions to treat a hugely diverse group of patients.

the patients Being a ship's doctor involves contact with a wide assortment of patients. Passengers and crew come from all four corners of the globe and present the full range of clinical problems. Gone are the days of cruising being a pastime purely for the recently retired; families with young children are now taking cruise holidays, as are people in their 80s and 90s.

the work Varied isn't really a good enough word to describe the work of a ship's doctor. They are true generalists but most have an emergency medicine background with either GP or anaesthetic experience. They see everything from common primary care ailments right through to critical illness and major medical emergencies. Any clinical scenario at sea can rapidly become complicated owing to the isolation from land-based hospital facilities. It is important to be resourceful enough to manage a spectrum of cases and yet know when to arrange emergency medical evacuations for patients who need shore-side attention urgently.

the job The medical team on board can be as many as two doctors and five nurses or as small as a single doctor and two nurses. In these smaller teams the doctor is always on-call, 24 hours a day, 7 days a week, while the larger teams have the luxury of a 1:2! However, the on-calls are usually not busy. Most of the medical work takes place in separate passenger and crew clinics. The ship's medical centres have fully equipped coronary care and intensive care beds as well as laboratory equipment for processing all the major blood analyses. X-rays and fractures are managed onboard and, on the larger ships, there is room for up to 7 inpatients. When medical disembarkation is needed, the doctor liaises with local shore-side hospital facilities and coordinates medical evacuation transport to ensure the safe transfer of patients.

extras There are many perks to being a cruise ship doctor. Food and accommodation is paid for, expenses are negligible and tax can be claimed back, allowing for ample saving on an already good salary. The opportunity for travel is unrivalled and there are chances to get off the ship and visit some wonderful places. Alongside the professional responsibilities as a doctor there are also the responsibilities to the ship as a senior Merchant Naval officer.

ℹ️ *For further information:*

Medical Recruitment Officer, Carnival UK, Richmond House, Terminus Terrace, Southampton, SO14 3PN
Tel: 02380 655186   Web: http://www.shipsdoctors.com

A day in the life ...

08:30	Morning crew clinic
09:45	Man overboard emergency drill exercise and stretcher party training
10:00	Passenger clinic
12:30	Lunch in the Officers' Mess
16:30	Afternoon clinics for passengers and crew
19:00	Captain's cocktail party
20:30	Dinner with passengers in the dining room
22:30	Called to assess passenger with chest pain in the ship's medical centre
00:00	Back to own cabin for a well-deserved sleep!

myth	All you see is motion sickness and care of the elderly
reality	A modern and dynamic specialty with enough variety to keep anyone satisfied and to maintain clinical skills
personality	Sociable, team player, easy-going, confident, calm in an emergency, able to cope with responsibility
best aspects	Fantastic travel opportunity; truly unique medical practice and life; 2 months of paid leave after each 4 months at sea
worst aspects	Paperwork involved in the public health element of the job
route	No specific training route; emergency experience is essential while general practice and anaesthetics helps; acute care common stem is a good starting point (p 28)
locations	On board a ship anywhere in the world; common locations include the Caribbean, Mediterranean, Alaska, South Pacific, Mexican Riviera, Australia and Asia

life						work
quiet on-call						busy on-call
boredom						burnout
uncompetitive						competitive
low salary						high salary

Spinal surgery

Spinal surgery is a rapidly growing and highly technical surgical field, but one where excellent communication skills and compassion are essential; think of a cross between a neurosurgeon and a clinical psychologist. Given that 80% of the population suffer from back pain at some time in their lives and 70% of people dying with a tumour have spinal metastases it is not surprising that this is an expanding field.

the patients The common misconception of spinal patients is that they are all 'malingerers' with back pain or simply complete nutters. While there are a few of these, the majority are everyday folk with serious symptoms. It is a patient population group that gets very poor support from employers, family and friends and even health professionals. Sensitivity, thorough and detailed history, examination (especially neuro exam) and explanation are paramount. The patients vary immensely in their presentation, ranging from the newborn with congenital scoliosis to the elderly lady with an osteoporotic fracture or metastasis from a breast primary. Many of them, such as spinal deformity patients, are known personally, as follow-up continues throughout growth.

the work The main pathologies are divided into deformity (adult and paediatric), degenerative, tumour, trauma and infection. Many surgeons will develop a particular interest in one of these fields. There is also an anatomical division; traditionally neurosurgeons looked after cervical spine conditions while orthopaedics cared for thoracolumbar. Increasingly, spinal surgeons look after the whole spine, front to back, top to bottom. Patients often rehabilitate quickly; in fact many cervical or lumbar disc patients hug you in the recovery room as they wake up with their crippling radicular pain gone!

the job is made up of inpatient and day case operating (not patients visiting for the day, but cases that take all day, e.g. front to back tumour excision/stabilisation or scoliosis correction); ward rounds (close post-op care is extremely important); adult and paediatric clinics; and several meetings. It is now a highly multidisciplinary field and relationships with oncologists, paediatricians, radiologists and pain specialists are paramount, as well as all the allied health professionals involved in rehab teams.

extras There are lots of opportunities for high quality research; *Spine* has the highest impact rating for any orthopaedic journal and teaching involves a wide range of health professionals, from chiropractors to neurosurgeons. Scarcity influences demand. This also means that private practice is large and growing. Most trainees do one or two years of fellowship, often abroad, at the end of the usual training programmes.

🛈 *For further information:*

British Association of Spinal Surgeons   Web: http://www.spinesurgeons.ac.uk

A day in the life ...

08:00	Trauma meeting or multidisciplinary meeting with therapists
09:00	Spinal deformity clinic
12:30	Ward round of post-op and emergency patients
13:00	Review a patient on the medical wards with cord compression from a prostate metastasis
14:00	Elective operating session—anterior cervical discectomy and fusion followed by lumbar spinal stenosis decompression
17:30	Post-op reviews
18:00	Emergency operation on the patient with cord compression from earlier
20:00	Home

myth	All mad back pain patients
reality	Ever had back pain? Did you see a psychiatrist?
personality	Meticulous, obsessional attention to detail
best aspects	Operating through almost every region of the body, on a vast range of pathology, in interesting and challenging patients
worst aspects	'Snake oil' treatments for spinal pain in alternative medicine and primary care; misconception that 'there's nothing we can do'; frequent and busy on-calls (some 1 in 2's still exist)
route	ST1 Surgery in general, trauma and orthopaedic surgery (p 48) then ST3 Trauma and orthopaedic surgery; MRCS exam; alternative route via Neurosurgery (p 50)
locations	Hospital-based in teaching hospitals and large district general hospitals

life						work
quiet on-call						busy on-call
boredom						burnout
uncompetitive						competitive
low salary						high salary

Sport and exercise medicine

Sport and exercise medicine (SEM) is one of the newest and most exciting of specialties: it was granted specialty status in 2005. The jobs are diverse, ranging from exercise prescription for those with chronic disease to looking after athletes with gold medal aspirations.

the patients The public health aspects of the job mean that the patients may include communities wishing to exercise for health promotion or individuals managing their chronic problems, for example obesity, cardiac and respiratory diseases or psychiatric problems. The sporting side of the job could involve tending to the 'weekend warriors' playing sport on a Sunday afternoon or looking after an elite athlete at a major championship. Overall the patients tend to be younger and healthier than in many medical specialties.

the work Sport and exercise medicine is about advising on injury prevention, managing acute injuries like anterior cruciate ligament (ACL) ruptures and advising on chronic injuries such as Achilles tendonosis. This requires an understanding of the interaction between exercise and illness, doping issues, sports psychology, ethics in sport, nutrition, biomechanics and physiology. It can involve anything from using exercise to help unhealthy people improve fitness through to maximizing performance in an elite athlete.

the job could be clinic-based in a hospital, community or sports institute. There are opportunities to work with many sporting teams, often part-time but increasingly full-time with professional teams. Most sports governing bodies will have chief medical officers and all major sporting events require medical teams of doctors and physiotherapists. The job can therefore involve travel all over the world working closely with physiotherapists, exercise scientists, sports psychologists, coaches and athletes.

extras As a new specialty the mainstay of SEM has previously been in private practice. One needs recognition from the private insurance companies which can be difficult to achieve. There are a limited number of research fellowships but some opportunities for teaching on diploma and masters courses.

ℹ️ *For further information:*

British Association of Sport and Exercise Medicine, BASEM Central Office, 15 Hawthorne Avenue, Norton, Doncaster, DN6 9HR
Tel: 01302 709342   Web: http://www.basem.co.uk

A day in the life of an international football team doctor ...

08:00	Wake up call
08:15	Assist exercise scientist assess players' urine osmolality for hydration
09:15	Assess injuries prior to training then accompany team on morning training
14:00	Assess injuries prior to afternoon training
15:00	Accompany team for afternoon training session
16:30	Go with player to MRI unit; need to obtain report immediately
18:00	Evening treatment session with physiotherapist
20:00	Player educational meeting on nutrition
21:00	Further treatments/assessments
22:00	Staff meeting: manager needs update on fitness of players for next game

myth	Sports doctors touring the world looking after elite athletes
reality	There are many weekend warriors who need specialist advice and SEM has a big role to play in promoting health
personality	Sense of humour, sense of adventure, passion for sport and exercise, sociable, flexible
best aspects	Watching some great sport and helping people achieve their dream, whether that is being able to run around with their kids in the park or win the FA cup!
worst aspects	Travelling and not seeing the world; looking after athletes when they lose
route	ST3 in Sports and exercise medicine; prior training is not specified; consider emergency medicine (p 28) or general practice (p 32); diploma or masters in sports medicine helps
locations	Mixture of hospitals, general practice, sports institutes and national governing bodies

life		work
quiet on-call		busy on-call
boredom		burnout
uncompetitive		competitive
low salary		high salary

Transfusion medicine

Transfusion medicine is usually a subspecialty of haematology (p 158) or immunology (p 166), however it also includes any other doctor with a special interest in the transfusion of blood products, e.g. epidemiologists. The majority of specialties require blood product transfusion in the treatment of their patients so there is great scope for contact with other specialists.

the patients Transfusion recipients range from fetuses to those undergoing palliative care, including every age group and stage of life in between. They include neonates, surgical patients, obstetric patients, trauma victims and those with neurological, haematological and immunological conditions. The recipient is rarely seen by the transfusion medicine specialist, however most practitioners maintain a degree of clinical practice alongside their transfusion medicine activities (e.g. haematology or immunology clinics).

the work can involve any aspect of the 'journey' of the blood products, from ethical issues and means of attracting donors, through the laboratory purification, storage and cross-matching, to the giving of the transfusion and managing possible reactions. Much of the workload entails ensuring that 'routine' blood transfusion services are available; transfusion specialists are also involved with difficult cases requiring specialist transfusions, e.g. unusual antibodies or unusual blood products. Finally stem cell (bone marrow) transplants are often managed by transfusion medicine specialists. Like other areas of haematology, biomedical scientists manage much of the routine laboratory work.

the job The majority of transfusion medicine specialists are laboratory-based, however some work with inpatients or outpatients. Those interested in the epidemiological side usually work in an office-based environment. Specialists work as part of a varied team including academics, nurse practitioners, infectious disease specialists, epidemiologists, surgeons, physicians, haematologists, immunologists, anaesthetists, intensive care physicians and paediatricians of all disciplines. The majority do not have on-call commitments.

extras The wide impact of blood products provides many opportunities to develop expertise in a specific area which may be nationally and even internationally valued. Research opportunities abound and flexible training is easy to accommodate. There are also travel opportunities ranging from conferences to giving advice to developing countries and even in humanitarian crises or war zones. Private practice is uncommon but not precluded.

ℹ *For further information:*

British Society for Haematology, 100 White Lion Street, London, N1 9PF
Tel: 020 7713 0990   Web: http://www.b-s-h.org.uk

09:00	Reporting results referred to the regional reference laboratory and giving medical advice to obstetricians, midwives and physicians looking after the patients requiring the tests
10:00	Laboratory meeting with the hospital laboratory manager discussing difficult transfusion issues in the hospital
11:00	Review notes for clinic in the afternoon
13:30	Outpatient haematology clinic
16:00	Meeting with maternal and fetal medicine consultants, trainees and midwives to discuss ongoing difficult cases of fetal anaemia and low platelet counts
17:00	Home to finish article on novel transfusion procedure

myth	Backroom doctors who delight in rejecting poorly labelled blood tubes
reality	Diverse range of roles that can be tailored to the individual's desires; provide a vital life-saving service
personality	Differing roles suit a wide range of different personalities; tend to be academic, happy away from direct patient contact and meticulous
best aspects	Outcomes are often very positive with infrequent need to give bad news (with the exception of some immunological conditions)
worst aspects	By necessity much of the practice is highly regulated, which can limit creativity; it can be difficult to avoid becoming superspecialized
route	CT1 Core medical training (p 34) followed by ST3 Haematology; MRCP and FRCPath exams; range of alternative routes e.g. paediatrics, public health
locations	Hospital- or blood centre-based with some options of working from home

life					work
quiet on-call					busy on-call
boredom					burnout
uncompetitive					competitive
low salary					high salary

Transplantation surgery

Solid organ transplantation encompasses surgeons of different specialties who, as part of their work, retrieve and transplant organs. Few other surgical specialties offer the opportunity to perform operations that provide cost-effective treatment for both chronic and acute organ failure with proven benefits in life-expectancy and quality of life, all steeped in Nobel Prize-winning scientific achievement. However, no-one goes into this specialty for the private work and a quiet time on-call.

the patients In February 2007, over 7000 people were waiting for a transplant in the UK, the majority of whom had chronic organ failure (kidney, pancreas, liver, lung and heart). This figure is growing by 5% per year. Organ failure is often a consequence of systemic disease, so the patients present numerous problems distinct from the organ requiring transplantation. Furthermore, immunosuppression following transplantation brings with it further challenges. It is often transplant surgeons who treat these patients' varied surgical problems.

the work Approximately 1800 kidney, 600 liver, 120 pancreas, 150 heart and 120 lung transplants are performed in the UK each year. Organs may be transplanted from living (kidney and liver-lobe) or deceased donors. Whilst retrieval is mainly performed by multi-organ retrieval teams, all transplant surgeons may at some time be involved in retrieval of organs from deceased donors; these often occur out of hours. The development of laparoscopic donor nephrectomy for living kidney donors and split-liver transplantation allowing living liver donation has kept transplantation at the forefront of surgical innovation.

the job Transplant units are based in tertiary referral centres and, like all surgical specialties, the work is a mixture of wards, outpatients, paperwork and theatre. Surgeons work closely with individual medical specialties relating to the organ the surgeon transplants (hepatology, nephrology, cardiology etc.) and the rest of the multidisciplinary team, in particular the transplant coordinator. It is consultant-led so out-of-hours work remains common, especially as organs for transplant often become available at night and have limited shelf-life. Traditionally most kidney transplant surgeons maintain another specialty (e.g. vascular or endocrine surgery), continue general surgery on-call and perform vascular access procedures for haemodialysis.

extras Transplantation provides huge opportunities for surgical and scientific innovation in all aspects of organ failure; as such many surgeons have active roles in research. Private practice and flexible training are virtually non-existent due to the nature of the job.

ℹ️ *For further information:*

The British Transplantation Society, Association House, South Park Road, Macclesfield, Cheshire, SK11 6SH
Tel: 01625 504060   Fax: 01625 267879   Web: http://www.bts.org.uk

08:15	X-ray meeting: review live donor CT scans and renal vascular problems
08:45	Ward round: 16 vascular patients, 10 with renal failure
10:45	Multidisciplinary team meeting
11:30	Liaise with transplant coordinators and renal physicians about living kidney donors
12:30	Lunch on the go amidst paperwork
13:00	See patients prior to afternoon operating list
13:30	Perform a couple of small cases and a living donor nephrectomy in a young boy's mother
15:30	Travel to children's hospital to transplant the kidney into the child
18:30	Home, trying to ignore the phone and pager

myth	Nocturnal creatures, found in theatre coffee rooms waiting for brainstem-dead young people to be brought from ITU
reality	Surgical heroes who save lives; the number of potential patients is increasing despite deceased donation, while elective in-hours living donor transplants are increasing rapidly
personality	Hard-working, high stamina, calm in stressful situations
best aspects	Hugely rewarding; life-changing for patients and their families
worst aspects	Out-of-hours commitment; emotionally draining organ retrieval; very little private work
route	CT1 Surgery in general, general surgery (p 48) then ST3 in General surgery; FRCS exam; a dedicated ST3 path to transplantation surgery has been proposed
numbers	270 of which 5% are women
locations	Hospital-based in dedicated transplantation units (28 for kidneys, 7 for livers and 7 cardiothoracic units)

life						work
quiet on-call						busy on-call
boredom						burnout
uncompetitive						competitive
low salary						high salary

Trauma surgery

Trauma surgery is the care of the acutely injured and critically unwell as a result of motor vehicle collisions, industrial accidents, assault with a knife or gun and deliberate self-harm. The patient may be the sickest in the hospital and requires timely investigation and treatment to stop them dying in the resuscitation room. Is the patient stable enough for a CT scan or do they need a life-saving laparotomy to pack a bleeding liver or an immediate emergency room thoracotomy to repair a stab wound to the heart? Trauma surgery is becoming its own specialty and by 2020 injury is likely to be the second most common cause of death in all age groups.

the patients Receiving trauma tends to be a young man's game, but expect a variety of patients who have suffered many different injuries (sometimes all at once). For some, their hospital stay is brief, but others require repeat operations and long-term rehabilitation so the doctor–patient relationship can be very gratifying. Patients are followed up in clinic and it can be very rewarding to see them back at work and playing sport or seeing an amputee walking upright unaided using a prosthetic limb.

the work includes timely decision-making in the emergency department (ED), interpreting investigations and deciding on conservative or surgical treatments for life-threatening injuries. Operations include damage control surgery in the chest and abdomen on hollow and solid organs as well as surgery in the neck and the extremities. The body is capable of withstanding terrible injuries, but you can't save everyone.

the job Work in the ED, operating theatre, intensive care and ward. A busy unit could have more than five trauma team activations a day. Some patients tend to suffer their injuries in the middle of the night. The surgeon is an integral member of the trauma team and works with ambulance staff, pre-hospital care specialists, ED physicians, anaesthetists, intensivists and other surgical specialties, physiotherapists and occupational health staff. They also oversee the referral of patients to other surgical specialties for expert advice and surgical intervention. Despite its exciting and acute nature the job requires a holistic approach, considering the emotional and psychological needs of the traumatized, often multiply injured patient.

extras The career offers lots of teaching opportunities to medical students and other members of the trauma team. Research, publications, audit and a genuine interest in trauma are beneficial; there are also many trauma conferences. There is some private practice, mostly in orthopaedics.

For further information:

British Orthopaedic Association, 35–43 Lincoln's Inn Fields, London, WC2A 3PE
Tel: 020 7405 6507   Fax: 020 7831 2676   Web: http://www.boa.ac.uk
An excellent website for trauma surgeons: http://www.trauma.org

A day in the life ...

08:00 Handover of patients from on-call team, review of imaging

09:00 Trauma ward round

10:00 'Trauma team to resus': attend a trauma call, conservatively manage a splenic injury while being filmed for a trauma documentary

11:00 Finish ward round

12:00 Weekly trauma meeting: present morbidity and mortality statistics

13:00 Trauma clinic or elective list

18:00 A road traffic accident sees two patients arrive simultaneously; manage a flail chest and pneumothorax with an intercostal drain

23:00 Another call and the pre-hospital team bring in a patient with stab wounds to the chest and abdomen

myth	Shouting type-A personalities who love wading in blood
reality	Emergency, damage-control surgery on the sickest patients in the hospital can be hugely rewarding and exciting
personality	Team player, able to converse across the blood–brain barrier and work with the anaesthetist during emergency surgery
best aspects	Working to avoid the lethal triad and the trimodal distribution of death; people like making documentaries about trauma
worst aspects	Terrible injuries can be psychologically draining; do you want to be getting up in the middle of the night when in your 50s?
route	ST1 Surgery in general, trauma and orthopaedic surgery (p 48) then ST3 Trauma and orthopaedic surgery; MRCS exam; period of training in the USA/South Africa is common
numbers	3200 (combined with orthopaedics) of which 3.5% are women
locations	Mainly teaching hospitals with a move towards large multispecialty regional trauma centres

life						work
quiet on-call						busy on-call
boredom						burnout
uncompetitive						competitive
low salary						high salary

Urogynaecology

Urogynaecology is a surgical subspecialty of gynaecology (p 156) dedicated to the treatment of women with pelvic floor disorders such as urinary or fecal incontinence and prolapse of the vagina, bladder and/or the uterus. Urinary incontinence is a very common condition affecting at least 10–20% of women under age 65 and up to 56% of women over the age of 65. Most urogynaecologists continue to work as general gynaecologists as well, some even continuing to work in obstetrics too.

the patients are similar to those in general gynaecology, i.e. women from reproductive age to the postmenopausal and elderly, though the average patient tends to be older. There is a good mixture of simple problems that require minimal interventions then discharge and complex problems requiring long-term follow-up and continuity of care. An understanding of the effects of pelvic floor problems on a woman's mental and physical health is required. It is important to think holistically about an individual's needs, particularly her sex life, when considering any surgical intervention.

the work includes both medical and surgical approaches. Common presentations include urinary stress incontinence, detrusor overactivity, pelvic organ prolapse, lower urinary and gastrointestinal fistulae and post-partum incontinence. Relatively minor interventions (e.g. pelvic floor stimulation and education) can make a big difference to a woman's quality of life, so most urinary problems are referred to physio and nursing specialists before invasive investigations such as urodynamics (bladder pressure studies). There are a diverse range of effective surgical procedures; most of these require a vaginal approach. Most urogynaecologists participate in the general gynaecology on-call rota—there is minimal need for on-call specific to urogynaecology.

the job necessitates a multidisciplinary approach working with clinical nurse specialists and physiotherapists. Liaison (and sometimes joint operations) with other surgical specialties is may be required, particularly urologists and colorectal surgeons. The working week often includes two outpatient sessions, with one or two theatre sessions and the ensuing ward rounds for post-operative care. While most urogynaecologists are found in larger hospitals some also hold clinics and theatre lists at peripheral hospitals. The general gynaecology on-calls are usually relatively mild, mostly requiring telephone advice.

extras There is huge scope for research and attendance at national and international conferences. Urogynaecology offers a lucrative private practice for those who are interested. Flexible training is possible and well-established.

ℹ️ *For further information:*

The British Society of Urogynaecology, 27 Sussex Place, Regents Park, London, NW1 4RG
Tel: 020 7772 6211   Web: http://www.rcog.org.uk/bsug

A day in the life ...

08:00	Ward round of post-op patients
09:00	Outpatient clinic: often busy, as urinary/prolapse symptoms are very common; may include multidisciplinary team of physiotherapists and nurse specialists within the clinic
12:30	Free lunch courtesy of drug company advertising latest incontinence medication
13:30	Pre-operative review of patients for afternoon lists
14:00	Theatre list: often a mixture of urethral tape procedures and pelvic floor repairs; occasionally more complex procedures take up a large part of the list
17:30	Go home: if on-call may occasionally be telephoned for advice on the management of acute gynaecological problems

myth	Experts in prescribing disposable knickers
reality	A rapidly developing specialty offering a wide range of treatments to relieve urinary symptoms that often trouble women greatly
personality	Sympathetic ear, good communication, enjoyment of practical procedures
best aspects	Simple procedures that dramatically improve quality of life
worst aspects	Procedures that fail to improve patient's symptoms or even make things worse; changing pessaries can be unpleasant too...
route	ST1 Obstetrics and gynaecology (p 36) then subspecialization into Urogynaecology at ST6; MRCOG exam
numbers	140 of which 33% are women
locations	Hospital-based in larger district general hospitals and teaching hospitals

life						work
quiet on-call						busy on-call
boredom			☺			burnout
uncompetitive						competitive
low salary						high salary

Urology

This job is for people with a diverse surgical interest. On offer is the possibility of major surgery, lasers, robotic operations, keyhole surgery, microscopic suturing, cutting-edge research and more! Furthermore, there are opportunities to attend and present at meetings all around the world. Initially, all doctors are trained as general urologists with a limited competitive entry into fellowship programmes for those who want to be a super-specialist. With an ageing population, the urological workload is expanding.

the patients Urology covers all ages and both sexes but most of urology deals with the ageing male. However, it is possible to specialize in paediatric or female aspects of urology. Generally, old men are very interesting and have many stories to tell—sometimes a problem in a busy clinic! Some of them will have lived through or been involved in major world events from the history books. Aside from their urological disease they are often relatively healthy.

the work Urologists manage disease of the renal tract including the kidney, ureters, bladder, prostate and penis. Common diseases include prostatic enlargement, renal stones and cancer. Prostate cancer is the number one urological cancer with an excellent prognosis in the vast majority of men. Patients requiring chemotherapy, radiotherapy or palliation are generally managed by the oncologists (medical p 196 and clinical p 118). The surgery is very variable, from transurethral resection of the prostate (TURP) to advanced endoscopic techniques to complicated resections and reconstructions. On-call emergencies include renal colic and urinary retention.

the job A normal week may comprise operative surgery, diagnostic tests (keyhole examinations of the bladder, urodynamics, ultrasound guided prostate biopsies, etc.), clinics, ward work and administration. While the days are usually busy, the nights are generally quiet with few urgent interventions requiring a consultant urologist's expertise. Urologists work closely with oncologists, gynaecologists and renal physicians.

extras There are plenty of research opportunities in urology if you are interested. Teaching of nurses, hospital doctors, GPs, medical students and other urologists is part of the normal teaching hospital urologist's programme. Most urologists will attend two or more meetings a year including annual meetings of the BAUS (British Association of Urological Surgeons), EAU (European Association of Urology) and AUA (American Urological Association). Subspecialization is common (e.g. urological oncology, renal transplant, stone disease). Private practice is readily available and pays well.

🛈 *For further information:*

British Association of Urological Surgeons, 35–43 Lincoln's Inn Fields, London, WC2A 3PE
Tel: 020 7869 6950   Fax: 020 7404 5048   Web: http://www.baus.org.uk

A day in the life ...

08:00	Handover from junior doctors covering the previous night
08:15	Cancer multidisciplinary team meeting: discuss patient management
09:00	Clinic: 16 patients seen, good mix of new and follow-ups
12:30	Consent patients for theatre then quick lunch
13:30	Operating theatre
17:00	Post-operative ward round
18:00	On-call but non resident
Night	Two calls for advice; occasionally need to go into hospital for a urological emergency

myth	Penis doctors
reality	Massively varied specialty with a good balance of operative, diagnostic, clinical, administrative and social sessions
personality	Outgoing, confident, sense of humour, both feet placed firmly on the ground, good practical skills and visuospatial awareness
best aspects	The patients, surgery, colleagues and no shift work
worst aspects	Getting called in to change suprapubic catheters
route	CT1 Surgery in general, urology (p 48) then ST3 Urology; FRCS exam; limited number of subspecialty fellowships
numbers	1000 of which 4% are women
locations	Hospital-based, found in most hospitals

life		work
quiet on-call		busy on-call
boredom		burnout
uncompetitive		competitive
low salary		high salary

Vascular surgery

Vascular surgery is one of the most challenging branches of surgery, integrating procedures from ancient Egyptian times (e.g. lower limb amputations) with cutting-edge technologies (e.g. endoluminal abdominal aortic aneurysm stent insertion). When blood starts to pour, the vascular surgeon becomes everyone's best friend, offering vital control and emergency replumbing.

the patients Vascular surgeons meet a huge range of patients in daily practice. Unsurprisingly, many patients have significant cardiovascular risk factors (smoking, age, diabetes, etc.); these can result in patients with low physiological reserves making for a challenge both medically and surgically. However, anyone, anytime and anywhere can get into life- or limb-threatening trouble and with the right management a vascular surgeon can save both. There is a good mix between 'quick fixes' (i.e. patients who just need a one-off operation) and chronic care (e.g. diabetic feet requiring multiple interventions over time).

the work is much more varied than most surgical specialties. Peripheral vascular disease contributes a large fraction in the form of angioplasties, stents, bypasses and the occasional amputation where these have not worked. Carotids often require dextrous attention to prevent strokes and vascular surgeons also electively treat aortic aneurysms. Venous disorders are also important; varicose vein surgery improves quality of life for many patients. The vascular surgeon is also the last port of call for vascular access including arteriovenous fistulae for dialysis and Hickman lines. One of the greatest satisfactions is integrating drug treatments, minimally invasive radiological techniques and old-fashioned surgery. On-call emergencies can be daunting including leaking abdominal aortic aneurysms and saving life and limb following trauma. No job is too big!

the job is split roughly 40% surgery, 40% clinic and meetings and 20% on the ward. Surgery takes place within a multidisciplinary team and includes trainees, anaesthetists, intensivists, vascular technicians, and vascular nurse specialists. Close working relations with other specialties (including radiologists, endocrinologists, cardiologists, oncologists, neurologists and the renal teams) are essential. On-call can be onerous and require frequent unscheduled hospital visits. There are often one or two long emergency cases each day and juniors need supervising in person for every arterial case.

extras Teaching is important for trainees and students. Research is strongly encouraged and can range from new endovascular techniques to cerebral perfusion at altitude. Private practice is reasonable, mostly in the form of varicose veins. The high out-of-hours component makes flexible training difficult.

ℹ️ *For further information:*

The Vascular Society, 35–43 Lincoln's Inn Fields, London, WC2A 3PE
Tel: 020 7973 0306   Web: http://www.vascularsociety.org.uk
An excellent website for vascular surgeons is: http://www.carotidsurgeon.com

07:45	Try to park in wonderful new private finance initiative (PFI) hospital car park
08.00	Paperwork/emails
08:30	Send for first patient, wait while an HDU bed is found; mini round of sickest patients while waiting
09.30	Say hello to patient for surgery, confirming consent/side etc., then coffee and paperwork for 45 minutes whilst anaesthetist puts lines in.
10:15	Start surgery: peace, quiet and in control at last!
13:30	Close up, write notes, fill in audit sheets, send for next patient and grab lunch while waiting
13:45	Operate until further patients have been cancelled due to bed shortage, an emergency intervenes or, least likely, the list ends
18:00	Mini-ward round of sickies/post-op patients
18:30	Home for family time, unless there is an emergency or post-op problem...

myth	Death by a thousand amputations
reality	Most patients do well and amputations are a last resort
personality	Hard-working, dynamic, enthusiastic, does not tolerate fools readily, excellent practical skills, calm in an emergency, decisive
best aspects	Good colleagues; saving the odd life or limb
worst aspects	NHS Bureaucracy
route	CT1 Surgery in general, general surgery (p 48) then ST3 General surgery; FRCS exam; a period of research and higher degree will increase job choice
numbers	1300 of which 3% are women (with the dubious honour of being the lowest of any specialty)
locations	Hospital-based in large district general hospitals and teaching hospitals

life						work
quiet on-call						busy on-call
boredom						burnout
uncompetitive						competitive
low salary						high salary

Virology

Clinical virology is an exciting, relatively new specialty that is rarely out of the news these days. There is a good mix of clinical work, laboratory liaison, research, development and teaching. The job ranges from investigating an outbreak to advising on the management of potential avian influenza and troubleshooting viral assays to interpreting results in the laboratory. Interpreting and understanding the relevance of certain viral infections in a variety of clinical situations makes the job both satisfying and rewarding.

the patients The virology lab offers diagnostic tests to clinicians throughout the hospital and community so the patients cover the complete range of age, ethnicity and background. Virologists also see some patients directly; for example unusual infections, immunocompromise or chronic viral infections (e.g. HIV, hepatitis).

the work The main role is providing a clinical diagnostic service for the local patient population and a reference service for other hospitals that carry out more routine virological tests. The virologist oversees the laboratory including interpreting and authorizing assay results (e.g. viral loads and antiviral resistance tests), planning service developments, liaising with laboratory staff and supervising research. Liaison with health protection units is also a key role and virologists are important advisors on local public health issues. There is also a clinical role acting as an interface between specialists and the laboratory, attending specific ward rounds (e.g. haematology–oncology, immunocompromised patients). For complicated cases the virologist might review the patients and their notes in person. A few virologists also see patients in clinic (e.g. chronic hepatitis, HIV).

the job The multidisciplinary nature of the job involves daily contact with a variety of health care professionals including microbiologists, trainees, infection control nurses, health care and clinical scientists and public health doctors. Much of the work takes place in the laboratory, but clinical experience is essential for interpreting results. On-call includes dealing with blood-borne virus exposure incidents (e.g. needle-sticks), rabies exposures, transplant donor screening results, and potential viral haemorrhagic fever infections in travellers returning home. Most of these can be handled over the phone.

extras There is a lot of potential for carrying out research, attending conferences, and teaching and training in different settings. There is little, if any, private practice. Flexible training is well established and respected.

ℹ️ *For further information:*

The Royal College of Pathologists, 2 Carlton House Terrace, London, SW1Y 5AF
Tel: 020 7451 6700   Fax: 020 7451 6701   Web: http://www.rcpath.org
UK Clinical Virology Network: http://www.clinical-virology.org

08:45	Handover from the previous day, authorize and discuss test results where clinically relevant
10:30	Haemato–oncology ward round
12:00	Review a paediatric inpatient with an Epstein–Barr virus driven lymphoma following a liver transplant
13:00	Lunch
13:45	Outpatient clinic e.g. HIV, sexual health, viral hepatitis depending on clinical experience
16:00	Laboratory authorization, review molecular test results and discuss with clinical teams
17:30	Go home; might be on-call

myth	Stuck in laboratory not interacting with staff or seeing patients
reality	Often see patients in the wards and in clinics
personality	Approachable, calm, academic, meticulous, logical
best aspects	Job diversity; tend to get interesting questions in grey areas that you might not have considered previously
worst aspects	As with any job there is a certain amount of routine work
route	ST1 Medical microbiology/virology, virology (p 40); FRCPath exam
numbers	50 of which 45% are women
locations	Teaching hospital or regional laboratory

life						work
quiet on-call						busy on-call
boredom						burnout
uncompetitive						competitive
low salary						high salary

Voluntary Services Overseas (VSO)

Voluntary Services Overseas is not so much a career as an opportunity: an opportunity to use skills and knowledge that have been gathered through the sweat and tears of medical school and the demoralizing hike through foundation posts, etc. These skills are an exceptionally valuable commodity and can be pivotal in the health and development of a resource-poor community. Many doctors choose to work outside the UK at some point in their career, so why VSO? Hopefully this chapter will provide some food for thought

the patients VSO works in 34 countries throughout Africa and Asia. Medical staff volunteers come from all walks of life so their patient base will depend on their specialty skills (e.g. paediatrics, gynaecology). Most placements will also include some general clinical care, e.g. primary care clinics or emergency medicine. Volunteers meet and work with an incredibly diverse range of people from a local nomadic tribesman (whose only health concern is that he is strong enough to herd his cattle) to a politician involved in shaping health policy at a national level. The translator is also a very useful friend in this field.

the work As opposed to shorter-term relief work that other development organisations offer (e.g. Merlin p 200), VSO placements are usually 2 years long and focus on developing/supporting a process or a service along with local colleagues. Each volunteer is matched to a suitable placement based on their previous experience and skills but the doctor does have some control over this. Once in the field, the placement can go many ways; sometimes it will follow the initial plan, other times it won't. The volunteer has to be aware of the need for flexibility, a lot of lateral thinking and the ability to expect the unexpected.

the job The objective is to impart skills to the local community to enable a service to continue once the volunteer has left. Achieving this can often take several volunteer placements. The job is usually in a resource-limited setting (even by NHS standards). This may be a hospital where the mattresses are laid on the floor, university buildings where simply getting a pencil from the stores needs to be agreed, signed and stamped by the Chancellor of the university or planning training sessions under the large marula tree to ensure enough shade.

extras There are so many: the travel, the teaching opportunities, the new experiences, the culture, the challenges, the frustrations, the new friends... and the chance to return to work in the UK with a whole new lease of life and outlook. There are many international development career options, such as posts with the World Health Organisation and International Red Cross, that rely on a period of overseas work as experience before recruitment. VSO is a fabulous and very well respected route into these opportunities

ⓘ *For further information:*

Voluntary Service Overseas, 317 Putney Bridge Road, London, SW15 2PN
Tel: 020 8780 720   Web: http://www.vso.org.uk

A day in the life in Namibia...

06:00	Sun's up but it's still cool...useful time to get things done
08:00	Morning meeting – outline the day's plan
08:30	Ward round: review of 30 inpatients (more in malaria season) with translator in tow, procedures done straight away (e.g. bloods, LP's)
10:30	Universal tea time, often rigidly adhered to regardless of workload
11:00	Deliver training session to local HIV counsellors; food provided otherwise it will be poorly attended (just like the NHS!)
13:00	Lunchtime
14:00	HIV clinic in decommissioned operating theatre, improvised space!
16:30	Home though this is still on the hospital compound
18:00	Socialise with colleagues – maybe a game of pool at the local bottle store or a walk into the bush as the sun goes down
21:30	Bedtime; it's easy to get an early night when life isn't so complicated

myth	Doctors hacking through jungles in linen suits
reality	Challenging jobs in places where a doctor can make a real difference to the community and to individuals
personality	Down to earth, easy-going, open-minded, flexible, enjoy new experiences, lateral thinking, a wee bit of wanderlust
best aspects	Diversity and unpredictability; challenge of improvising ways around cultural barriers and resource limitations; the travel
worst aspects	Being so far from the known support network; reverse culture shock of coming home
route	At least ST3/post-membership in a specific specialty; diploma of tropical medicine and hygiene is useful but not mandatory
locations	Overseas in remote settings in hospitals, clinics, laboratories, schools, communities, under trees, on the back of a truck, etc.

life					work
quiet on-call					busy on-call
boredom					burnout
uncompetitive					competitive
low salary					high salary

Index